INTERNATIONAL REVIEW OF CHILD NEUROLOGY SERIES

Leukodystrophies

Edited by

Gerald V. Raymond
Florian Eichler
Ali Fatemi
Sakkubai Naidu

© 2011 Mac Keith Press

6 Market Road, London N7 9PW, UK

Editor: Hilary Hart
Managing Director: Caroline Black
Production Manager: Udoka Ohuonu
Project Manager: Andrew Colborne
Indexer: Jill Halliday

First published in this edition 2011

British Library Cataloguing-in-Publication data:
A catalogue record for this book is available from the British Library

ISBN: 978-1-907655-09-8

Typeset by Keystroke Typesetting and Graphic Design Ltd, 6 Station Road,
Codsall, Wolverhampton, UK
Printed by Latimer Trend and Company Ltd, Plymouth, UK

Cover image: T2-weighted MRI in adrenoleukodystrophy showing hyperintensity
of the posterior white matter with involvement of the splenium of the corpus
callosum and symmetrical parieto-occipital disease. See Chapter 5, Figure 5.1.

INTERNATIONAL REVIEW OF CHILD NEUROLOGY SERIES

Leukodystrophies

Edited by

GERALD V. RAYMOND
Kennedy Krieger Institute, Baltimore, MD, USA

FLORIAN EICHLER
Massachusetts General Hospital, Harvard Medical School,
Boston, MA, USA

ALI FATEMI
Kennedy Krieger Institute, Baltimore, MD, USA

SAKKUBAI NAIDU
Kennedy Krieger Institute, Baltimore, MD, USA

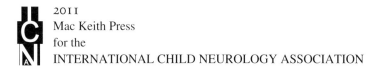
2011
Mac Keith Press
for the
INTERNATIONAL CHILD NEUROLOGY ASSOCIATION

CONTENTS

AUTHORS' APPOINTMENTS

Genila Bibat

Research Associate, Neurogenetics Unit, The Hugo W. Moser Research Institute, Kennedy Krieger Institute, Baltimore, MD, USA; *and* Research Associate, Department of Pediatrics, Johns Hopkins School of Medicine, Baltimore, MD, USA

Michael Brenner

Professor, Department of Neurobiology, Evelyn F. McKnight Brain Institute *and* The Center for Glial Biology in Medicine, University of Alabama at Birmingham, Birmingham, AL, USA

Ajit Singh Dhaunchak

Postdoctoral Fellow, Department of Neurology and Neurosurgery, Montreal Neurological Institute, McGill University, Montreal, Canada *and* Max-Planck Institute for Experimental Medicine, Goettingen, Germany

Jörg Dietrich

Instructor in Neurology, Department of Neurology, Massachusetts General Hospital, Center for Neuro-Oncology and Center for Regenerative Medicine, Harvard Medical School, Boston, MA, USA

Florian Eichler

Assistant Professor, Department of Neurology, Massachusetts General Hospital, Harvard Medical School, Boston, MA, USA

Ali Fatemi

Attending Pediatric Neurologist, Neurogenetics Research Center, The Hugo W. Moser Research Institute, Kennedy Krieger Institute, Baltimore, MD, USA; *and* Assistant Professor of Neurology and Pediatrics, Johns Hopkins School of Medicine, Baltimore, MD, USA

Daniel Flint
Department of Neurobiology, Evelyn F. McKnight Brain Institute *and* The Center for Glial Biology in Medicine, University of Alabama at Birmingham, Birmingham, AL, USA

Volkmar Gieselmann
Professor, Institute for Biochemistry and Molecular Biology, Rheinische Friedrich Wilhelms University, Bonn, Germany

Grahame Kidd
Project Staff, Department of Neurosciences, Cleveland Clinic, Cleveland, OH, USA

Ingeborg Krägeloh-Mann
Professor, Clinic for Child and Youth Medicine, Eberhard Karls University, Tübingen, Germany

Doris Lin, MD
Assistant Professor of Radiology, Department of Radiology, Division of Neuroradiology, Johns Hopkins University School of Medicine, Baltimore, MD, USA

Reuben Matalon
Professor, Pediatrics and Human Biological Chemistry and Genetics, Department of Pediatrics, University of Texas Medical Branch, Galveston, TX, USA

Kimberlee Michals
Associate Professor of Nutrition, Department of Health and Human Performance, University of Houston, Houston, TX, USA

Ann Moser
Lab Manager, Peroxisomal Diseases Lab, The Hugo W. Moser Research Institute, Kennedy Krieger Institute, Baltimore, MD USA; *and* Research Associate, Department of Neurology, Johns Hopkins School of Medicine, Baltimore, MD, USA

Hugo Moser†
Director of Neurogenetics Research, Kennedy Krieger Institute, Baltimore, MD, USA; *and* University Professor of Neurology,

	Johns Hopkins School of Medicine, Baltimore, MD, USA
Patricia Musolino	Pediatric Neurology Fellow, Department of Neurology, Massachusetts General Hospital, Harvard Medical School, Boston, MA, USA
Sakkubai Naidu	Director, Neurogenetics Unit, The Hugo W. Moser Research Institute, Kennedy Krieger Institute, Baltimore, MD, USA; *and* Professor of Neurology and Pediatrics, Johns Hopkins School of Medicine, Baltimore, MD, USA
Klaus-Armin Nave	Professor of Biology, Department of Neurogenetics, Max-Planck Institute for Experimental Medicine, Goettingen, Germany
Charles Peters	Pediatric Hematology/Oncology, Sanford Children's Specialty Clinic, Sioux Falls, SD, USA
Christoph Pröschel	Assistant Professor of Genetics, Department of Biomedical Genetics, Institute for Stem Cell and Regenerative Medicine, University of Rochester, Rochester, NY, USA
Gerald V. Raymond	Director, Neurogenetics Research Center, The Hugo W. Moser Research Institute, Kennedy Krieger Institute, Baltimore, MD, USA; *and* Professor of Neurology, Johns Hopkins School of Medicine, Baltimore, MD, USA
Bruce D. Trapp	Chairman, Department of Neurosciences, Cleveland Clinic, Cleveland, OH, USA
David A. Wenger	Professor, Department of Neurology, Thomas Jefferson University, Jefferson Medical College, Philadelphia, PA, USA

DEDICATION AND ACKNOWLEDGMENT

This book is dedicated to the memory of Hugo Moser who inspired researchers worldwide in disorders of white matter.

We, the Editors, would like to acknowledge the United Leukodystrophy Foundation in DeKalb, Illinois, USA for their dedication to the cause of leukodystrophies.

FOREWORD

From 1955 to 1957 Hugo Moser was a National Multiple Sclerosis Research Fellow in Biochemistry in the laboratory of Manford Karnovsky at Harvard. Their studies of the biosynthesis of glycolipids and other lipids of the brain were published in the *Journal of Biological Chemistry* in 1959. In 1961 he received a grant to study brain lipids in autopsy specimens from patients with leukodystrophies in laboratory space at the Research Laboratory of McLean Hospital directed by Jordi Folch Pi and his associate, Marjorie Lees. The neurochemical techniques employed by these mentors and other colleagues led to the discovery of changes in brain lipids and to a better understanding of the pathogenesis of inherited diseases of the brain.

With the need for early diagnosis, Hugo established the biochemical test for metachromatic leukodystrophy developed by Jim Austin, which led to the confirmatory diagnosis of two cases of this disease and one case of multiple sulfatase deficiency, which were clinically diagnosed at Massachusetts General Hospital. Together with his colleague at this hospital, Guy McKhann, he tried therapy using a low-sulfate diet on these three patients, without success; however, these research studies early in his scientific career set the path for Hugo's lifelong commitment to the diagnosis, understanding, and therapy of metabolic diseases of the brain. The disorders included lysosomal diseases such as metachromatic leukodystrophy, Krabbe disease, and Tay–Sachs disease; also the peroxisomal diseases, X-linked adrenoleukodystrophy, and the Zellweger spectrum disorders. The following excerpt from Hugo is the mission statement for the 2003 scientific meeting at the United Leukodystrophy Foundation:

> Advances in our understanding of leukodystrophies usually begin with the clinical delineation of the diseases. The subsequent discovery of genetic or biochemical markers often leads to the development of new methods for the detection of these diseases and raises the potential for new therapeutic approaches. The leukodystrophies, caused by enzyme deficiencies of the various organelles may be among the first to have effective treatment modalities available. Recent advances in enzyme replacement therapy, metabolic inhibitors, bone marrow transplantation, stem cell therapy and genetic viral vectors show promise for the treatment of a variety of the leukodystrophies, not just those caused by any one particular enzymatic defect.

Hugo would have been pleased to know that the work on leukodystrophies that he fostered is being carried forward by his colleagues and those whom he mentored as residents and

xi

postdoctoral fellows. I extend my thanks and gratitude to each and every one who contributed to the book. You have honored his memory by participating and sharing your knowledge and expertise in this book on leukodystrophies.

Ann Moser

1
LEUKODYSTROPHY AND MYELIN

Hugo Moser and Gerald V. Raymond

Introduction

There are many disorders that affect myelin in both children and adults. The increasingly widespread use of neuroimaging techniques – particularly magnetic resonance imaging (MRI), magnetic resonance spectroscopy (MRS), and diffusion tensor imaging (DTI) – provides a powerful new resource for the study of myelin. Various abnormalities of myelin are reported frequently, even when they had not been suspected clinically, so that disorders of myelin need to be included in the differential diagnosis – more than had been true in the past. Their etiology, clinical significance, and therapeutic implications vary greatly, and precise definition of etiology is essential.

This applies particularly to the leukodystrophies, which are serious and progressive disorders that should be distinguished as quickly as possible from other conditions that involve myelin. Not so long ago, a period of clinical observation could be allowed, but this is no longer appropriate. Minimal delay in diagnosis is particularly important, so that therapies that have emerged in recent years can be applied when they are most effective, in the early stage of the illness and, when possible, presymptomatically. Prompt and accurate diagnosis is also essential for genetic counseling. These goals can be achieved by careful correlation of clinical features, analysis of radiological findings, and the targeted application of biochemical and molecular diagnostic techniques. The purpose of this book is to facilitate and speed the accomplishment of these goals.

Definition of leukodystrophies

The term leukodystrophy (*leuko* – white, *dystrophy* – defective nutrition) was introduced by Bielschowsky and Henneberg (1928). In this book we use the definition proposed by Powers (2004) who classified leukodystrophies as disorders that are known or presumed to have (1) a genetic causation, (2) a progressive clinical course, (3) a predominant and usually confluent involvement of the central nervous system (CNS) white matter, and (4) a primary lesion of myelin or myelinating cells. The latter may be manifested by either a loss or failed development of the CNS white matter due to a biochemical abnormality or a molecular abnormality of a myelinating cell.

The first three criteria are relatively clear-cut and separate the leukodystrophies from a large number of conditions that affect myelin and are not genetically determined, which include multiple sclerosis, infectious disorders, nutritional disorders, acquired toxic–metabolic disorders, and disturbances of blood flow (see Table 1.1).

TABLE 1.1
Disorders of myelin that are not mainly genetically determined

Demyelinating diseases
- Multiple sclerosis
- Acute disseminated encephalomyelitis

Infectious diseases
- HIV vacuolar myelopathy
- Progressive multifocal leukoencephalopathy
- Subacute sclerosing panencephalitis
- Postinfectious encephalomyelitis
- Postvaccinial encephalomyelitis

Nutritional diseases of myelin
- Vitamin B12 deficiency
- Marchiafava–Bignami disease
- Central pontine myelinolysis

Acquired toxic–metabolic disorders
- Hypoxic encephalopathy
- Carbon monoxide poisoning
- Hexachlorophene poisoning
- Triethyl tin poisoning
- Posterior leukoencephalopathy syndrome
- Blood flow disturbances
- Binswanger microangiopathic leukoencephalopathy
- Leukoararaiosis

Traumatic diseases of myelin
- Pressure release

Criterion 4 is the most difficult to apply precisely, is the cause of some controversy, and subject to change as the understanding of genetic disorders of myelin increases. The basic nature of the problem was stated well by Raymond D. Adams and Charles Kubic in their 1952 review (Adams and Kubic 1952), who wrote:

> It has long been the practice to set apart a group of diseases in which demyelination is a prominent feature. They are believed to possess characteristics that point to a unique etiology and pathogenesis as yet unknown. To state these characteristics in an exact definition is, however, difficult if not impossible. Neuropathologists pretend to know what a demyelinative disease is, yet have found it hard to describe in a few simple words. The actual difficulty is . . . that there is probably no disease in which myelin destruction is the primary or exclusive pathological change. The whole idea of a demyelinative disease is more or less of an abstraction which serves to focus attention on one of the more striking and distinctive features of a pathological process. . . . The commonly accepted criteria of a demyelinative disease are: (1) destruction of the myelin sheaths of the nerve fibers; (2) relative sparing of the other elements of nervous tissue, i.e., axis cylinders of the other elements of nervous tissue.

2

The science is now catching up with these prescient words. The interaction of the axon, and by extension the neuron, with the glia and myelin sheath is now well established, and it is becoming very apparent that the injury to myelin or the oligodendrocyte does not occur in isolation.

It has been argued that classification as leukodystrophy should be reserved for disorders in which the primary lesion affects myelin or myelination cells. Adherence to this criterion leads to the exclusion of certain genetically determined disorders that meet the first three criteria listed above and resemble the leukodystrophies in respect to clinical and radiological features. An example of this is CADASIL (cerebral autosomal-dominant arteriopathy with subcortical infarcts and leukoencephalopathy) in which the primary defect, a mutation of *Notch3*, affects the endothelium of small arteries, and the fundamental abnormality is ischemia. Other disorders that have been excluded from the leukodystrophy category are those which involve the neuron primarily, such as Tay–Sachs disease, or those such as Refsum disease and Charcot–Marie–Tooth disease, which affect peripheral nerves primarily. Disorders of amino acids, mucopolysaccharides, and gangliosides, which do not appear to affect myelin primarily, are also typically excluded, although myelin abnormalities have been clearly associated with many of them. Perhaps with less justification, mitochondrial disorders and the disorders of peroxisome biogenesis have been excluded because these disorders appear to affect many components of the nervous system and not myelin primarily.

However, in fairness, limits do need to be set, and so the main focus of this work is on disorders that affect CNS myelin or myelinating cells primarily, and for which the gene defect has been defined. These disorders are listed in Table 1.2.

Finally, with the use of new genetic tools, disorders are rapidly being identified, but more importantly, also rapidly being genetically clarified (Table 1.3). With this new information, previously undiagnosed leukodystrophies can now be diagnosed. The challenge remains to disseminate these developments clinically, and to further the care and treatment of this rapidly expanding group of patients. Clearly, important work still needs to be done.

TABLE 1.2
Examples of genetic disorders that affect myelin or myelinating cells mainly,
and in which the gene defect has been defined

- X-linked adrenoleukodystrophy
- Metachromatic leukodystrophy
- Globoid leukodystrophy
- Pelizaeus–Merzbacher disease
- Canavan disease
- Alexander disease

TABLE 1.3
Recently identified genetic disorders affecting myelin

Disease	Gene where known	Reference
Leukoencephalopathy with brainstem involvement and high lactate	*DARS2*	Van der Knaap et al. 2003
Cystic leukoencephalopathy without megalencephaly	*RNASE 2*	Henneke et al. 2005
Hereditary leukoencephalopathy with spheroids		Van der Knaap et al. 2000
Progressive cavitating leukoencephalopathy		Naidu et al. 2005
Hereditary leukoencephalopathy and palmoplantar keratoderma		Lossos et al. 1995
Oculodentodigital dysplasia	*GJA1*	Norton et al. 1995
Hereditary adult-onset leukodystrophy	*Lamin B1*	Eldridge et al. 1984

REFERENCES

Adams RD, Kubik CS. (1952) The morbid anatomy of the demyelinative diseases. Am J Med 12: 510–546.

Bielschowsky M, Henneberg R. (1928) Ueber familiare diffuse Sklerose (Leukodystrophia cerebri progressive hereditaria). J Psychol Neurol (Lpz) 36: 131–181.

Eldridge R, Anayiotos CP, Schlesinger S, et al. (1984) Hereditary adult-onset leukodystrophy simulating chronic progressive multiple sclerosis. N Engl J Med 311: 948–953.

Henneke M, Preuss N, Engelbrecht V, et al. (2005) Cystic leukoencephalopathy without megalencephaly: a distinct disease entity in 15 children. Neurology 64: 1411–1416.

Lossos A, Cooperman H, Soffer D, et al. (1995) Hereditary leukoencephalopathy and palmoplantar keratoderma: a new disorder with increased skin collagen content. Neurology 45: 331–337.

Naidu S, Bibat G, Lin D, et al. (2005) Progressive cavitating leukoencephalopathy: a novel childhood disease. Ann Neurol 58: 929–938.

Norton KK, Carey JC, Gutmann DH. (1995) Oculodentodigital dysplasia with cerebral white matter abnormalities in a two-generation family. Am J Med Genet 57: 458–461.

Powers JM. (2004) The leukodystrophies: overview and classification. In: Lazzarini RA, Ed. Myelin Disorders and Classification. London: Elsevier / Academic Press, pp. 663–690.

van der Knaap MS, Naidu S, Kleinschmidt-Demasters BK, Kamphorst W, Weinstein HC. (2000) Autosomal dominant diffuse leukoencephalopathy with neuroaxonal spheroids. Neurology 54: 463–468.

van der Knaap MS, van der Voorn P, Barkhof F, et al. (2003) A new leukoencephalopathy with brainstem and spinal cord involvement and high lactate. Ann Neurol 53: 252–258.

2
MYELINATION IN HEALTH AND DISEASE

Grahame Kidd and Bruce D. Trapp

Introduction

It is more than 50 years since the pioneering work of Geren (1954) and others (Peters 1964, Bunge 1968) demonstrated that myelin was part of a living cell. Subsequent investigation of the cellular nature of myelin has continually provided surprising insights into the process of myelination and myelin diseases. These early electron microscopy (EM) studies were pivotal for several reasons. Demonstration of myelination by spiral wrapping of the oligodendrocyte plasma membrane around the axon explained both the ordered structure of myelin and the mechanisms of myelin biosynthesis. Tracing the processes from myelin internodes to oligodendrocytes definitively identified them as the sole cells responsible for myelination in the central nervous system (CNS). The idea that myelin is a dynamic part of a living cell also has ramifications that continue to shape myelin research. Recent studies of transgenic mice and human populations have shown that in both structure and function, myelin is surprisingly fault tolerant. Loss of major lipids and even the most abundant structural proteins produces comparatively minor neurological phenotypes. CNS myelination represents a phenomenal feat of membrane biosynthesis, and it should not be surprising that oligodendrocytes are susceptible to genetic defects that interfere with the cell biology of myelination. Thus many myelin-related diseases stem from defects in protein folding, trafficking, and degradation. Furthermore, as with all cells, oligodendrocytes are in constant communication with the adjacent cellular environment and disruption of the cell–cell interactions underlies axonal degeneration in diseases affecting oligodendrocytes. In this chapter we provide a general overview of the cellular events that impact myelination in health and disease, including oligodendrocyte lineage, myelin structure, the cell biology of myelin biogenesis, and oligodendrocyte interaction with the axon. Later chapters focus in detail on the genetics, pathology, neurology, and cell biology of specific inherited diseases affecting myelin.

Oligodendrocytes have a highly polarized shape

Few cell types have the extreme morphological appearance of myelinating oligodendrocytes. It is important to have an appreciation of the overall structure of oligodendrocytes and their myelin membranes. The cell bodies of mature oligodendrocytes are moderately sized (Fig. 2.1a), with variable numbers of extending cytoplasmic processes. These fine processes were first demonstrated in preparations by delRio Hortega and Penfield (Penfield 1924), and the use of confocal microscopy and enhanced green fluorescent protein (EGFP)-expressing mouse oligodendrocytes (Fig. 2.1a) now permits tracing these processes in three dimensions. The processes branch frequently and provide cytoplasmic connections with each myelin internode produced by that cell. The quantity and orientation of oligodendrocyte processes depend largely on the type of axons being myelinated. For example, an oligodendrocyte producing a single myelin internode on a large spinal motor axon will have only a single process that wraps helically around the internode, superficially resembling Schwann cell myelination. On the other hand, oligodendrocytes in the corpus callosum and optic nerves produce 20 to 30 myelin internodes and have numerous processes (Fig. 2.1b). The major biosynthetic organelles of the secretory pathway, such as the rough endoplasmic reticulum and Golgi apparatus, are concentrated in the cell body and proximal processes (Peters et al. 1991).

Myelin sheaths, or "internodes," are extensions of the oligodendrocyte plasma membrane, which is partitioned into a systematic patchwork of biochemically and functionally diverse membrane domains. Compact myelin comprises the majority of the myelin internode and contains no cytoplasm (Fig. 2.2a). Non-compact myelin encompasses several different membrane domains. These include the adaxonal membrane and inner mesaxon, which is where inner membrane leaflets are apposed and begin the myelin spiral, the abaxonal membrane and outer mesaxon of the outer tongue process, and the paranodal loops (Fig. 2.2b). Non-compact regions all retain cytoplasm organelles and are continuous from the cell body, along the inner and outer margins of compact myelin and along the processes that extend to the myelin internode. These channels are sites for protein synthesis by free ribosomes and conduits for vesicular transport. Understanding the complex interrelationships between regions of the internode and the oligodendrocyte soma can be accomplished by considering an artificial "unrolled" membrane expansion configuration (Fig. 2.1b) that does not occur in vivo but does allow for easy visualization. Here each internode is a large, sheet-like expansion of the oligodendrocyte plasma membrane. A central region devoid of cytoplasm forms the compact myelin. Around its exterior, cytoplasm-filled channels form inner and outer tongue processes and paranodal loops. Paranodal loops are so-named because they appear as loops when rolled around the axon cylinder and examined by EM in longitudinal sections (Fig. 2.2b). The outer tongue process connects to a somatic branch from the oligodendrocyte cell body along the internode. This allows newly synthesized molecules and organelles such as mitochondria to be transported to different areas of the myelin internode using the cytoplasmic channels. These channels may also participate in ion and metabolite distribution. Partitioning of the plasma membrane into different domains is not unique to oligodendrocytes, but most other cell types are restricted to two types of surfaces (e.g., apical and basolateral in epithelial cells). Oligodendrocytes are therefore unusual because of the membrane domains produced.

Oligodendrocytes synthesize remarkable amounts of surface membrane. Figure 2.1b shows an oligodendrocyte producing 25 myelin internodes around axons approximately 2 μm in diameter. The size and area of each oligodendrocyte ultimately depend on the quantity of internodes produced and the size of the internode. Oligodendrocytes myelinating small axons (1.5 μm) produce internodes with a length of approximately 200 μm with about 20 lamellae. These oligodendrocytes typically myelinate 30 to 40 axons and may have a total myelin surface area of 1.5 mm^2 (Blakemore 1981, Hildebrand et al. 1993). Oligodendrocytes

a

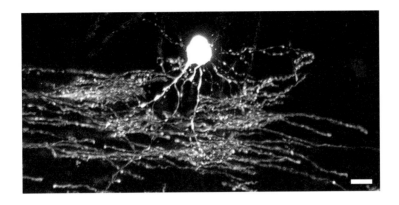

b

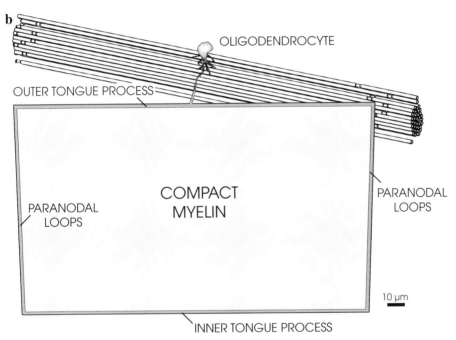

OLIGODENDROCYTE

OUTER TONGUE PROCESS

PARANODAL
LOOPS

COMPACT
MYELIN

PARANODAL
LOOPS

10 µm

INNER TONGUE PROCESS

Fig. 2.1. Oligodendrocytes synthesize and maintain large volumes of surface membranes. A confocal image of an oligodendrocyte that expresses enhanced green fluorescent protein from the proteolipid protein promoter (**a**) illustrates the main processes and numerous fine processes that extend to and along axons. The schematic diagram (**b**) highlights the size and complex organization of mature oligodendrocyte and myelin internodes (drawn to scale). Scale bars: 10 µm.

ensheathing larger (10 µm) axons produce a single internode that many be up to 1250 µm long with more than 120 wraps and a total surface area of approximately 14 mm^2 (Blakemore 1981, Hildebrand et al. 1993). In sharp contrast, absorptive epithelial cells have surface areas of approximately 0.002 mm^2. The number of internodes formed by each oligodendrocyte is regulated by several factors, including myelin length and thickness and the axons

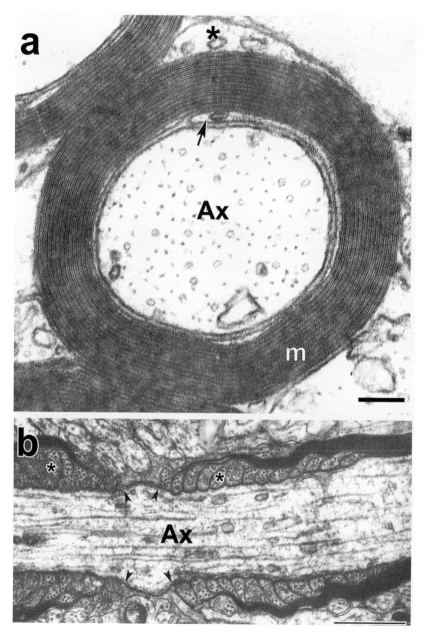

Fig. 2.2. Electron micrographs of CNS myelin internodes in transverse (**a**) and longitudinal (**b**) orientations. In cross-section, the axon (Ax) is surrounded by compact myelin (m), except at the outer (*) and inner tongue processes (arrow). At the node of Ranvier (**b**), compact myelin lamellae terminate in paranodal loops (*). The nodal axolemma (between arrowheads) is characteristically demarcated by dense undercoating. Scale bars: **a**, 0.1 μm; **b**, 1 μm. Reproduced from Tabira et al. (1978) (**a**) and Peters et al. (1991) (**b**) with permission.

being ensheathed (Blakemore 1981, Fanarraga et al. 1998). This is in stark contrast to Schwann cells, which produce only a single internode. This regulatory capacity greatly reduces the number of cells required for myelination of the CNS, minimizing the space occupied by oligodendrocyte nuclei and cell bodies.

Schwann cell internodes also have prominent and regularly spaced cytoplasmic channels that traverse compact myelin and connect outer and inner margins of the myelin internode called Schmidt-Lantermann incisures. Structures that resemble peripheral nervous system (PNS) incisures have been identified in some larger CNS myelin internodes (Blakemore 1969) but generally are not found among smaller CNS internodes. The molecular composition of these incisure-like structures has not been extensively characterized.

Molecular composition of myelin and oligodendrocyte membranes

Myelin, like all plasma membranes, is composed of a lipid bilayer that is enhanced by intrinsic and extrinsic proteins. CNS myelin membranes are biochemically unique, however. Purified myelin (mainly compact myelin) has 50% less total protein than plasma membranes from erythrocytes and 75% less total protein than liver cells (Guidotti 1972). Products of two genes (PLP and MBP, see below) make up approximately 80% of total (dry weight) protein. Given that the primary function of myelin is insulation, one might envision a lipid-rich membrane with a few small proteins and no bulky ion pumps, metabolite transporters, or cytoskeletal-anchoring proteins. Compact myelin indeed fits this characterization.

Myelin also has a unique lipid composition. Myelin is enriched in galactose-containing glycolipids and contains more cholesterol (up to 50% more) than most plasma membranes (Norton and Cammer 1984). Roughly 20 to 30% of the myelin membrane is composed of galactosylceramide (GalC; cerebroside) (Norton and Cammer 1984). Myelin galactolipids also contain saturated very long chain fatty acids (VLCFAs) of 22 to 25 carbons, which balance the effects of cholesterol and other unsaturated lipids by reducing membrane fluidity. Galactosyl lipids are not essential for compact myelin formation, as mice that are null for galactoseceramide galactosyl-transferase (GCT) produce ample amounts of compact myelin. Paranodal abnormalities and neurological deficits were reported in these GCT-null mice, indicating an essential function in myelin function (Bosio et al. 1998, Dupree et al. 1998, Marcus et al. 2000, Honke et al. 2002). While immunocytochemistry has described the distributions of myelin proteins in detail, the distributions of lipids are less amenable to staining in vivo. Because of this, detailed lipid distributions in specific membrane domains are currently lacking. In most plasma membranes, lipids are distributed with a "sidedness," and in myelin it is believed that galactolipids and cholesterol are likely to be enriched in the outer, extracellular-facing leaflet of the bilayer, whereas negatively charged lipids are oriented toward the cytoplasmic surface.

Compact Myelin and Roles of the Major Myelin Proteins

The vast majority of the myelin internode consists of compact myelin, which is characterized by a lamellar structure of alternating dark and light lines that spiral around the axon (Fig. 2.2a). In the compacted spiral, apposing extracellular leaflets called intraperiod or intermediate lines (IPLs) are separated by 2.0 nm in the CNS (Fig. 2.3a,b). The cytoplasmic leaflets appear fused and form the major dense lines (MDLs). The spiral membranes of compact myelin have a periodicity (distance from dense line to dense line) of 13 to 14 nm when fixed with aldehydes (Fernandez-Moran and Finean 1957, Kirschner and Hollingshead 1980), which is slightly smaller than in myelin of the PNS. Extracellular spacing of compact myelin is much less than sites of cell–cell contact, which are normally 20 nm or more. This reflects, in part, the absence of large carbohydrate-containing proteins on the compact myelin membrane surface. The extreme regularity of the lamellar spacing suggests adhesion between proteins in extracellular leaflets. In peripheral nerves and in the CNS of lower vertebrates, homotypic adhesion of immunoglobulin gene (Ig) superfamily adhesion molecule P0 in both *cis* and in *trans* binds apposing membrane leaflets together at both extracellular and cytoplasmic faces. In oligodendrocyte myelin, a combination of proteins performs a similar, though not identical, role.

The most abundant CNS myelin protein is the *proteolipid protein* (PLP). The PLP is relatively small, with a molecular weight of approximately 30 kDa. It is a hydrophilic protein

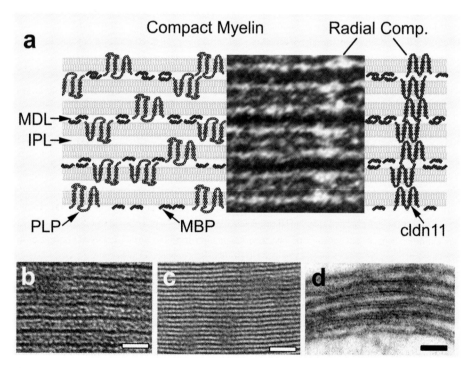

Fig. 2.3. Molecular localization of major CNS myelin proteins. **a:** Myelin basic protein (MBP) is concentrated at the major dense line (MDL), while proteolipid protein (PLP) spans the lipid bilayer of the myelin membrane and contributes to the intraperiod line (IPL). Claudin-11 (cldn11) is concentrated in the radial component (Comp.). As compared to normal myelin (**b**), myelin lacking PLP has a narrowing or fusion of the IPL and reduced lamellar thickness (**c**). Myelin lacking MBP (**d**) exhibits characteristic widening of the MDL. Scale bars: 25 nm. Reproduced from Duncan et al. (1988) (**b, c**) and Stoffel et al. (1997) (**d**) with permission.

with four membrane-spanning domains. Both the amino and carboxy termini reside in the cytoplasm (reviewed by Lees 1998, and Griffiths et al. 1998a). The *PLP* gene also has alternative transcription start sites. An alternative splice variant named DM20 is predominant during the early phases of myelin wrapping, but is much less abundant than PLP in mature compact myelin. DM20 lacks a 35 amino acid segment of the internal peptide loop (Macklin et al. 1987a, Nave et al. 1987). Additional hydrophobicity of PLP and DM20 is produced by the addition of oleate or stearate fatty acids or by acylation through palmitoylation (Agrawal et al. 1982, Bizzozero et al. 1986). PLP has six acylation sites (Weimbs and Stoffel 1992), two of which are not present in DM20, as they are in the sequence that is lacking in the internal loop. Fatty acylation might regulate the targeting of proteins to compact myelin and may facilitate the orientation of other membrane lipids. Its prominence in CNS myelin initially suggested that PLP may have adhesive functions, but in-vitro adhesion studies and protein structure comparisons indicate that PLP is not an obligatory adhesion protein (Timsit et al. 1992). Furthermore, rodents lacking the *PLP* gene (Duncan et al. 1988, 1989) produce compact myelin where the extracellular leaflets appear fused (Fig. 2.3c) (Klugmann et al. 1997, Griffiths et al. 1998b). The primary structural role of PLP in compact myelin appears to maintain tight juxtaposition between extracellular leaflets, which may involve weak electrostatic interactions (Rosenbluth et al. 2009). PLP loss in oligodendrocytes results in extensive detrimental effects in axons, ultimately leading to axonal degeneration (Klugmann et al. 1997, Griffiths et al. 1998b, Garbern et al. 2002, Edgar et al. 2004, Yin et al. 2006). The role and extent of PLP involvement in axonal maintenance are discussed in the "Reciprocal interactions between axons and oligodendrocytes" section below.

Myelin basic proteins (MBPs) are the other major protein component of compact myelin. MBPs are a family of small proteins ranging from 14 to 21.5 kDa (Barbarese et al. 1978, Zeller et al. 1984) and are generated from a single gene by alternative splicing. MBPs are extrinsic membrane proteins and are localized at the cytoplasmic surface of compact myelin in both the CNS (Fig. 2.3a) and the PNS (Omlin et al. 1982). The cytoplasmic leaflets of compact CNS myelin are not fused in MBP-deficient *shiverer* mice (Fig. 2.3d) (Privat et al. 1979). This indicates that MBPs maintain the major dense line of myelin in the CNS. MBPs have a high percentage of charged amino acids with a net excess of basic amino acids regardless of splicing (see review by Boggs 2006; and Greenfield et al. 1973, Zeller et al. 1984). MBPs may interact with the membrane via negatively charged inner leaflets. The MBPs are heavily phosphorylated along most of their lengths (Carnegie et al. 1974, Miyamoto et al. 1974), and methylation, arginylation and citrullination have all been described (see review by Boggs 2006). Thus MBPs have charges and phosphorylation sites that permit interaction with charged proteins. MBPs appear to be the myelin proteins that are most important for sustained spiral myelin growth, as genetic defects that prevent MBP synthesis result in axonal ensheathment with minimal spiral wrapping of myelin membranes (Fig. 2.3d) (Privat et al. 1979, Readhead et al. 1987, Kwiecien et al. 1998). In support of this concept, a single MBP cDNA transgene rescues the mouse *shiverer* phenotype (Kimura et al. 1989).

Other less abundant proteins are also enriched in compact myelin. *Myelin-oligodendrocyte basic proteins* (MOBPs) are a family of small (7–14 kDa) proteins produced by a single gene

(Yamamoto et al. 1994, Holz et al. 1996). They are positively charged and located at the MDL, similar to the MBPs. Though MOBPs are relatively abundant, their functions remain unclear and they are unable to compensate for the loss of MBPs (see review by Montague et al. 2006). P_2 *protein* is another extrinsic protein enriched at the MDL in PNS myelin. P_2 protein is not present in the CNS of mice or rats, but is present in CNS myelin of rabbits, humans, cattle, and horses, where it is more abundant in spinal cord and brainstem myelin than in cerebral cortex myelin (Trapp et al. 1983). P_2 is a member of a family of proteins that functions in fatty acid transport (Uyemura et al. 1984). The functions of P_2 in myelin and the factors underlying its heterogenous distribution remain unknown. *Myelin and lymphocyte* (MAL) protein is a tetraspan-like protein enriched in compact myelin (Schaeren-Wiemers et al. 1995, Frank 2000) and expressed by other cell types. In epithelial cells it associates with glycolipid-rich membranes and contributes to protein targeting (Cheong et al. 1999). Its role in compact myelin, however, is unknown.

RADIAL COMPONENT OF COMPACT CNS MYELIN

The radial component of compact CNS myelin is often overlooked at the ultrastructural level because it is not readily apparent in conventional EM preparations. However, when the preparation is optimized (Peters 1961, Tabira et al. 1978) it appears in transverse sections as registered lines of intralammelar junctional complexes that extend partially or completely across the thickness of the myelin sheath (Fig. 2.4a). Radial components resemble tight junctions in that extracellular leaflets appear fused (Fig. 2.3a). Radial components are also in register and extend from paranode to paranode when visualized in a longitudinal orientation. Freeze-fracture analysis shows intramembranous particles typical of tight junctions in compact myelin distributed identically to the radial components. The MDL shows little variation in the radial component. In the mature myelin internode, radial components are common beneath the outer tongue process and often extend to the inner tongue process, which frequently lies in the same quadrant. Radial components can also appear elsewhere and seem to align with each other between internodes at locations where adjacent myelin internodes make contact. In certain pathological conditions such as hexachlorophene or triethyl tin intoxication, white matter edema develops and large intramyelinic vacuoles appear from the splitting of the extracellular leaflets of compact CNS myelin (Fig. 2.4c). These myelin vacuoles remain tethered to the axons in the area of the inner tongue process where the tight junction-like radial component is present (Tabira et al. 1978). Therefore it appears that the molecules comprising the radial component provide focal points of lamellar adhesion that extend longitudinally along the compact myelin.

Radial component assembly depends on *claudin-11* (also called oligodendrocyte specific protein, OSP), a 22-kDa protein that constitutes about 7% of CNS myelin protein (Fig. 2.3a) (Bronstein et al. 1997, Gow et al. 1999, Morita et al. 1999). Like PLP, the claudins are integral membrane proteins with four transmembrane domains and cytoplasmically oriented N- and C-termini. Unlike PLP, the claudins adhere to one another between adjacent plasma membranes, binding both homotypically and heterotypically (Krause et al. 2008). Claudins are also common components of tight junctions, and claudin-11 is also found in tight junctions between oligodendrocyte cell bodies (Gow et al. 1999) and between para-

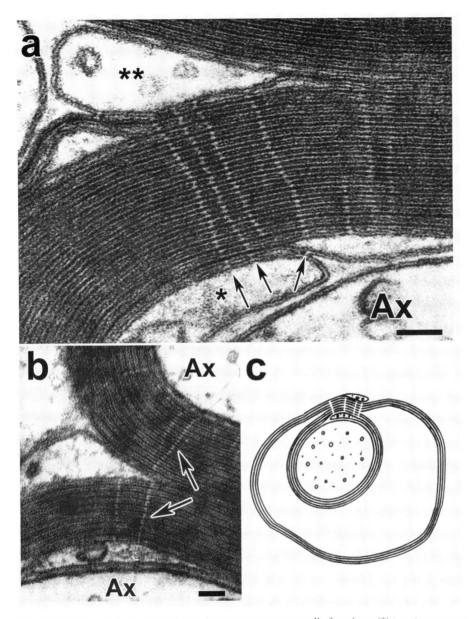

Fig. 2.4. (a) The radial component (arrows) traverses compact myelin from inner (*) to outer mesaxon (**). **(b)** Radial components in adjacent internodes are aligned (arrows). In hexachlorophene intoxication **(c)**, the radial components help tether the vacuolated myelin internode to the axon (Ax). Scale bars: 0.1 μm. Reproduced from Tabira et al. (1978) with permission.

nodal loops (below). It is also found in other cell types, including epithelial cells of the ependyma and testis (Gow et al. 1999). Despite superficially resembling a tight junction, an ultrastructural cytoplasmic plaque and tight junction complex proteins such as ZO-1 are not detectable elements of the radial component. The close registration of radial components between myelin lamellae of even different internodes suggests that the protein interacts both extracellularly and cytoplasmically. Claudin-11-null mice exhibit no significant discernible phenotype or myelin defects (Gow et al. 1999), but mice that lack both claudin-11 and PLP/DM20 have a severe phenotype (Chow et al. 2005) characterized by prominent IPL separation, suggesting that one of these two proteins is necessary for stabilization of compact myelin during spiral growth.

NON-COMPACT MYELIN DOMAINS AND AXONAL ORGANIZATION AT THE NODE
Non-compact myelin membrane domains consist of the periaxonal membrane, paranodal loops, and the outer tongue process. Non-compact membranes are key sites of interaction with the axonal surface. Although contiguous with compact myelin, non-compact membranes have distinct mutually exclusive protein compositions. While compact myelin consists of small four-pass proteins with moderately sized extracellular domains, large adhesion molecules with substantial extracellular projections are often present in non-compact myelin domains. Proteins normally do not mix between compact and non-compact domains. Functionally, some non-compact myelin proteins serve in a more general capacity and are enriched in multiple non-compact membranes, while others perform specialized functions at one particular location.

One extrinsic membrane protein common to all non-compact myelin regions is *2´, 3´-cyclic nucleotide 3´-phosphodiesterase* (CNP) (Fig. 2.5a) (Braun et al. 1988, Trapp et al. 1988). CNP consists of two highly basic proteins of 46 kDa (CNP1) and 48 kDa (CNP2) produced by alternative splicing as multiple transcripts from a single gene. Post-translational modifications of these proteins include C-terminal isoprenylation and fatty acylation, and these mediate interaction with the inner leaflet of the non-compact membranes (Braun et al. 1991). As its name implies, CNP is capable of catalyzing the hydrolysis of 2´, 3´-nucleotides into corresponding 2´-nucleotides (Drummond et al. 1962, Sprinkle et al. 1978); however, a substrate for this enzymatic activity has yet to be identified in the CNS. CNP may interact with cytoskeletal components, and it promotes process outgrowth when transfected into some cell lines (Lee et al. 2005). Absence of CNP expression does not inhibit CNS myelination or disrupt the ultrastructure of compact and non-compact membranes (Lappe-Siefke et al. 2003). As discussed latter in this chapter, absence of CNP does cause extensive axonal pathology (Lappe-Siefke et al. 2003). When over-expressed, CNP is mislocalized to compact CNS myelin membranes and compaction is prevented (Yin et al. 1997). These membranes are deficient in MBP and do not form MDLs (Yin et al. 1997). Taken together, this evidence suggests that CNP may serve to prevent compaction of an MDL in regions where cytoplasm is required and to help target MBP to compacting myelin membranes.

Non-compact CNS myelin membranes also contain *connexins,* which are channel-forming proteins found in gap junctions. Connexins are the products of several different

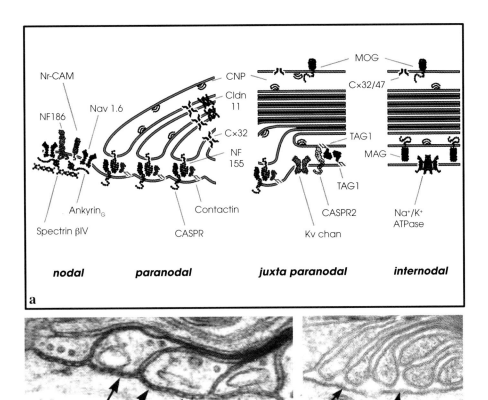

Fig. 2.5. Localization of proteins in non-compact CNS myelin membranes and axonal binding partners (**a**). Electron microscopy of a wild-type node (**b**) illustrates septate paranodal junctions (arrows) and corresponding loss in contactin-null mice (**c**). Scale bar: 0.1 μm. Reproduced from Bosio et al. (1998) (**b**) and Boyle et al. (2001) (**c**) with permission. For abbreviations and symbols, see text.

genes and are four-pass transmembrane proteins, which have cytoplasmically oriented C- and N-termini. Connexins can homodimerize and heterodimerize into connexons, which are hemi-junctional complexes that have the capacity to bind other connexons in apposing membranes to form gap junctions between cells (Orthmann-Murphy et al. 2008). Oligodendrocytes express at least three connexins: Cx32, Cx47, and Cx29. Each connexin has a different distribution pattern in oligodendrocytes. Cx32 is the best characterized and is found on the membranes of the oligodendrocyte cell body, at the paranodes and on abaxonal membranes (Fig. 2.5a) (Kleopa et al. 2004, Kamasawa et al. 2005). Cx47 localizes to cell bodies, processes, and the outer tongue process (Kleopa et al. 2004, Kamasawa et al. 2005). Although mutations in Cx32 result in X-linked Charcot–Marie–Tooth disease (Bergoffen et al. 1993, Bruzzone et al. 1994), an inherited dysmyelination of the human PNS, CNS myelin appears unaffected by the absence of Cx32 or mutations that cause the disease (Scherer et al. 1998, Menichella et al. 2003). Animals lacking both Cx32 and Cx47,

15

on the other hand, have thin or absent CNS myelin sheaths and die as neonates (Menichella et al. 2003). Cx32 and Cx47 are present in ultrastructurally defined gap junctions between oligodendrocytes and astrocytes and reflexive junctions between apposing paranodal loops (Kamasawa et al. 2005). It is generally believed that they mediate the exchange of ions and small molecules between oligodendrocytes and astrocytes. This is likely to be critical for oligodendrocytes in particular, as there is little extracellular space around individual internodes in white matter tracts which presumably would impede ion and metabolite exchange via extracellular pathways. It is hypothesized that gap junctions may also create a shortcut between paranodal loops, which could promote rapid intracellular passage of ions such as K^+ between the juxtaparanode and the node.

Nodal region

As illustrated in Fig. 2.5, the nodal axolemma contains voltage-gated Na^+ channels and is particularly enriched in the Nav1.6 isoform (Black et al. 1990). In response to an action potential, Na^+ enters through these channels, generating a sudden voltage drop resulting in channel-opening at the next node, thereby propagating the action potential along the axon. Nodal membranes also contain many other proteins (Fig. 2.5a), including the adhesion protein neurofascin-186 (Ariyasu and Ellisman 1987, Davis et al. 1996, Tait et al. 2000). Upon examination by EM, the nodal axolemma presents as a dense coating (20nm thick) beneath the axolemma (Fig. 2.2b) (Ellisman and Levinson 1982, Caldwell et al. 2000). This submembranous cytoskeleton contains spectrin ßIV (Berghs et al. 2000, Lacas-Gervais et al. 2004), f-actin (Kordeli et al. 1990) and two alternately spliced isoforms of ankyrin$_G$ (270 kD and 480 kD) (Kordeli et al. 1990, 1995). Ankyrin$_G$ associates with Na^+ channels in the neuronal soma and assists in targeting Na^+ channels to the node (Kordeli et al. 1995, Bennett and Lambert 1999). Oligodendrocyte contact is essential for node formation and maintenance. Following demyelination, the nodal channels diffuse laterally into the internodal plasma membrane and Nav1.6 is replaced by Nav1.2 as saltatory conduction is lost (Black et al. 1990, Craner et al. 2003, 2004).

Paranodal loops

As compact myelin approaches the node, the MDL "opens up" to accommodate cytoplasm (Fig. 2.2b). A characteristic lateral spacing of 12 to 14 nm is maintained between paranodal loop extracellular leaflets. The underlying molecular basis for this is unclear. CNP is present in paranodal loops and may contribute to loop maintenance (Rasband et al. 2005), but it is not essential for paranodal loop formation (Lappe-Siefke et al. 2003). On the other hand, GalC and/or sulfatide are important for paranodal loop formation, as GCT-null and CST-null mice have major paranodal abnormalities, including reversed paranodal loops, nodal widening, and heminode formation (Dupree et al. 1998, 1999), a lack of paranodal septate junctions (see below, Fig. 2.5c) with the axonal surface, and are unable to make one or both glycolipids. It has been proposed that glycolipids act as ligands for axonal receptors, as mediators of protein targeting (see below) or as structural lipids, but their precise functions are currently unknown. Autotypic reflexive junctions are present between adjacent paranodal loops (Fig. 2.5a). Claudin-11-containing tight junctions tether apposing paranodal loop membranes together (Schnapp and Mugnaini 1976, Gow et al. 1999, Morita et al. 1999) and also contain other tight junction-associated proteins, including ZO. Tight junctions are assumed to prevent extracellular entry of ions into compact myelin, and they may also structurally support the paranodal loops. The gap junction protein Cx32 is also present and forms Cx32/Cx32 channels (Kleopa et al. 2004, Kamasawa et al. 2005) between adjacent paranodal loops. The significance of these gap junctions has been debated, but evidence suggests that they facilitate the passage of small ions between adjacent loops, creating a direct route between the juxtaparanodal and nodal compartments (Kleopa et al. 2004, Kamasawa et al. 2005).

Evenly spaced densities connect the paranodal loops and axolemma (Fig. 2.5b). These densities were originally referred to as transverse bands and represent a septate-like junctional complex that is the major adhesive apparatus between axons and myelin (Peters et al. 1991, Einheber et al. 1997). The septate axoglial junctions between the axolemma and paranodal loops have two important functions. First, they create a diffusion barrier that impedes passage of nodal ions into the internodal periaxonal space. Second, they compartmentalize the molecules in the axonal surface. The major oligodendrocyte component of the axoglial septate junctions is *neurofascin 155* (NF155), which is also found at Schwann cell paranodal loop membranes (Tait et al. 2000, Charles et al. 2002). NF155 is a single-pass transmembrane protein with an extensive extracellular domain containing multiple Ig-like repeats and fibronectin-type III repeats. As a 155-kDa member of the Ig superfamily of adhesion molecules, NF155 structurally resembles primitive septate junction proteins in drosophila, and has homology with the neural adhesion molecule L1 (Tait et al. 2000). NF155 is produced by alternate splicing of the neurofascin gene, which also produces neuronal NF186. The extracellular domain of NF155 interacts with its axonal binding partners *contactin* and *Caspr* (contactin-associated protein, also called paranodin) on the axon surface at septate junctions (Fig. 2.5a) (Einheber et al. 1997, Menegoz et al. 1997, Rios et al. 2000, Tait et al. 2000, Charles et al. 2002). Contactin is a neural Ig superfamily cell adhesion molecule of 135 kDa that is anchored to the axonal surface through a glycosylphosphatidylinositol (GPI)-link (Ranscht and Dours 1988). It interacts in *cis* with Caspr (Cross et al. 1994, Menegoz et al. 1997, Einheber et al. 1997), which is a single-pass transmembrane protein of 180 kDa. All three molecules form a trimeric adhesion complex across the axoglial space (Fig. 2.5a) and have homologues associated with septate junctions in invertebrates. In animals with complete deficiency of Caspr or contactin, axoglial junctions are abnormal or missing (Bhat et al. 2001, Boyle et al. 2001). Protein 4.1B is also a cytoskeletal protein that binds to Caspr, and it may serve as an intracellular scaffolding protein because it is required for normal paranodal structure (Gollan et al. 2002, Denisenko-Nehrbass et al. 2003).

Juxtaparanodal region
This region is defined as the 10 to 15 µm of the myelin internode that lies adjacent to the paranodal loops. Though this region is not distinguished by transmission EM, freeze fracture EM can identify clusters of intramembranous particles in the juxtaparanodal axolemma (Rosenbluth 1976). These correspond to the location of shaker-type delayed rectifier K^+

channels as identified by immunostaining. K$^+$ channels in myelinated axons include Kv1.1, Kv1.2 and their associated subunit ß$_2$ (Rasband et al. 1998). Some evidence suggests that an additional axoglial complex may participate in the localization of Kv channels.

Transient axonal glycoprotein-1 (TAG-1) is a GPI-anchored Ig superfamily protein related in structure to contactin (Furley et al. 1990) that co-localizes with K$^+$ channels. TAG-1 is present at juxtaparanodal membranes in both oligodendrocytes and axons and appears to interact homotypically in *trans* between the membranes. TAG-1 interacts with another Caspr isoform, Caspr2, which is also restricted to the juxtaparanodal region, within the axolemma (Poliak et al. 1999, Traka et al. 2002). Caspr2 failed to localize to juxta-paranodal regions and K$^+$ channels had a less restricted, paranodal distribution and were reduced in concentration in mice deficient in TAG-1 (Traka et al. 2003). In the juxtapara-nodal region, K$^+$ channels are thought to play a role in saltatory conduction by facilitating rapid, repetitive firing by rectifying the membrane potential after Na$^+$ channel opening during action potential propagation. They may also play a prominent role in preventing retrograde propagation of the action potential.

Adaxonal inner tongue membrane and internodal axolemma
A single oligodendrocyte cytoplasmic channel is present at the inner surface of CNS internodes and extends longitudinally for the entire internode. It includes the inner mesaxon, cytoplasm, and some organelles. This inner rim of cytoplasm extends around the entire circumference in developing CNS fibers, but much of the inner myelin wrap forms a MDL with the compact myelin lamellae in mature CNS fibers. The inner surface of CNS myelin internodes is separated from the axon by a periaxonal space of 12 to 14 nm. The inner tongue process is best characterized by the presence of *myelin associated glycoprotein* (MAG) (Fig. 2.5a) (Sternberger et al. 1979, Trapp et al. 1989) and is also enriched in CNP and microfilaments (Trapp et al. 1988).

MAG is a type I integral membrane glycoprotein consisting of a single transmembrane domain, a cytoplasmic C-terminal, and five immunoglobulin-like domains. MAG is alter-natively spliced to generate two developmentally regulated polypeptides of molecular weight 72 kDa (L-MAG) and 67 kDa (S-MAG) (Arquint et al. 1987), which differ at the C-terminal whereby S-MAG lacks 44 amino acids found in L-MAG and has a C-terminal decapeptide that is not present in L-MAG. Therefore, L-MAG and S-MAG have different cytoplasmic domains which probably contain protein targeting or sorting sequences, as discussed in the "Molecular mechanisms of myelin membrane formation" section below. Glycosylation gives the mature proteins a molecular weight of about 100 kDa. In the CNS, L-MAG is more abundant than S-MAG during the early stages of myelination, whereas they are both present in approximately equal quantities in mature CNS myelin internodes. MAG-containing membranes are characterized by the absence of an MDL and by 12 to 14 nm apposition with other membranes. Thus MAG is positioned to interact with the axon and to help maintain the periaxonal compartment. Structurally, MAG is a cell adhesion molecule of the Ig superfamily (Salzer et al. 1987) and is also a member of the siglec family of sialic acid binding proteins (Kelm et al. 1994). MAG binds sialyated glycans (Kelm et al. 1994), including axonal gangliosides. MAG-null mice (Li et al. 1994, Montag et al. 1994) have modest morphological changes, but show little initial phenotype. The periaxonal collar is lost from CNS internodes except at the inner tongue process (Li et al. 1994, Montag et al. 1994, Bartsch et al. 1995). Mice lacking neuronal GM2/GD2 synthase, an enzyme required for ganglioside GD1a and GT1b production, have similar phenotypes to MAG-deficient mice (Sheikh et al. 1999).

The underlying internodal axolemma is enriched for Na^+/K^+ ATPases $\alpha1$ and $\alpha3$ (Fig. 2.5a) (Mata et al. 1991, Young et al. 2008). These pumps are not enriched in the paranodal or nodal axolemma (Young et al. 2008). Following demyelination, these ATPases are distributed along the entire demyelinated axolemma, suggesting that oligodendrocytes play a role in restricting ATPase from nodal axolemma. Na^+/K^+ ATPases are essential for normal neuronal functioning because they restore the gradients of Na^+ and K^+ across the plasma membrane after action potential firing, by exporting three Na^+ ions and importing two K^+ ions from the extracellular environment. Internodal localization places them beneath compact myelin, similar to Kv channels. While this provides an ideal mechanism for K^+ exchange into the axon, it does not address the fate of the Na^+ pumped into the periaxonal space, suggesting that oligodendrocytes have a mechanism for Na^+ uptake and redistribution to the node, possibly through paranodal gap junctions.

Abaxonal membrane and outer tongue process
CNS myelin internodes have an outer tongue process, which is a single external cytoplasmic channel that occupies 5 to 20% of the outer (abaxonal) myelin internode circumference (Figs. 2.1b, 2.2a) and runs the length of the internode. The remaining circumference of the outer myelin spiral includes a MDL and appears identical to all other compact myelin lamellae. In addition, the outer membrane can form an IPL with adjacent neighboring internodes (Fig. 2.2a). This arrangement is in sharp contrast to that of the Schwann cell outer membrane, which secretes and attaches to basal lamina and collagen-rich extracellular matrix. Thus, oligodendrocyte myelination requires significantly less extracellular space and makes more efficient use of space than peripheral nerve myelination.

The *myelin oligodendrocyte (glyco)protein* (MOG) is present in the abaxonal membrane (Fig. 2.5a). MOG is a glycoprotein of about 25 kDa that has an extracellular N-terminal Ig-like domain, a hydrophobic C-terminal domain, and a transmembrane domain (Linnington et al. 1984, Kroepfl et al. 1996). MOG was originally discovered as an autoantigen and immunogen for inducing demyelination (Linnington et al. 1984), and continues to be widely used to induce experimental allergic encephalomyelitis. MOG is not present in paranodal loops, but is concentrated on the outer surface of the myelin internode (Brunner et al. 1989), almost mirroring the internal distribution of MAG. MOG-null mice have no obvious phenotypes (Delarasse et al. 2003). Consequently, the function of MOG is unknown.

Molecular mechanisms of myelin membrane formation

In rodents, oligodendrocytes produce significant amounts of myelin membranes by the end of the third postnatal week. During this period, oligodendrocytes produce an estimated $>10^4 \mu m^2$ myelin membrane surface area per cell per day (Pfeiffer et al. 1993). Myelin formation involves more than just simple membrane biogenesis, however, and special mechanisms are utilized for spiral and longitudinal myelin membrane extension along the axon and site-specific targeting of myelin proteins to compact and non-compact myelin membrane domains. Myelination requires specialized microtubule networks, which serve as the "railroad tracks" for transportation of myelin components to the developing internode. Spiral myelin growth is actin-dependent and locally regulated at axonal contact sites. Surprisingly, spiral myelin growth can occur in the absence of individual myelin proteins including MAG, PLP and CNP. How spiral growth and myelin membrane assembly are regulated remains a critical question for understanding myelination in development and disease.

OLIGODENDROCYTE PRODUCTION

Oligodendrocytes are produced by oligodendrocyte progenitor cells (OPCs) (Fig. 2.6). OPCs originate in the subventricular zone (SVZ) and can be identified by their expression of the sulfated proteoglycan NG2 and the platelet-derived growth factor receptor alpha (PDGFαR). OPCs colonize the developing CNS as bipolar migratory cells and establish a network of stellate-shaped, process-bearing cells throughout the white and gray matter. Processes of neighboring OPCs are closely apposed, but rarely overlap. OPCs are the

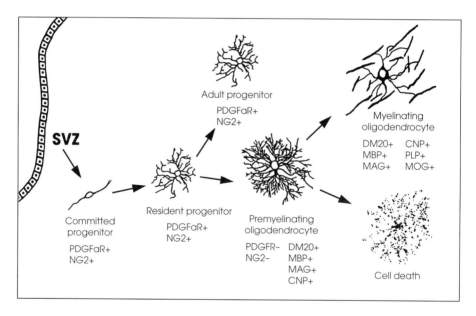

Fig. 2.6. Cells of the oligodendrocyte lineage and the proteins expressed during various differentiation states. Subventricular zone (SVZ) cells produce migratory oligodendrocyte progenitor cells (OPCs) which colonize the central nervous system and become resident progenitor cells. During development, OPCs differentiate into premyelinating oligodendrocytes, which myelinate axons or undergo apoptosis. A substantial population of OPCs also persists into adulthood, which in demyelinating diseases can divide and differentiate into remyelinating oligodendrocytes. Adapted from Trapp et al. (1997) with permission. For other abbreviations and symbols, see text.

only known source of oligodendrocytes and the transition from an OPC to a myelinating oligodendrocyte occurs in two stages. OPCs initially differentiate into a premyelinating oligodendrocyte. This cell is negative for NG2 and PDGFαR. It extends multiple processes which are usually more abundant and often longer than OPC processes. These processes contain myelin proteins but do not appear to have any obvious association with axons. The premyelinating oligodendrocyte has a limited lifespan (a few days in rodents) and either proceeds to myelinate axons or dies by programmed cell death. Myelin proteins are detected in all premyelinating oligodendrocyte surface membranes. OPC differentiation into a premyelinating oligodendrocyte does not dependent on the axon, as it occurs in neuron-free cultures and in the absence of axons in vivo (Ueda et al. 1999). Premyelinating oligoden-drocytes differentiate into myelinating oligodendrocytes. This switch involves ensheathment of axons and targeted delivery of myelin proteins to discrete membrane domains.

SPECIALIZED CYTOSKELETAL NETWORKS UNDERLIE OLIGODENDROCYTE MYELINATION

Expansion, reorganization, and specialization of the microtubule network underlie the gen-eration of complex shapes in many large cells, including myelin-forming cells. Microtubules provide essential "railroad tracks" for transport of myelin components and organelles (see reviews by Goldstein and Yang 2000, Schliwa and Woehlke 2003). Microtubules are polar filamentous structures with fast-growing "plus" ends – at which dimers of α and ß tubulins are added or removed – and slow-growing "minus" ends. The kinesin family of proteins helps propel vesicles and organelles toward microtubule plus-ends, while dynein-family motors mediate minus-end directed transport. The Golgi apparatus, endoplasmic reticulum, intermediate filaments, and endosome distributions are mediated by interactions with microtubules. Depolymerization of microtubules caused by experimental toxins (Jacobs et al. 1972) or genetic mutations that affect microtubule organization (Duncan et al. 1992, Song et al. 1999) have dramatic, negative impacts on myelination, and can be lethal.

Migrating cells have a dynamic microtubule network organized with plus-ends uni-formly oriented toward the cell periphery and minus-ends anchored at a central *microtubule organizing center* containing the centrioles and termed the centrosome. Migrating OPCs have a uni- or bipolar shape and share this kind of microtubule organization (Simpson and Armstrong 1999). Many complex cells generate a network featuring highly stable micro-tubules that are not attached to the centrosome. The oligodendrocyte microtubule network undergoes substantial transformation during differentiation (Kachar et al. 1986, Wilson and Brophy 1989), which includes development of a dispersed, non-centrosomal microtubule network (Lunn et al. 1997, Song et al. 2001, Terada et al. 2005). Consistent with a non-centrosomal microtubule organization, the minus-end tethered Golgi apparatus appears as scattered "biosynthetic stations" throughout the perinuclear cytoplasm and proximal processes (Sternberger et al. 1979, Terada et al. 2005). Microtubules in oligodendrocyte processes have a mixed polarity (Song et al. 2001), similar to Schwann cells (Kidd et al. 1996). The microtubule binding and stabilizing protein tau is enriched in oligodendrocytes and co-localizes with microtubules (LoPresti et al. 1995, Richter-Landsberg and Gorath 1999, Gorath et al. 2001). Levels of tau are developmentally regulated in oligodendrocytes

(Richter-Landsberg and Gorath 1999, Gorath et al. 2001) and antisense inhibition of tau expression dramatically inhibits oligodendrocyte process outgrowth (Gordon et al. 2008).

Several other microtubule activating proteins (MAPs) and microtubule modulating proteins are expressed by oligodendrocytes and contribute to microtubule assembly, stabilization, and organization during myelination. These include MAP1B (Fischer et al. 1990), MAP4 (Vouyiouklis and Brophy 1995) and MAP2C (Vouyiouklis and Brophy 1995, Richter-Landsberg and Gorath 1999). Oligodendrocyte-specific STOP (stable tubule only polypeptide) isoforms (Galiano et al. 2004) have also been described which, like tau and other MAPs, may promote microtubule stabilization. The microtubule destabilizing protein stathmin-1 is expressed early in myelinogenesis and has been suggested to destabilize microtubules at paranodal sites (Southwood et al. 2007). Sirtuin 2 is a deacetylase enriched in myelin membranes (Roth et al. 2006, Southwood et al. 2007), including paranodal loops, and may reduce microtubule acetylation. Acetylated α-tubulin is common in stable microtubules and may enhance MAP and motor binding (Fukushima et al. 2009).

MYELIN PROTEIN TARGETING

Greater than 50% of myelin proteins are synthesized in the rough endoplasmic reticulum and processed through the Golgi apparatus. How the integral membrane proteins – including PLP, MAG, MOG, claudin-11 and NF155 – become targeted to different myelin membrane domains is not known, although parallels with the secretory pathways in smaller polarized cells such as Madin–Darby canine kidney (MDCK) cells have provided some clues. Domain-specific targeting begins within the terminal Golgi compartment (Fig. 2.7a), called the trans-Golgi network, where different protein subsets are segregated into separate carrier vesicles. In oligodendrocytes, PLP and MAG are transported to myelin in different vesicles (Trapp et al. 1989). From the trans-Golgi network, myelin proteins travel along microtubules (Fig. 2.7b) directly to their target membrane (Fig. 2.7c) or follow indirect routes involving insertion, endocytosis, and insertion into another membrane domain (transcytosis). These pathways and molecular targeting signals have been documented in epithelial cells (Weimbs et al. 1997, Mostov et al. 2000). In oligodendrocytes, L-MAG is enriched in endosomes during early stages of CNS myelination (Trapp et al. 1989). Endosomes enriched for L-MAG were detected in cytoplasmic domains of the myelin internode, oligodendrocyte processes and oligodendrocyte perinuclear cytoplasm. Since MAG is only detected in the periaxonal membrane of CNS myelin internodes (Fig. 2.7d), it seems unlikely that L-MAG is transcytosed. The most likely explanation is that endocytosed L-MAG is taken up during spiral growth of the periaxonal membrane (Fig. 2.7e) and recycled back to growing MAG-containing regions or degraded in the endosomal/lysosomal system (Fig. 2.7f). PLP is not abundant in endosomes (Bo et al. 1995), indicating that MAG enrichment in endosomes is not simply part of a mechanism for removal of nonpolarized delivery of myelin proteins to the early oligodendrocyte plasma membrane.

Unfolded protein response

When conditions interfere with protein folding in the lumen of the endoplasmic reticulum, the accumulation of unfolded or misfolded proteins causes stress. To alleviate this stress,

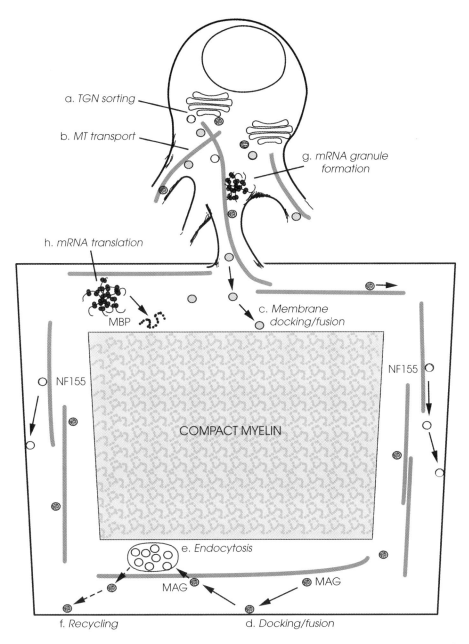

Fig. 2.7. Summary diagram of protein trafficking to different myelin domains through the secretory (a–f) and mRNA trafficking pathways (g, h) (described in detail in the text). MAG, myelin associated protein; MBP, myelin basic protein; MT, microtubule; NF, neurofascin; PLP, proteolipid protein; TGN, trans-Golgi network.

cells activate the "unfolded protein response", which affects nearly every level of the secretory pathway (Schroder and Kaufman 2005). If the unfolded protein response fails to decrease the unfolded protein load, then apoptosis can result. Missense point mutations, deletions, and duplications of the *PLP* gene cause developmental diseases of myelin, referred to as Pelizaeus–Merzbacher disease. A number of experimental animal models for this disease have also been produced or arose spontaneously (Macklin et al. 1987b, Gencic and Hudson 1990, Griffiths et al. 1998b). Most of these PLP-related mutations produce oligodendrocyte apoptosis. Mutated and misfolded proteins are retained in the endoplasmic reticulum rather than being transported to the plasma membrane (Gow et al. 1994, 1998). In vivo, the intracellular accumulation of PLP is minimal but may be sufficient to cause apoptosis of oligodendrocytes via an unfolded protein response. Over-expression of PLP can also kill oligodendrocytes by a similar mechanism (Kagawa et al. 1994, Readhead et al. 1994).

SPIRAL MYELIN GROWTH

Spiral and longitudinal growth of myelin depend upon actin-based mechanisms. Filamentous actin is abundant in the processes and non-compact regions of the growing myelin internode. A large repertoire of actin binding proteins regulates the assembly and spatial organization of actin filaments in growing cells. Actin filaments (f-actin, microfilaments) assemble spontaneously from free actin in the cytoplasm (g-actin). Actin-associated proteins direct and modulate actin assembly in several ways. Some promote actin filament nucleation, including the Arp2/3 complex and the formins. Some initiate filament depolymerization, including the actin-depolymerizing factor (ADF/cofilin) family and filament-severing proteins like gelsolin. Others scavenge monomeric actin and regulate its availability for filament assembly; profilin is one such protein. Proteins such as the WAVE (Wiskott-Aldrich syndrome protein family verprolin-homologous protein) complexes serve to cap and protect the ends of filaments, impeding disassembly. Many actin-associated proteins are targets of diverse signaling pathways involving receptor tyrosine kinases affected through Rho GTPase family members. An oligodendrocyte-enriched isoform (Kim et al. 2006) of WAVE1 is present at the actin-enriched leading edge of cultured oligodendrocytes. Mice deficient for WAVE1 have "patchy" hypomyelination, which entails reductions in the number of axons that are myelinated and in oligodendrocyte number, but where myelination occurs, internode thickness and length appear normal. This indicates that WAVE1 is not indispensable for spiral growth but suggests that WAVE is important prior to spiral growth, such as in process outgrowth, and may affect premyeli-nating oligodendrocyte survival.

Cytoplasmic myosin II is an actin motor that assembles into filaments upon phospho-rylation of the regulatory light chain. These filaments pull against actin microfilaments in an ATP-dependent manner and provide tension at sites such as focal adhesion complexes. A recent paper (Wang et al. 2008) indicates that activation of myosin II promotes Schwann cell myelination. In vitro, however, activation of myosin II regulatory chain retarded oligo-dendrocyte process outgrowth and myelination. Inhibition of myosin II activation promoted extensive process outgrowth and increased the number of internodes formed 3- to 4-fold over control cultures (Wang et al. 2008). Myosin II regulatory light chain becomes less phosphorylated, and thus less active, during myelination in rat brain lysates (Wang et al. 2008), and the oligodendrocyte-enriched myosin isoform myosin IIB is also reduced in concentration. These data suggest that myosin II may act as a brake, preventing oligodendrocyte processes from selecting and myelinating axons, and signaling pathways that modulate myosin regulatory light chain phosphorylation may be important in myelination.

Gelsolin is an 82-kDa microfilament severing protein implicated in lamellipodial movement of many cells. In oligodendrocytes, gelsolin is selectively enriched in the cell body, processes, and in paranodal cytoplasm (Legrand et al. 1986, Tanaka and Sobue 1994). Gelsolin is one of a family of actin-severing and actin-capping proteins, which break actin filaments and cap the fast-growing end of the filament upon Ca^{2+} binding. They also bind monomers to inhibit actin growth. Phosphoinositide binding releases gelsolin from the filament ends and promotes rapid actin reassembly. Gelsolin is also regulated by Rac GTPases. Gelsolin-null BalbC or C57/BL mice die in utero or in the immediate postnatal period (Kwiatkowski 1999). In mixed-background mice, however, lack of gelsolin produces very subtle phenotypes (Kwiatkowski 1999). Although in-vivo roles for gelsolin in myelination have yet to be determined, its distribution in paranodal loops and central role in actin cytoskeletal dynamics in cell movement make it a likely component of the spiral growth machinery.

Reciprocal interactions between axons and oligodendrocytes

Axons are the principal regulator of myelination. Although oligodendrocytes produce myelin-like membranes when isolated in vitro, they myelinate only axons and a small population of dendrites in vivo (Peters et al. 1991). Furthermore, there is a quantitative geometric relationship (or g-ratio) between axonal diameter and myelin internode thickness. The axonal diameter expressed as a fraction of the total myelinated fiber diameter is a relatively constant 0.6–0.7 for most CNS axons (Peters et al. 1991, Hildebrand et al. 1993). G-ratios are a useful measure for identifying aberrant myelination. The molecular basis for axonal modulation of myelination has been investigated for many years. Because large and small axons may lie in close proximity to one another, it is generally accepted that axons modulate oligodendrocyte myelination through physical contact or by secreting molecules with limited diffusion; longer range factors would have bystander effects on nearby myelin internodes. Likely scenarios entail activation of receptors in the oligodendrocyte by ligands attached to or shed from the axonal surface, which activate signaling cascades that modify f-actin-based membrane growth. Hypotheses in which axonal diameter provides direct mechanical cues for myelination have also been proposed and do not necessarily exclude such molecular scenarios. Some recently identified components of axon-myelin signaling are described below.

AXONAL REGULATORS OF MYELIN THICKNESS

In the PNS, axonal neuregulin 1 (NRG1) regulates Schwann cell–axon ensheathment (Taveggia et al. 2005) and myelin sheath thickness (Michailov et al. 2004, Taveggia et al. 2005; also see reviews by Corfas et al. 2004, Nave and Trapp 2008). NRG1 and ErbB receptor signaling does not appear to be essential for CNS myelin, but NRG1 enhances the proliferation and survival of oligodendrocyte precursors (see Nave and Trapp 2008). Reduced expression of type III NRG1 in CNS axons (Taveggia et al. 2008) resulted in myelin thinning in the forebrain but did not alter myelination in the optic nerve or spinal cord. Three principal NRG1 forms exist (types I–III) and all contain an epidermal growth factor domain that interacts with the ErbB family of receptor tyrosine kinases. NRGs are synthesized as single-pass transmembrane proteins and can be released from the membrane by proteolytic cleavage. NRG1 type III is cleaved by the beta-amyloid converting enzyme 1 (BACE1) (Hu et al. 2006). BACE1-null mice exhibited reduced rates of NRG1-cleavage in the CNS (Hu et al. 2006), less secreted/cleaved NGR1, higher levels of NRG1 tethered to the transmembrane domain, and hypomyelination of optic nerve axons (Hu et al. 2006). These results implicate BACE1 substrates in regulating myelin thickness and support a role of cleaved NRG1.

Myelin thickness can be modulated by other mechanisms. For example, integrins have also been implicated as regulators of CNS myelination. Comprised of α and ß subunits, integrins are activated by extracellular matrix components. OPCs express several integrins in vitro (Milner and Ffrench-Constant 1994). Oligodendrocyte expression of a dominant negative ß1 integrin (Lee et al. 2006) resulted in hypomyelination and fewer myelinated axons in spinal cords and optic nerves. Corpus callosum axons were myelinated normally. The axonal ligand for oligodendrocyte integrins remains to be identified.

Other studies investigating the regulation of myelin thickness have demonstrated hypermyelination. For example, over-expression of insulin-like growth factor (IGF)-1 (Ye et al. 1995) resulted in hypermyelination of CNS axons. Constructs driven by the MBP promoter yielded similar results (Luzi et al. 2004). Oligodendrocytes express IGF receptors and IGF increases OPC proliferation (Carson et al. 1993). Oligodendrocyte expression of a constitutively active form of the signaling kinase Akt caused a significant increase in myelin sheath thickness (Flores et al. 2008). Overstimulation of Akt signaling pathways did not alter oligodendrocyte numbers or axonal diameters (Flores et al. 2008). Akt is a downstream signaling component of receptor tyrosine kinases. ErbB receptors, IGF receptors and integrins mediate their intracellular effects through PI3 kinase activity. Recent studies suggest that mTOR (mammalian target of rappamycin) may lie downstream of Akt signaling in myelinating oligodendrocytes (Narayanan et al. 2009). Further elucidation of the upstream and downstream pathways of Akt activation is likely to be important in unraveling the mechanisms regulating CNS myelination.

OLIGODENDROCYTES MODULATE AXONAL DIAMETER AND SURVIVAL

Myelination increases axonal calibre. Increases in axonal diameter with Schwann cell myelination correlate with increases in axonal intermediate filament packing density (deWaegh et al. 1992, Hsieh et al. 1994). Phosphorylation of neurofilament (NF)-M and NF-H increases neurofilament sidearm extension, which in turn increases both the distance between neurofilaments and the axonal diameter. Loss of MAG results in minor myelin defects but substantial changes in PNS axonal diameter, neurofilament phosphorylation, and neurofilament spacing (Yin et al. 1998). Similar axonal defects in MAG-null mice and mice unable to synthesize complex axonal gangliosides (Sheikh et al. 1999, Pan et al. 2005) suggests that MAG–glycolipid interactions may play a role in modulating axonal diameter Dashiell et al. (2002) correlated decreased activities of extracellular-signal regulated kinases (ERK1/2) and cyclin-dependent kinase-5 (cdk5) with reduced neurofilament phosphorylation in MAG-deficient axons. The effects of myelin protein loss on CNS axonal diameter appear to be less dramatic than those in the PNS, although this may reflect the overall smaller sizes of CNS axons. X-irradiation of the optic nerve to remove OPCs and oligodendrocytes resulted in reduced axonal diameters (Colello et al. 1994). Loss of MBP in *shiverer* mice results in reduced optic nerve axonal diameter, reduced neurofilament concentration, and reduced neurofilament phosphorylation (Kirkpatrick et al. 2001). Partial rescue of the *shiverer* phenotype by transgenic expression of 25% of wild-type MBP levels resulted in thin myelin and a partial restoration of axonal diameter (Kirkpatrick et al. 2001). These studies support the possibility that CNS myelination modulates axonal caliber by modulating both concentration and phosphorylation of neurofilaments.

While myelination and increased axonal diameter are important to axonal electrophysiology, far more devastating changes occur in axons following demyelination and dysmyelination. In multiple sclerosis, exposure of the axon to the acute inflammatory demyelinating environment can result in axonal transection (Trapp and Stys 2009). Late-onset degeneration of demyelinated and dysmyelinated axons (Nave and Trapp 2008, Trapp and Nave 2008) indicates that ongoing interactions between oligodendrocytes and axons are essential for long-term axonal survival. Although the precise nature of these interactions remains to be determined, maintenance of axonal integrity requires the expression of MAG, PLP and CNP. For example, axons in PLP-null mice develop normally, but eventually undergo a late-onset (>12 months) degeneration (Fig. 2.8) that preferentially occurs in long-projecting, small-caliber axons (Griffiths et al. 1998b). Axonal transport is impaired by loss of PLP (Edgar et al. 2004) and beginning at P90, pronounced swellings containing mitochondria, amyloid precursor protein (Fig. 2.8a–c), and membranous organelles occur in myelinated axons, particularly at distal paranodes. This axonal pathology appears to be regulated at the level of individual internodes, as chimeric mice in which 50% of the oligodendrocytes lack PLP had only half the swellings of PLP-null mice (Edgar et al. 2004). Interestingly, replacement of PLP with P0, the major structural protein of mammalian PNS myelin, resulted in PNS-like compact myelin, but accelerated axonal defects and resulted in reduced lifespans compared with PLP-null mice (Fig. 2.8c,d) (Yin et al. 2006). Targeted disruption of the *CNP1* gene did not affect myelination but did induce an early onset of axonal swellings, axonal degeneration (Lappe-Siefke et al. 2003), and early death. While MAG, PLP and CNP are required for long-term myelinated axonal survival, none is necessary for myelin assembly. Thus, the role of these myelin proteins in maintaining axonal integrity and survival is independent of their role in myelination. Further characterization of how myelin maintains axonal integrity should provide therapeutics that delay axonal degeneration and neurological disability in individuals with primary diseases of myelin.

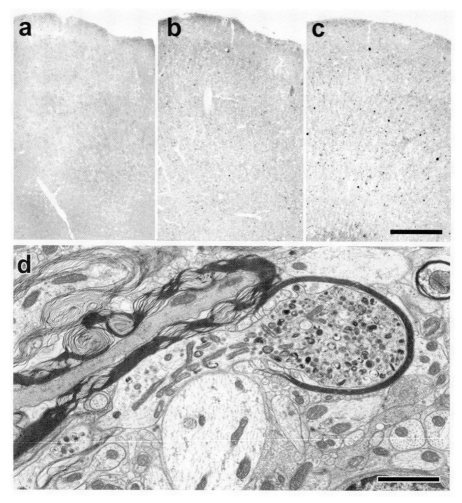

Fig. 2.8. Loss of proteolipid protein (PLP) impairs axonal function. Impaired axonal function results in accumulation of the amyloid precursor protein (APP), which appears as dots of staining that are absent from wild-type mouse cortex (**a**). At 12 months of age, APP accumulations are common in cortex of PLP-null mice (**b**), and abundant in P0-CNS mice (**c**), in which PLP is replaced by the peripheral nerve myelin protein P0. By electron microscopy (**d**), APP staining corresponds with intra-axonal accumulation of mitochondria and other membranous organelles that are pronounced at distal paranodes. Scale bars: **a–c**, 200 μm; **d**, 2.5 μm. Reproduced from Yin et al. (2006) with permission.

Summary and conclusions

Oligodendrocytes generate prodigious expanses of well-ordered spiralled myelin membrane around multiple axons and participate dynamically in organizing the axonal surface and cytoskeleton. Our current knowledge of how myelin and oligodendrocyte molecules achieve these functions has expanded our understanding of what myelination is and achieves.

Oligodendrocyte and myelin proteins are as important to the structural organization, function and survival of the axon as they are for the formation and maintenance of the myelin internode. Future advances in high-throughput genomics and proteomics approaches, manipulation of the mouse myelin genome, and critical analysis of human myelin diseases will continue to delineate the molecular mechanisms of myelination and the pathogenesis of neurological disability associated with myelin disease.

Acknowledgments

The authors thanks Dr Chris Nelson for assistance in preparing the manuscript, and Ms Jacqueline Stern for assistance with the Figures.

REFERENCES

Agrawal HC, Randle CL, Agrawal D. (1982) In vivo acylation of rat brain myelin proteolipid protein. J Biol Chem 257: 4588–4592.

Ariyasu RG, Ellisman MH. (1987) The distribution of (Na+ + K+)ATPase is continuous along the axolemma of unensheathed axons from spinal roots of "dystrophic" mice. J Neurocytol 16: 239–248.

Arquint M, Roder J, Chia L-S, et al. (1987) Molecular cloning and primary structure of myelin-associated glycoproteins. Proc Natl Acad Sci USA 84: 600–604.

Barbarese E, Carson JH, Braun PE. (1978) Accumulation of the four myelin basic proteins in mouse brain during development. J Neurochem 31: 779–782.

Bartsch U, Montag D, Bartsch S, Schachner M. (1995) Multiply myelinated axons in the optic nerve of mice deficient for the myelin-associated glycoprotein. Glia 14: 115–122.

Bennett V, Lambert S. (1999) Physiological roles of axonal ankyrins in survival of premyelinated axons and localization of voltage-gated sodium channels. J Neurocytol 28: 303–318.

Berghs S, Aggujaro D, Dirkx R, Jr et al. (2000) betaIV spectrin, a new spectrin localized at axon initial segments and nodes of ranvier in the central and peripheral nervous system. J Cell Biol 151: 985–1002.

Bergoffen J, Scherer SS, Wang S, et al. (1993) Connexin mutations in X-linked Charcot–Marie–Tooth disease. Science 262: 2039–2042.

Bhat MA, Rios JC, Lu Y, et al. (2001) Axon–glia interactions and the domain organization of myelinated axons requires neurexin iv/caspr/paranodin. Neuron 30: 369–383.

Bizzozero OA, McGarry JF, Lees MB. (1986) Acylation of rat brain myelin proteolipid protein with different fatty acids. J Neurochem 47: 772–778.

Black JA, Kocsis JD, Waxman SG. (1990) Ion channel organization of the myelinated fiber. Trends Neurosci 13: 48–54.

Blakemore WF. (1969) Schmidt–Lantermann incisures in the central nervous system. J Ultrastruct Res 29: 496–498.

Blakemore WF. (1981) Observations on myelination and remyelination in the central nervous system. In: Garrod DR, Feldman JD, eds. Development in the Nervous System. Cambridge: Cambridge University Press, pp. 289–308.

Bo L, Quarles RH, Fujita N, Bartoszewicz Z, Sato S, Trapp BD. (1995) Endocytic depletion of L-MAG from CNS myelin in quaking mice. J Cell Biol 131: 1811–1820.

Boggs JM. (2006) Myelin basic protein: a multifunctional protein. Cell Mol Life Sci 63: 1945–1961.

Bosio A, Bussow H, Adam J, Stoffel W. (1998) Galactosphingolipids and axono-glial interaction in myelin of the central nervous system. Cell Tissue Res 292: 199–210.

Boyle ME, Berglund EO, Murai KK, Weber L, Peles E, Ranscht B. (2001) Contactin orchestrates assembly of the septate-like junctions at the paranode in myelinated peripheral nerve. Neuron 30: 385–397.

Braun PE, De Angelis D, Shtybel WW, Bernier L. (1991) Isoprenoid modification permits 2', 3'-cyclic nucleotide 3'-phosphodiesterase to bind to membranes. J Neurosci Res 30: 540–544.

Braun PE, Sandillon F, Edwards A, Matthieu J-M, Privat A. (1988) Immunocytochemical localization by electron microscopy of 2', 3'-cyclic nucleotide 3'-phosphodiesterase in developing oligodendrocytes of normal and mutant brain. J Neurosci 8: 3057–3066.

Bronstein JM, Micevych PE, Chen K. (1997) Oligodendrocyte-specific protein (OSP) is a major component of CNS myelin. J Neurosci Res 50: 713–720.

Brunner C, Lassmann H, Waehneldt TV, Matthieu J, Linington C. (1989) Differential ultrastructural localization of myelin basic protein, myelin/oligodendroglial glycoprotein, and 2', 3'-cyclic nucleotide 3'-phosphodiesterase in the CNS of adult rats. J Neurochem 52: 296–304.

Bruzzone R, White TW, Scherer SS, Fischbeck KH, Paul DL. (1994) Null mutations of connexin32 in patients with X-linked Charcot–Marie–Tooth disease. Neuron 13: 1253–1260.

Bunge RP. (1968) Glial cells and the central myelin sheath. Physiol Rev 48: 197–251.

Caldwell JH, Schaller KL, Lasher RS, Peles E, Levinson SR. (2000) Sodium channel Na(v)1.6 is localized at nodes of ranvier, dendrites, and synapses. Proc Natl Acad Sci USA 97: 5616–5620.

Carnegie PR, Dunkley PR, Kemp BE, Murray AW. (1974) Phosphorylation of selected serine and threonine residues in myelin basic protein by endogenous and exogenous protein kinases. Nature 249: 147–150.

Carson MJ, Behringer RR, Brinster RL, McMorris FA. (1993) Insulin-like growth factor I increases brain growth and central nervous system myelination in transgenic mice. Neuron 10: 729–740.

Charles P, Tait S, Faivre-Sarrailh C, et al. (2002) Neurofascin is a glial receptor for the paranodin/Caspr–contactin axonal complex at the axoglial junction. Curr Biol 12: 217–220.

Cheong KH, Zacchetti D, Schneeberger EE, Simons K. (1999) VIP17/MAL, a lipid raft-associated protein, is involved in apical transport in MDCK cells. Proc Natl Acad Sci USA 96: 6241–6248.

Chow E, Mottahedeh J, Prins M, Ridder W, Nusinowitz S, Bronstein JM. (2005) Disrupted compaction of CNS myelin in an OSP/Claudin-11 and PLP/DM20 double knockout mouse. Mol Cell Neurosci 29: 405–413.

Colello RJ, Pott U, Schwab ME. (1994) The role of oligodendrocytes and myelin on axon maturation in the developing rat retinofugal pathway. J Neurosci 14: 2594–2605.

Corfas G, Velardez MO, Ko CP, Ratner N, Peles E. (2004) Mechanisms and roles of axon–Schwann cell interactions. J Neurosci 24: 9250–9260.

Craner MJ, Lo AC, Black JA, Waxman SG. (2003) Abnormal sodium channel distribution in optic nerve axons in a model of inflammatory demyelination. Brain 126: 1552–1561.

Craner MJ, Newcombe J, Black JA, Hartle C, Cuzner ML, Waxman SG. (2004) Molecular changes in neurons in multiple sclerosis: altered axonal expression of Nav1.2 and Nav1.6 sodium channels and Na$^+$/Ca^{2+} exchanger. Proc Natl Acad Sci USA 101: 8168–8173.

Cross D, Farias G, Dominguez J, Avila J, Maccioni RB. (1994) Carboxyl terminal sequences of beta-tubulin involved in the interaction of HMW-MAPs. Studies using site-specific antibodies. Mol Cell Biochem 132: 81–90.

Dashiell SM, Tanner SL, Pant HC, Quarles RH. (2002) Myelin-associated glycoprotein modulates expression and phosphorylation of neuronal cytoskeletal elements and their associated kinases. J Neurochem 81: 1263–1272.

Davis JQ, Lambert S, Bennett V. (1996) Molecular composition of the node of Ranvier: identification of ankyrin-binding cell adhesion molecules neurofascin (mucin+/third FNIII domain-) and NrCAM at nodal axon segments. J Cell Biol 135(5): 1355–1367.

Delarasse C, Daubas P, Mars LT, et al. (2003) Myelin/oligodendrocyte glycoprotein-deficient (MOG-deficient) mice reveal lack of immune tolerance to MOG in wild-type mice. J Clin Invest 112: 544–553.

Denisenko-Nehrbass N, Oguievetskaia K, et al. (2003) Protein 4.1B associates with both Caspr/paranodin and Caspr2 at paranodes and juxtaparanodes of myelinated fibres. Eur J Neurosci 17: 411–416.

deWaegh SM, Lee VMY, Brady ST. (1992) Local modulation of neurofilament phosphorylation, axonal caliber, and slow axonal transport by myelinating Schwann cells. Cell 68: 451–463.

Drummond GI, Lyer NT, Keith J. (1962) Hydrolysis of ribonucleoside 2', 3' cyclic phosphates by a diesterase from brain. J Biol Chem 237: 3535–3539.

Duncan ID, Hammang JP, Goda S, Quarles RH. (1989) Myelination in the jimpy mouse in the absence of proteolipid protein. Glia 2: 155–160.

Duncan ID, Hammang JP, Trapp BD. (1988) Abnormal compact myelin in the myelin-deficient rat: absence of proteolipid protein correlates with a defect in the intraperiod line. Proc Natl Acad Sci USA 84: 6287–6291.

Duncan ID, Lunn KF, Holmgren B, Urba-Holmgren R, Brignolo-Holmes L. (1992) The Taiep rat; a myelin mutant with an associated oligodendrocyte microtubulin defect. J Neurocytol 12: 870–874.

Dupree JL, Coetzee T, Blight A, Suzuki K, Popko B. (1998) Myelin galactolipids are essential for proper node of Ranvier formation in the CNS. J Neurosci 18: 1642–1649.

Dupree JL, Girault JA, Popko B. (1999) Axo-glial interactions regulate the localization of axonal paranodal proteins. J Cell Biol 147: 1145–1152.

Edgar JM, McLaughlin M, Yool D, et al. (2004) Oligodendroglial modulation of fast axonal transport in a mouse model of hereditary spastic paraplegia. J Cell Biol 166: 121–131.

Einheber S, Zanazzi G, Ching W, et al. (1997) The axonal membrane protein Caspr, a homologue of neurexin IV, is a component of the septate-like paranodal junctions that assemble during myelination. J Cell Biol 139: 1495–1506.

Ellisman MH, Levinson SR. (1982) Immunocytochemical localization of sodium channel distributions in the excitable membranes of *Electrophorus electricus*. Proc Natl Acad Sci USA 79: 6707–6711.

Fanarraga ML, Griffiths IR, Zhao M, Duncan ID. (1998) Oligodendrocytes are not inherently programmed to myelinate a specific size of axon. J Comp Neurol 399: 94–100.

Fernandez-Moran H, Finean JB. (1957) Electron microscope and low-angle x-ray diffraction studies of the nerve myelin sheath. J Biophys Biochem Cytol 3: 725–748.

Fischer I, Konola J, Cochary E. (1990) Microtubule associated protein (MAP1B) is present in cultured oligodendrocytes and co-localizes with tubulin. J Neurosci Res 27: 112–124.

Flores AI, Narayanan SP, Morse EN, et al. (2008) Constitutively active Akt induces enhanced myelination in the CNS. J Neurosci 28: 7174–7183.

Frank M. (2000) MAL, a proteolipid in glycosphingolipid enriched domains: functional implications in myelin and beyond. Prog Neurobiol 60: 531–544.

Fukushima N, Furuta D, Hidaka Y, Moriyama R, Tsujiuchi T. (2009) Post-translational modifications of tubulin in the nervous system. J Neurochem 109: 683–693.

Furley AJ, Morton SB, Manalo D, Karagogeos D, Dodd J, Jessell TM. (1990) The axonal glycoprotein TAG-1 is an immunoglobulin superfamily member with neurite outgrowth-promoting activity. Cell 61: 157–170.

Galiano MR, Bosc C, Schweitzer A, Andrieux A, Job D, Hallak ME. (2004) Astrocytes and oligodendrocytes express different STOP protein isoforms. J Neurosci Res 78: 329–337.

Garbern JY, Yool DA, Moore GJ, et al. (2002) Patients lacking the major CNS myelin protein, proteolipid protein 1, develop length-dependent axonal degeneration in the absence of demyelination and inflammation. Brain 125: 551–561.

Gencic S, Hudson LD. (1990) Conservative amino acid substitution in the myelin proteolipid protein of jimpymsd mice. J Neurosci 10: 117–124.

Geren BB. (1954) The formation from the Schwann cell surface of myelin in the peripheral nerves of chick embryos. Exp Cell Res 7: 558–562.

Goldstein LS, Yang Z. (2000) Microtubule-based transport systems in neurons: the roles of kinesins and dyneins. Annu Rev Neurosci 23: 39–71.

Gollan L, Sabanay H, Poliak S, Berglund EO, Ranscht B, Peles E. (2002) Retention of a cell adhesion complex at the paranodal junction requires the cytoplasmic region of Caspr. J Cell Biol 157: 1247–1256.

Gorath M, Stahnke T, Mronga T, Goldbaum O, Richter-Landsberg C. (2001) Developmental changes of tau protein and mRNA in cultured rat brain oligodendrocytes. Glia 36: 89–101.

Gordon D, Kidd GJ, Smith R. (2008) Antisense suppression of tau in cultured rat oligodendrocytes inhibits process formation. J Neurosci Res 86: 2591–2601.

Gow A, Friedrich VL, Jr., Lazzarini RA. (1994) Many naturally occurring mutations of myelin proteolipid protein impair its intracellular transport. J Neurosci Res 37: 574–583.

Gow A, Southwood CM, Lazzarini RA. (1998) Disrupted proteolipid protein trafficking results in oligodendrocyte apoptosis in an animal model of Pelizaeus–Merzbacher disease. J Cell Biol 140: 925–934.

Gow A, Southwood CM, Li JS, et al. (1999) CNS myelin and sertoli cell tight junction strands are absent in Osp/claudin-11 null mice. Cell 99: 649–659.

Greenfield S, Brostoff S, Eylar HH, Morell P. (1973) Protein composition of myelin of the peripheral nervous system. J Neurochem 20: 1207–1216.

Griffiths I, Klugmann M, Anderson T, Thomson C, Vouyiouklis D, Nave KA. (1998a) Current concepts of PLP and its role in the nervous system. Microsc Res Tech 41: 344–358.

Griffiths I, Klugmann M, Anderson T, et al. (1998b) Axonal swellings and degeneration in mice lacking the major proteolipid of myelin. Science 280: 1610–1613.

Guidotti G. (1972) Membrane proteins. Annu Rev Biochem 41: 731–752.

Hildebrand C, Remahl S, Persson H, Bjartmar C. (1993) Myelinated nerve fibres in the CNS. Prog Neurobiol 40: 319–384.

Holz A, Schaeren-Wiemers N, Schaefer C, Pott U, Colello RJ, Schwab ME. (1996) Molecular and developmental characterization of novel cDNAs of the myelin-associated/oligodendrocytic basic protein. J Neurosci 16: 467–477.

31

Honke K, Hirahara Y, Dupree J, et al. (2002) Paranodal junction formation and spermatogenesis require sulfoglycolipids. Proc Natl Acad Sci USA 99: 4227–4232.

Hsieh S-T, Kidd GJ, Crawford TO, et al. (1994) Regional modulation of neurofilament organization by myelination in normal axons. J Neurosci 14: 6392–6401.

Hu X, Hicks CW, He W, et al. (2006) Bace1 modulates myelination in the central and peripheral nervous system. Nat Neurosci 9: 1520–1525.

Jacobs JM, Cavanagh JB, Chen FCK. (1972) Spinal subarachnoid injection of colchicine in rats. J Neurol Sci 17: 461–480.

Kachar B, Behar T, Dubois-Dalcq M. (1986) Cell shape and motility of oligodendrocytes cultured without neurons. Cell Tissue Res 244: 27–38.

Kagawa T, Ikenaka K, Inoue Y, et al. (1994) Glial cell degeneration and hypomyelination caused by over-expression of myelin proteolipid protein gene. Neuron 13: 427–442.

Kamasawa N, Sik A, Morita M, et al. (2005) Connexin-47 and connexin-32 in gap junctions of oligodendrocyte somata, myelin sheaths, paranodal loops and Schmidt–Lanterman incisures: implications for ionic homeostasis and potassium siphoning. Neuroscience 136: 65–86.

Kelm S, Pelz A, Schauer R, et al. (1994) Sialoadhesin, myelin-associated glycoprotein and CD22 define a new family of sialic acid-dependent adhesion molecules of the immunoglobulin superfamily. Curr Biol 4: 965–972.

Kidd GJ, Andrews SB, Trapp BD. (1996) Axons regulate the distribution of Schwann cell microtubules. J Neurosci 16: 946–954.

Kim HJ, DiBernardo AB, Sloane JA, et al. (2006) WAVE1 is required for oligodendrocyte morphogenesis and normal CNS myelination. J Neurosci 26: 5849–5859.

Kimura M, Sato M, Akatsuka A, et al. (1989) Restoration of myelin formation by a single type of myelin basic protein in transgenic shiverer mice. Proc Natl Acad Sci USA 86: 5661–5665.

Kirkpatrick LL, Witt AS, Payne HR, Shine HD, Brady ST. (2001) Changes in microtubule stability and density in myelin-deficient shiverer mouse CNS axons. J Neurosci 21: 2288–2297.

Kirschner DA, Hollingshead CJ. (1980) Processing for electron microscopy alters membrane structure and packing in myelin. J Ultrastruct Res 73: 211–232.

Kleopa KA, Orthmann JL, Enriquez A, Paul DL, Scherer SS. (2004) Unique distributions of the gap junction proteins connexin29, connexin32, and connexin47 in oligodendrocytes. Glia 47: 346–357.

Klugmann M, Schwab MH, Puhlhofer A, et al. (1997) Assembly of CNS myelin in the absence of proteolipid protein. Neuron 18: 59–70.

Kordeli E, Davis JD, Trapp BD, Bennett V. (1990) An isoform of ankyrin is localized at nodes of Ranvier in myelinated axons of central and peripheral nerves. J Cell Biol 110: 1341–1352.

Kordeli E, Lambert S, Bennett V. (1995) AnkyrinG. A new ankyrin gene with neural-specific isoforms localized at the axonal initial segment and node of Ranvier. J Biol Chem 270: 2352–2359.

Krause G, Winkler L, Mueller SL, Haseloff RF, Piontek J, Blasig IE. (2008) Structure and function of claudins. Biochim Biophys Acta 1778: 631–645.

Kroepfl JF, Viise LR, Charron AJ, Linington C, Gardinier MV. (1996) Investigation of myelin/oligodendrocyte glycoprotein membrane topology. J Neurochem 67: 2219–2222.

Kwiatkowski DJ. (1999) Functions of gelsolin: motility, signaling, apoptosis, cancer. Curr Opin Cell Biol 11: 103–108.

Kwiecien JM, O'Connor LT, Goetz BD, Delaney KH, Fletch AL, Duncan ID. (1998) Morphological and morphometric studies of the dysmyelinating mutant, the Long Evans shaker rat. J Neurocytol 27: 581–591.

Lacas-Gervais S, Guo J, Strenzke N, et al. (2004) ßIVΣ1 spectrin stabilizes the nodes of Ranvier and axon initial segments. J Cell Biol 166: 983–990.

Lappe-Siefke C, Goebbels S, et al. (2003) Disruption of Cnp1 uncouples oligodendroglial functions in axonal support and myelination. Nat Genet 33: 366–374.

Lee J, Gravel M, Zhang R, Thibault P, Braun PE. (2005) Process outgrowth in oligodendrocytes is mediated by CNP, a novel microtubule assembly myelin protein. J Cell Biol 170: 661–673.

Lee KK, de RY, Saulnier R, Rippstein P, Macklin WB, Kothary R. (2006) Dominant-negative beta1 integrin mice have region-specific myelin defects accompanied by alterations in MAPK activity. Glia 53: 836–844.

Lees MB. (1998) A history of proteolipids: a personal memoir. Neurochem Res 23: 261–271.

Legrand C, Ferraz C, Clavel MC, Rabie A. (1986) Immunocytochemical localisation of gelsolin in oligoden-droglia of the developing rabbit central nervous system. Brain Res 395: 231–235.

Li C, Tropak MB, Gerial R, et al. (1994) Myelination in the absence of myelin-associated glycoprotein. Nature 369: 747–750.

Linnington C, Webb M, Woodhams PL. (1984) A novel myelin-associated glycoprotein defined by a mouse monoclonal antibody. J Neuroimmunol 6: 387–396.

LoPresti P, Szuchet S, Papasozomenos SC, Zinkowski RP, Binder LI. (1995) Functional implications for the microtubule-associated protein tau: localization in oligodendrocytes. Proc Natl Acad Sci USA 92: 10 369–10 373.

Lunn KF, Baas PW, Duncan ID. (1997) Microtubule organization and stability in the oligodendrocyte. J Neurosci 17: 4921–4932.

Luzi P, Zaka M, Rao HZ, Curtis M, Rafi MA, Wenger DA. (2004) Generation of transgenic mice expressing insulin-like growth factor-1 under the control of the myelin basic protein promoter: increased myelination and potential for studies on the effects of increased IGF-1 on experimentally and genetically induced demyelination. Neurochem Res 29: 881–889.

Macklin WB, Campagnoni CW, Deininger PL, Gardinier MV. (1987a) Structure and expression of the mouse myelin proteolipid gene. J Neurosci Res 18: 383–394.

Macklin WB, Gardinier MV, King KD, Kampf K. (1987b) An AG–GG transition at a splice site in the myelin PLP gene in jimpy mice results in the removal of an exon. FEBS Lett 223: 417–421.

Marcus J, Dupree JL, Popko B. (2000) Effects of galactolipid elimination on oligodendrocyte development and myelination. Glia 30: 319–328.

Mata M, Fink DJ, Ernst SA, Siegel GJ. (1991) Immunocytochemical demonstration of $Na^+,K(^+)$-ATPase in internodal axolemma of myelinated fibers of rat sciatic and optic nerves. J Neurochem 57: 184–192.

Menegoz M, Gaspar P, Le Bert M, et al. (1997) Paranodin, a glycoprotein of neuronal paranodal membranes. Neuron 19: 319–331.

Menichella DM, Goodenough DA, Sirkowski E, Scherer SS, Paul DL. (2003) Connexins are critical for normal myelination in the CNS. J Neurosci 23: 5963–5973.

Michailov GV, Sereda MW, Brinkmann BG, et al. (2004) Axonal neuregulin-1 regulates myelin sheath thickness. Science 304: 700–703.

Milner R, Ffrench-Constant C. (1994) A developmental analysis of oligodendroglial integrins in primary cells: changes in α v-associated ß subunitsduring differentiation. Development 120: 3497–3506.

Miyamoto E, Kakiuchi S, Kakimoto Y. (1974) In vitro and in vivo phosphorylation of myelin basic protein by cerebral protein kinase. Nature 249: 150–151.

Montag D, Giese KP, Bartsch U, et al. (1994) Mice deficient for the myelin-associated glycoprotein show subtle abnormalities in myelin. Neuron 13: 229–246.

Montague P, McCallion AS, Davies RW, Griffiths IR. (2006) Myelin-associated oligodendrocytic basic protein: a family of abundant CNS myelin proteins in search of a function. Dev Neurosci 28: 479–487.

Morita K, Sasaki H, Fujimoto K, Furuse M, Tsukita S. (1999) Claudin-11/OSP-based tight junctions of myelin sheaths in brain and Sertoli cells in testis. J Cell Biol 145: 579–588.

Mostov KE, Verges M, Altschuler Y. (2000) Membrane traffic in polarized epithelial cells. Curr Opin Cell Biol 12: 483–490.

Narayanan SP, Flores AI, Wang F, Macklin WB. (2009) Akt signals through the mammalian target of rapamycin pathway to regulate CNS myelination. J Neurosci 29: 6860–6870.

Nave KA, Lai C, Bloom FE, Milner RJ. (1987) Splice site selection in the proteolipid protein (PLP) gene transcript and primary structure of the DM-20 protein of central nervous system myelin. Proc Natl Acad Sci USA 84: 5665–5669.

Nave K-A, Trapp BD. (2008) Axon-glial signaling and the glial support of axon function. Annu Rev Neurosci 31: 535–561.

Norton WT, Cammer W (1984) Isolation and characterization of myelin. In: Morell P, ed. Myelin. New York: Plenum Press, pp. 146–196.

Omlin FX, Webster Hd, Palkovits CG, Cohen SR. (1982) Immunocytochemical localization of basic protein in major dense line regions of central and peripheral myelin. J Cell Biol 95: 242–248.

Orthmann-Murphy JL, Abrams CK, Scherer SS. (2008) Gap junctions couple astrocytes and oligodendrocytes. J Mol Neurosci 35: 101–116.

Pan B, Fromholt SE, Hess EJ, et al. (2005) Myelin-associated glycoprotein and complementary axonal ligands, gangliosides, mediate axon stability in the CNS and PNS: neuropathology and behavioral deficits in single- and double-null mice. Exp Neurol 195: 208–217.

Penfield W. (1924) Oligodendroglia and its relation to classical neuroglia. Brain 47: 430–452.

Peters A. (1961) A radial component of central myelin sheaths. J Biophys Biochem Cytol 11: 733–735.

Peters A. (1964) Observations on the connexions between myelin sheaths and glial cells in the optic nerves of young rats. J Anat 98: 125–134.

Peters A, Palay SL, Webster HD. (1991) The Fine Structure of the Nervous System: Neurons and their Supporting Cells. New York: Oxford University Press.

Pfeiffer SE, Warrington AE, Bansal R. (1993) The oligodendrocyte and its many cellular processes. Trends Cell Biol 3: 191–197.

Poliak S, Gollan L, Martinez R, et al. (1999) Caspr2, a new member of the neurexin superfamily, is localized at the juxtaparanodes of myelinated axons and associates with K+ channels. Neuron 24: 1037–1047.

Privat A, Jacque C, Bourre JM, Duponey P, Baumann N. (1979) Absence of the major dense line in myelin of the mutant mouse "Shiverer." Neurosci Lett 12: 107–112.

Ranscht B, Dours MT. (1988) Sequence of contactin, a 130-kD glycoprotein concentrated in areas of interneuronal contact, defines a new member of the immunoglobulin supergene family in the nervous system. J Cell Biol 107: 1561–1573.

Rasband MN, Tayler J, Kaga Y, et al. (2005) CNP is required for maintenance of axon–glia interactions at nodes of Ranvier in the CNS. Glia 50: 86–90.

Rasband MN, Trimmer JS, Schwarz TL, et al. (1998) Potassium channel distribution, clustering, and function in remyelinating rat axons. J Neurosci 18: 36–47.

Readhead C, Popko B, Takahashi N, et al. (1987) Expression of a myelin basic protein gene in shiverer transgenic mice: Correction of the dysmyelinating phynotype. Cell 48: 703–712.

Readhead C, Schneider A, Griffiths I, Nave K-A. (1994) Premature arrest of myelin formation in transgenic mice with increased proteolipid protein gene dosage. Neuron 12: 583–595.

Richter-Landsberg C, Gorath M. (1999) Developmental regulation of alternatively spliced isoforms of mRNA encoding MAP2 and tau in rat brain oligodendrocytes during culture maturation. J Neurosci Res 56: 259–270.

Rios JC, Melendez-Vasquez CV, Einheber S, et al. (2000) Contactin-associated protein (Caspr) and contactin form a complex that is targeted to the paranodal junctions during myelination. J Neurosci 20: 8354–8364.

Rosenbluth J. (1976) Intramembranous particle distribution at the node of Ranvier and adjacent axolemma in myelinated axons of the frog brain. J Neurocytol 5: 731–745.

Rosenbluth J, Schiff R, Lam P. (2009) Effects of osmolality on PLP-null myelin structure: implications re axon damage. Brain Res 1253: 191–197.

Roth AD, Ivanova A, Colman DR. (2006) New observations on the compact myelin proteome. Neuron Glia Biol 2: 15–21.

Salzer JL, Holmes WP, Colman DR. (1987) The amino acid sequences of the myelin-associated glycoproteins: homology to the immunoglobulin gene superfamily. J Cell Biol 104: 957–965.

Schaeren-Wiemers N, Schaefer C, Valenzuela DM, Yancopoulos GD, Schwab ME. (1995) Identification of new oligodendrocyte- and myelin-specific genes by a differential screening approach. J Neurochem 65: 10–22.

Scherer SS, Xu YT, Nelles E, Fischbeck K, Willecke K, Bone LJ. (1998) Connexin32-null mice develop demyelinating peripheral neuropathy. Glia 24: 8–20.

Schliwa M, Woehlke G. (2003) Molecular motors. Nature 422: 759–765.

Schnapp B, Mugnaini E. (1976) Freeze-fracture properties of central myelin in the bullfrog. Neuroscience 1: 459–467.

Schroder M, Kaufman RJ. (2005) The mammalian unfolded protein response. Annu Rev Biochem 74: 739–789.

Sheikh KA, Sun J, Liu Y, Kawai H, Crawford TO, Proia RL, Griffin JW, Schnaar RL. (1999) Mice lacking complex gangliosides develop Wallerian degeneration and myelination defects. Proc Natl Acad Sci USA 96: 7532–7537.

Simpson PB, Armstrong RC. (1999) Intracellular signals and cytoskeletal elements involved in oligodendrocyte progenitor migration. Glia 26: 22–35.

Song J, Goetz BD, Baas PW, Duncan ID. (2001) Cytoskeletal reorganization during the formation of oligodendrocyte processes and branches. Mol Cell Neurosci 17: 624–636.

Song J, O'Connor LT, Yu W, Baas PW, Duncan ID. (1999) Microtubule alterations in cultured taiep rat oligodendrocytes lead to deficits in myelin membrane formation. J Neurocytol 28: 671–683.

Southwood CM, Peppi M, Dryden S, Tainsky MA, Gow A. (2007) Microtubule deacetylases, SirT2 and HDAC6, in the nervous system. Neurochem Res 32: 187–195.

Sprinkle TJ, Zaruba ME, McKhann GM. (1978) Activity of 2', 3'-cyclic nucleotide 3'-phosphodiesterase in regions of rat brain during development: quantitative relationship to myelin basic protein. J Neurochem 30: 309–314.

Sternberger NH, Quarles RH, Itoyama Y, Webster HD. (1979) Myelin-associated glycoprotein demonstrated immunocytochemically in myelin and myelin-forming cells of developing rats. Proc Natl Acad Sci USA 76: 1510–1514.

Stoffel W, Boison D, Bussow H. (1997) Functional analysis in vivo of the double mutant mouse deficient in both proteolipid protein (PLP) and myelin basic protein (MBP) in the central nervous system. Cell Tissue Res 289: 195–206.

Tabira T, Cullen MJ, Reier PJ, Webster Hd. (1978) An experimental analysis of interlamellar tight junctions in amphibian and mammalian CNS myelin. J Neurocytol 7: 489–503.

Tait S, Gunn-Moore F, Collinson JM, et al. (2000) An oligodendroctye cell adhesion molecule at the site of assembly of the paranodal axo-glial junction. J Cell Biol 150: 657-666.

Tanaka J, Sobue K. (1994) Localization and characterization of gelsolin in nervous tissues: gelsolin is specifically enriched in myelin-forming cells. J Neurosci 14: 1038–1052.

Taveggia C, Thaker P, Petrylak A, et al. (2008) Type III neuregulin-1 promotes oligodendrocyte myelination. Glia 56: 284–293.

Taveggia C, Zanazzi G, Petrylak A, et al. (2005) Neuregulin-1 type III determines the ensheathment fate of axons. Neuron 47: 681–694.

Terada N, Kidd GJ, Kinter M, Bjartmar C, Moran-Jones K, Trapp BD. (2005) Beta(IV) tubulin is selectively expressed by oligodendrocytes in the central nervous system. Glia 50: 212–222.

Timsit S, Sinoway MP, Levy L, et al. (1992) The DM20 protein of myelin: intracellular and surface expression patterns in transfectants. J Neurochem 58: 1936–1942.

Traka M, Dupree JL, Popko B, Karagogeos D. (2002) The neuronal adhesion protein TAG-1 is expressed by Schwann cells and oligodendrocytes and is localized to the juxtaparanodal region of myelinated fibers. J Neurosci 22: 3016–3024.

Traka M, Goutebroze L, Denisenko N, et al. (2003) Association of TAG-1 with Caspr2 is essential for the molecular organization of juxtaparanodal regions of myelinated fibers. J Cell Biol 162: 1161–1172.

Trapp BD, Andrews SB, Cootauco C, Quarles RH. (1989) The myelin-associated glycoprotein is enriched in multivesicular bodies and periaxonal membranes of actively myelinating oligodendrocytes. J Cell Biol 109: 2417–2426.

Trapp BD, Bernier L, Andrews SB, Colman DR. (1988) Cellular and subcellular distribution of 2', 3' cyclic nucleotide 3' phosphodiesterase and its mRNA in the rat nervous system. J Neurochem 51: 859–868.

Trapp BD, Itoyama Y, MacIntosh TD, Quarles RH. (1983) P2 protein in oligodendrocytes and myelin of the rabbit central nervous system. J Neurochem 40: 47–54.

Trapp BD, Nave K-A. (2008) Multiple sclerosis: an immune or neurodegenerative disorder? Annu Rev Neurosci 31: 247–269.

Trapp BD, Nishiyama A, Cheng D, Macklin W. (1997) Differentiation and death of premyelinating oligodendrocytes in developing rodent brain. J Cell Biol 137: 459–468.

Trapp BD, Stys PK. (2009) Virtual hypoxia and chronic necrosis of demyelinated axons in multiple sclerosis. Lancet Neurol 8: 280–291.

Ueda H, Levine JM, Miller RH, Trapp BD. (1999) Rat optic nerve oligodendrocytes develop in the absence of viable retinal ganglion cell axons. J Cell Biol 146: 1365–1374.

Uyemura K, Yoshimura K, Suzuki M, Kitamura K. (1984) Lipid binding activities of the P2 protein in peripheral nerve myelin. Neurochem Res 9: 1509–1514.

Vouyiouklis DA, Brophy PJ. (1995) Microtubule-associated proteins in developing oligodendrocytes: transient expression of a MAP2c isoform in oligodendrocyte precursors. J Neurosci Res 42: 803–817.

Wang H, Tewari A, Einheber S, Salzer JL, Melendez-Vasquez CV. (2008) Myosin II has distinct functions in PNS and CNS myelin sheath formation. J Cell Biol 182: 1171–1184.

Weimbs T, Low SH, Chapin SJ, Mostov KE. (1997) Apical targeting in polarized epithelial cells: there's more afloat than rafts. Trends Cell Biol 7: 393–399.

Weimbs T, Stoffel W. (1992) Proteolipid protein (PLP) of CNS myelin: positions of free, disulfide-bonded, and fatty acid thioester-linked cysteine residues and implications for the membrane topology of PLP. Biochemistry 31: 12 289–12 296.

Wilson R, Brophy PJ. (1989) Role of the oligodendrocyte cytoskeleton in myelination. J Neurosci Res 22: 439–448.

Yamamoto Y, Mizuno R, Nishimura T, et al. (1994) Cloning and expression of myelin-associated oligodendrocytic basic protein. A novel basic protein constituting the central nervous system myelin. J Biol Chem 269: 31 725–31 730.

Ye P, Carson J, D'Ercole AJ. (1995) In vivo actions of insulin-like growth factor-I (IGF-I) on brain myelination: studies of IGF-I and IGF binding protein-1 (IGFBP-1) transgenic mice. J Neurosci 15: 7344–7356.

Yin X, Baek RC, Kirschner DA, et al. (2006) Evolution of a neuroprotective function of central nervous system myelin. J Cell Biol 172: 469–478.

Yin X, Crawford TO, Griffin JW, et al. (1998) Myelin-associated glycoprotein is a myelin signal that modulates the caliber of myelinated axons. J Neurosci 18: 1953–1962.

Yin X, Peterson J, Gravel M, Braun PE, Trapp BD. (1997) CNP overexpression induces aberrant oligodendrocyte membranes and inhibits MBP accumulation and myelin compaction. J Neurosci Res 50: 238–247.

Young EA, Fowler CD, Kidd GJ, et al. (2008) Imaging correlates of decreased axonal Na^+/K^+ ATPase in chronic MS lesions. Ann Neurol 63: 428–435.

Zeller NK, Hunkeler MJ, Campagnoni AT, Sprague J, Lazzarini RA. (1984) Characterization of mouse myelin basic protein messenger RNAs with a myelin basic protein cDNA clone. Proc Natl Acad Sci USA 81: 18–22.

3
THE ROLE OF ASTROCYTES IN WHITE MATTER DISEASE

Jörg Dietrich and Chris Pröschel

Introduction

The proper functioning of the mammalian central nervous system (CNS) depends on a highly organized interaction between numerous cell types, including astrocytes, oligodendrocytes, and neurons (Fields and Stevens-Graham 2002, Miller 2005, Lichtman and Smith 2008, Allen and Barres 2009). Dysfunction of any particular cell type or cell population may result in aberrant nervous system function and manifestation of neurological disease. Recent advances in cell-biological analysis of the complex lineage relationships in the developing and adult nervous system have started to shed light on the mechanisms that may constitute the cellular basis for distinct neurological diseases.

Diseases of the white matter are common neurological conditions and may be caused by autoimmune demyelinating processes, neurotoxic syndromes, acute or chronic ischemia, inflammatory disease, and developmental or neurodegenerative disease. While the exact underlying mechanisms leading to white matter disruption may be quite different in each of these conditions, the consequences commonly are impaired myelin formation, enhanced myelin loss, disruption of myelin fiber tracts, and subsequent impairment of neurological function.

As all major cell lineage systems in the CNS are closely dependent on each other, it is not surprising that disruption of one particular lineage population or subpopulation may result in global neurological dysfunction. Consistent with clinical and radiographical observations, experimental studies have shown that oligodendrocytes – the myelin-forming cells of the CNS – and their progenitor cells (also known as oligodendrocyte precursor cells [OPCs], or oligodendrocyte-type 2 astrocytes progenitor cells [O-2As]) appear to be one of the most vulnerable cell populations to various neurotoxicants and oxidative stress (McDonald et al. 1998a, b, Noble et al. 2003, Dietrich et al. 2006, Li et al. 2007).

Astrocytes are the most abundant glial cells of the nervous system. For many years, following the original morphological description of the astrocyte as "neuroglia" (Cajal, 1913), these cells were long thought to play only a structural role in the CNS. However, this view has changed dramatically as multiple functions of these cells have been identified (Horner and Palmer 2003, Pekny and Pekna 2004, Nishiyama et al. 2005, Volterra and Meldolesi 2005, Allen and Barres 2009, Webster and Astrom 2009). There has been increasing appreciation that astrocytes may not only respond to injury or neurological disease as "reactive gliosis" or "reactive astrocytes," but also may be the primary cause of disease, and in fact may be indispensable for function and survival of oligodendrocytes and neurons (Nedergaard et al. 2003, Ransom et al. 2003). Astrocytes exert their critical cell-biological function in various ways, including: supply of energy substrates (Tsacopoulos and Magistretti 1996, Brown et al. 2004); neurotransmitter release and uptake (Nedergaard 1994, Kimelberg 1995, Porter and McCarthy 1997, Anderson and Swanson 2000); growth factor production (Zaheer et al. 1995); regulation of cerebral blood flow (Takano et al. 2006); immune modulation (Farina et al. 2007); modulation of synapse formation and transmission (Helmuth 2001, Newman 2003); blood–brain barrier maintenance (Abbott et al. 2006); and control of water and electrolyte homeostasis (Amiry-Moghaddam and Ottersen 2003, Verkman et al. 2006, De Keyser et al. 2008). Moreover, glial fibrillary acidic protein (GFAP)-expressing astrocytes are considered to be neural stem cells localized to the lateral subventricular zone (Doetsch et al. 1999, Doetsch 2003, Chojnacki et al. 2009).

Consistent with these diverse and yet fundamental cellular functions, there has been the increasing notion that astrocytes may be critical players in the pathogenesis of various neurological diseases, ranging from inflammatory–demyelinating diseases to neurodegenerative diseases and leukodystrophies. Growing understanding of astrocyte function in neurological diseases may in turn lead to new avenues and strategies to identify therapeutic targets. This chapter will focus on the role of astrocytes and their progenitors in leukodystrophies, with special emphasis on recent findings on the cell-biological pathogenesis of Vanishing White Matter Disease.

Cellular lineage systems in the mammalian brain

In order to understand how glial cells, such as astrocytes, or any other cell type may impair brain function, it is important to be familiar with the current understanding of the cellular lineage systems in the CNS, which is composed of various mature cell types and their distinct progenitors. Mature cell types, such as astrocytes, oligodendrocytes, and neurons, are generated from neural stem cells (NSCs) via lineage committed progenitor cells. While this hierarchical process of cell generation is of fundamental importance during development, it appears that NSCs and their progeny orchestrate cellular regeneration even throughout adult life. NSCs are defined by their self-renewal potential, their ability to proliferate extensively, and their multipotentiality, reflecting their capability of differentiating into multiple neuroectodermal lineages (Reynolds and Weiss 1992, Temple and Alvarez-Buylla 1999, Gage 2000). Through the hierarchical generation of intermediate glial and neuronal progenitor cells (Mayer-Proschel et al. 1997, Rao et al. 1998, Gregori et al. 2002), NSCs have the ability to subsequently generate all major cell types of the CNS (Fig. 3.1). Neural progenitor cells are considered more restricted in their differentiation potential, but may still be able to give rise to more than one lineage. For example, glial-restricted progenitor cells are able to give rise to both oligodendrocytes and astrocytes, but not neuronal lineage cells (Rao et al. 1998, Lee et al. 2000, Dietrich et al. 2002, Noble et al. 2004). NSCs and neural progenitor cells play an integral part in brain development, and also appear to be critical components in the physiology and integrity of the adult mammalian brain. Whereas progenitor cell populations are found abundantly throughout the CNS during

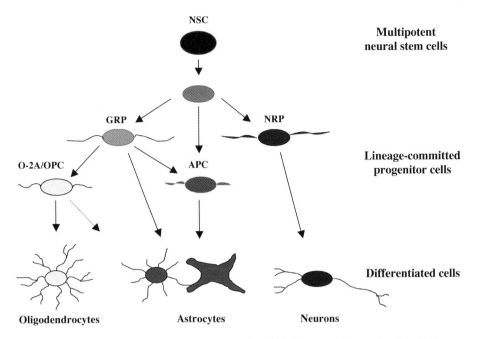

NSC

Multipotent
neural stem cells

GRP   NRP

O-2A/OPC   APC

Lineage-committed
progenitor cells

Differentiated cells

Oligodendrocytes   Astrocytes   Neurons

Fig. 3.1. Cellular lineage relationships in the mammalian CNS. Simplified diagram showing the lineage relationship between both immature and mature cell types. Multipotent neural stem cells (NSC) give rise to neurons, astrocytes, and myelin-forming oligodendrocytes through the generation of lineage-committed progenitor cell populations. Tripotential glial-restricted precursor cells (GRP) can differentiate into both astrocytes and oligodendrocytes through oligodendrocyte progenitor cells (OPC/O-2A) and astrocyte progenitor cells (APC). Mature neurons may be generated via neuron-restricted progenitor cells (NRP). Additional lineage-committed cell populations, such as putative oligodendrocyte–neuron progenitor cells, are not shown.

development and in adult life (Chang et al. 2000, Nishiyama et al. 2005), NSCs persist in the adult mammalian brain within specifically organized neurovascular niches (Palmer et al. 2000, Alvarez-Buylla and Lim 2004, Sanai et al. 2004, Shen et al. 2004, Quinones-Hinojosa et al. 2006), where they support ongoing neurogenesis and gliogenesis.

During development, stem cells are found in the ventricular zone of the CNS. In the adult brain, NSCs are primarily restricted to two brain areas: the subependymal zone of the lateral ventricles, and the subgranular zone of the dentate gyrus within the hippocampus (Eriksson et al. 1998, Gage 2000, Sanai et al. 2004). In the rodent brain, progeny of neural stem cells from the subventricular zone migrate along the rostral migratory stream to the olfactory bulb to differentiate into local interneurons (Luskin 1993, Lois et al. 1996). In the human brain, migration of neuroblasts toward the olfactory bulb appears to be orchestrated differently and occurs via alternate routes (Sanai et al. 2004, Quinones-Hinojosa et al. 2006, Curtis et al. 2007). In the hippocampus, NSCs give rise to new granule cells that are functionally integrated in the existing neuronal network (Altman and Das 1965, Kuhn et al. 1996, Cameron and McKay 2001, Hastings et al. 2002, van Praag et al. 2002).

In addition to the main germinal zones of the CNS – the lateral subventricular zone and the hippocampus – small numbers of NSCs have also been identified in other brain regions, such as the subcortical white matter (Nunes et al. 2003), cortex (Marmur et al. 1998, Arsenijevic et al. 2001), and retina (Coles et al. 2004), where they may give rise to progenitor populations, including glia-restricted cells and OPCs. It has been suggested that both cell intrinsic and local environmental signals contribute to the presence of regionally different NSC populations (Temple 2001, Hitoshi et al. 2002, Shen et al. 2006).

There is increasing evidence that the persistence of NSCs and their progeny, and the abundance of progenitor cell populations (e.g., oligodendrocyte precursor and astrocyte precursor cells) in the adult mammalian brain, reflects their role for endogenous repair mechanisms and maintenance of normal brain functions (Dietrich and Kempermann 2006). Glial and neuronal progenitor cells derived from multipotent stem cells will eventually differentiate in mature cell types of the CNS to replace existing astrocytes, oligodendrocytes, and neurons (Goldman et al. 1997, Marshall et al. 2003, Lie et al. 2004). Consequently, the disruption of either neural stem cells, or their progenitor cells, might result in critical impairment of neurological function and in distinct neurological disease.

Astrocytes in development and adult life

While it has been argued that a satisfactory definition of the term "astrocyte" remains elusive (Kimelberg 2004), the expressions of GFAP and S-100b proteins remain the key markers used to identify cells of the astrocytic lineage (Eng 1985, Boyes et al. 1986). Other markers that have also found to be co-expressed in astrocytes include glutamine synthetase (Norenberg 1979), aquaporin 4 (Nielsen et al. 1997, Vizuete et al. 1999), Ran-2 (Raff et al. 1984), the transcription factor Pax2 (Mi and Barres 1999), the glutamate transporters GLAST/EAAT1 (Lehre et al. 1995) and GLT-1/EAAT2 (Rothstein et al. 1994), as well as the intermediate filament protein vimentin (Bignami et al. 1972, Drager et al. 1984, Aloisi et al. 1992). However, these markers are either only expressed by certain astrocyte sub-populations, or are also expressed to varying degrees in cells of other neural lineages (Miller and Raff 1984, Tansey et al. 1991, Seidman et al. 1997, Meaney et al. 1998, Mennerick et al. 1998, Mi and Barres 1999, Rao 1999, Hartfuss et al. 2001).

ASTROCYTE DEVELOPMENT

Astrocytes may be derived from maturing radial glia (Voigt 1989), or from distinct astrocyte precursors. The latter have been identified in the brain by retroviral lineage studies, which identify astrocyte-only clones in-vivo (Lubetzki et al. 1992, Goldman et al. 1997) and by the isolation of putative astrocyte precursor cells from various rodent CNS tissues (Miller and Szigeti 1991, Fok-Seang and Miller 1992, Alfei et al. 1999, Mi and Barres 1999). Recently, expression of CD44 has been described as a possible marker of astrocyte precursors in the spinal cord (Alfei et al. 1999, Liu et al. 2002, 2004). These CD44-positive and GFAP-negative astrocyte precursors represent a transient population of cells that can in turn be derived in-vitro from glial restricted precursor (GRP) cells, and that can be induced to differentiate further to generate GFAP-positive / S-100b-positive astrocytes.

ASTROCYTE INDUCING SIGNALS

Several extrinsic signals have been identified that induce the development of astrocytes from neural precursor cells. These include leukemia inhibitory factor (LIF) (Nishiyama et al. 1993, Nakagaito et al. 1995), ciliary neurotrophic factor (CNTF) (Hughes et al. 1988, Lillien et al. 1988, Johe et al. 1996), cardiotrophin-1 (CT-1) (Barnabe-Heider et al. 2005), neuropoietin (Ohno et al. 2006), as well as bone morphogenetic proteins (BMPs) (Gross et al. 1996), and Notch receptor ligands (Morrison et al. 2000, Tanigaki et al. 2001, Ge et al. 2002). Studies in rodents reveal, that the in-vivo timing of astrocyte development is regulated by changes in ligand expression (Lillien et al. 1988, Stockli et al. 1991) and changes in the competence of progenitors to respond to these ligands (Burrows et al. 2000, Mehler et al. 2000, Molne et al. 2000, Sun et al. 2001, Viti et al. 2003, Fukuda et al. 2004).

CNTF, LIF and cardiotrophin belong to a class of signaling molecules that promote astrocyte generation through the gp130 cell surface receptor to cause signaling along the JAK-STAT pathway, which results in the induction of GFAP expression (Bonni et al. 1997). CNTF may play an important role in the induction of astrogliosis following injury to the CNS (Sendtner et al. 1994).

Activation of bone morphogenic protein receptor (BMP-R) by BMP-2, 4 or 7, which leads to activation of the SMAD signaling pathway, provides an alternative means of inducing generation of astrocytes. BMPs have been shown to promote astroglial differentiation in various culture systems (Gross et al. 1996, Mabie et al. 1997, Nakashima et al. 1999b, Grinspan et al. 2000). In addition, LIF and BMP-2, although each factor promotes generation of astrocytes with distinct morphology and self-renewal potential (Bonaguidi et al. 2005), may also synergize to induce astrocytes (Nakashima et al. 1999a, b, 2001, Yanagisawa et al. 2001, Weible and Chan-Ling 2007).

ASTROCYTIC SUBTYPES

Based on morphological criteria, two broad classes of astrocytes have been defined in normal brain (Privat and Rataboul 1986): (a) stellate astrocytes, also referred to as protoplasmic or type-1 astrocytes, and (b) fibrous astrocytes. A third category of astrocytes, referred to as reactive astrocytes is defined by the fact that they are formed in response to a large variety of different insults to the brain (Ridet et al. 1997, Ullian et al. 2001, Sofroniew 2005).

The relationship between these three classes of astrocytes is not clear. For example, type-1 astrocytes may develop a fibrous morphology in response to injury during the process of reactive gliosis, consistent with the observation that type-1 astrocytes undergo mitosis in response to CNS injury (Miller et al. 1986).

In-vitro studies using embryonic GRP cells have demonstrated, depending on the type of astrocyte-inducing factor used, that the differentiation of two phenotypically and functionally distinct astrocyte populations can be induced (Davies et al. 2008). Both astrocyte populations express aquaporin-4; however, induction with BMP-4 results in the formation of stellate astrocytes expressing low levels of GFAP, and CNTF promotes the generation of fibrous astrocytes that express high levels of GFAP and GLAST/EAAT1.

Astrocytes play an important role in response to injury (Ridet et al. 1997, Ullian et al. 2001, Sofroniew 2005). Traumatic injury to the CNS is associated with the generation of a dense network of hypertrophic astrocytes that express a variety of proteoglycans that inhibit neurite outgrowth (Ridet et al. 1997, Asher et al. 2001, Silver and Miller 2004). A rapid and dramatic upregulation of GFAP marks the appearance of reactive astrocytes, which are also observed in and around lesions of several forms of leukodystrophy (e.g., Hirato et al. 1994, Schiffmann et al. 1994, 1997, Knopman et al. 1996, Gieselmann et al. 2003, Suzuki 2003, Terada et al. 2004, Hagemann et al. 2006).

The role of astrocytes in determining the outcome of CNS injuries is further exemplified by the differential effects of BMP- and CNTF-induced astrocytes after transplantation into spinal cord injury lesion sites (Davies et al. 2008). Transplantation of astrocytes derived from GRP cells by induction with BMPs promotes extensive recovery (Davies et al. 2006), while CNTF-induced astrocytes do not (Davies et al. 2008), suggesting that different astrocyte subtypes may exhibit very different effects on the injury environment. Comparisons of astrocytes derived from different regions of the CNS also demonstrate different sensitivity toward oxygen and glucose deprivation, and in turn demonstrate that astrocytes themselves can be differentially affected by cytotoxic insults (Xu et al. 2001).

Leukodystrophies with distinct astrocyte pathology

ALEXANDER DISEASE

Initial insights into a possible connection between astrocyte pathology and white matter disease have come from studies on Alexander disease, which is a rare leukodystrophy characterized by progressive demyelination and megalencephaly and, clinically, by seizures, psychomotor retardation, paralysis, and spasticity. The disease was first described by the Australian pathologist Stewart Alexander as "progressive fibrinoid degeneration of fibrillary astrocytes" (Alexander 1949). Reporting on autopsy findings of a 15-month-old infant with seizures, megalencephaly, and developmental delay, Alexander identified prominent abnormalities in frontal and parietal lobes with abnormal myelin, and astrocytes characterized by degenerative and proliferative changes associated with "fuchsinophil" bodies – later recognized as Rosenthal fibers (Hallervorden 1961). The term "Alexander disease" was eventually coined in 1964, following the publication of a series of similar cases (Friede 1964). The clinical presentation of Alexander disease may show considerable variation, and consequently different forms have been distinguished based on clinical grounds and age at disease onset.

An infantile form of Alexander disease manifests in the first two years of life and is characterized by megalencephaly and/or hydrocephalus, seizures, psychomotor retardation, and spastic paresis. Death usually occurs within the first decade of life. Imaging and autopsy studies identify bilateral symmetrical white matter lesions primarily affecting the frontal lobes, subependymal and deep white matter, with occipital and parietal lobes being much less affected.

The juvenile form of the disease has a slower onset and usually manifests between age 4 and 10 years. Brainstem dysfunction, with dysphagia and ataxia, and psychiatric symptoms may dominate the clinical picture. Seizures are less common. Demyelination occurs predominantly in frontal lobes and is associated ex vacuo with dilatation of the ventricular system. Survival is variable and death usually occurs in the second or third decade of life.

An adult form of Alexander disease is much less frequent than either the infantile or juvenile form. Clinical symptoms are variable in presentation and severity and are less well defined. Patients may show bulbar or pseudobulbar symptoms, spastic paralysis, autonomic dysfunction, and varying degrees of cognitive dysfunction and psychiatric symptoms. The adult form is overall much less progressive, and even incidental findings of Alexander disease have been described in individuals who died from a different cause (Johnson 1996). Whether the infantile, juvenile, and adult forms of Alexander disease are fundamentally the same disease is not entirely clear.

Histopathologically, white matter tracts show progressive rarefaction and degeneration with little or no sparing of the arcuate fibers. Myelin degeneration is more prominent in younger patients (Klein and Anzil 1994). In older patients, patchy areas of demyelination and cavitation are frequent, whereas widespread myelin disruption is less commonly seen (Schwankhaus et al. 1995).

Most strikingly, Alexander disease is characterized by widespread accumulation of fibrous, eosinophilic deposits, so-called "Rosenthal fibers," within hypertrophied astrocytes. Rosenthal fibers are insoluble, rod-shaped aggregates of intermediate filaments containing GFAP, heat shock protein 27 (hsp 27), ubiquitin and a,b-crystallin (Iwaki et al. 1989, 1993, Tomokane et al. 1991, Head and Goldman 2000). These aggregates are one of the hallmarks of Alexander disease, although they can be found in other conditions as well, such as in reactive gliosis and pilocytic astrocytomas.

Pronounced gliosis, extensive myelin disintegration, and eventually axonal loss are other characteristic histological features. Abnormal and pleomorphic astrocytes are typically located in subpial, subependymal, and perivascular sites, but may also occur throughout the CNS, although their distribution and location does not strictly correlate with areas of myelin loss. In contrast to astrocytes, oligodendrocytes have been reported to appear histologically normal (Peiffer 1968, Mignot et al. 2004), supporting the concept that Alexander disease might be primarily an astrocyte disorder.

Previously, a firm diagnosis of Alexander disease was only possible following histopathological analysis of a biopsy or autopsy specimen. Advances in magnetic resonance imaging (MRI) have allowed establishment of radiographic criteria to diagnose the disease with high likelihood (van der Knaap et al. 2001), although atypical imaging findings in patients, later confirmed to have Alexander disease by genetic testing, have been described (van der Knaap et al. 2005, 2006).

The first suggestion that GFAP might play a fundamental role in the pathogenesis of the disease had come from studies using transgenic mice engineered to constitutively over-express wild-type GFAP. These mice died within a few weeks after birth and displayed histopathological features of Alexander disease with accumulation of protein aggregates indistinguishable from Rosenthal fibers (Messing et al. 1998).

Subsequent studies identified Alexander disease as the first disease caused by mutations in the coding region for GFAP, located on chromosome 17q21 (Brenner et al. 2001), and usually occurring as a sporadic mutation with an autosomal dominant pattern. With rare exceptions (van der Knaap et al. 2006), all cases of genetically assessed and reported patients have revealed heterozygous mis-sense mutations resulting in a change of a single amino acid residue (Rodriguez et al. 2001, Li et al. 2002, Gorospe and Maletkovic 2006).

The finding of GFAP gene mutations underlying Alexander disease supported the notion that this leukodystrophy is primarily a disease of astrocytes (Borrett and Becker 1985), as Alexander initially suspected in 1949, and that associated white matter loss occurs merely as a consequence of astrocytic dysfunction.

The mechanisms of how abnormal GFAP expression impairs astrocyte function and subsequently myelin generation and integrity remain largely unknown. GFAP is considered to be a major type-III intermediate filament protein in mature astrocytes throughout the brain. As discussed earlier, GFAP-positive cells have also been identified as neural stem cells located in the germinal zones of the CNS (Doetsch et al. 1999).

Upregulation of GFAP is seen usually in fully differentiated astrocytes (Dahl 1981, Bovolenta et al. 1984), whereas early astrocyte progenitor cells may lack GFAP expression (Liu et al. 2004, Liu and Rao 2004, Chan-Ling et al. 2009). Reactive gliosis as a response to CNS injury is characterized by upregulation of GFAP-positive hypertrophic astrocytes. In-vitro studies suggest that GFAP is involved in regulation of cell processes and cellular outgrowth (Hatten et al. 1991, Weinstein et al. 1991). Studies using genetically engineered GFAP-null mice revealed that GFAP is not strictly necessary for animal survival (Gomi et al. 1995, Pekny et al. 1995, Liedtke et al. 1996, McCall et al. 1996), although these mice exhibited abnormal astrocytes with thin and truncated processes, and impaired neuronal synaptic function (Liedtke et al. 1996, McCall et al. 1996, Shibuki et al. 1996).

While over-expression of GFAP in transgenic mice strikingly results in formation of intermediate filament aggregates consistent with Rosenthal fibers (Messing et al. 1998, 2001, Li et al. 2002), these models lack other key features of Alexander disease, such as significant white matter abnormalities, megalencephaly, ataxia, and seizures. In contrast, GFAP deficient mice were shown to develop myelin degeneration and hydrocephalus during adult life (Liedtke et al. 1996), although formation of Rosenthal fibers, developmental delay, and other clinical features of Alexander disease were missing in these models.

It is not entirely clear whether the mutations identified in the *GFAP* gene in affected individuals represent a gain or loss of protein function. Collective evidence suggests that both explanations may hold true and that heterozygous mis-sense mutations identified in patients possibly result in a toxic gain of GFAP function (Li et al. 2002, Hsiao et al. 2005). However, it seems that an abnormal function of GFAP with subsequent intermediate filament disorganization only partially explains the disease phenotype in humans, and additional factors are probably contributing to the disease manifestation.

The mechanisms by which GFAP mutations result in Rosenthal fiber formation and how Rosenthal fibers contribute to the disease pathology are not known. A recent study revealed that wild-type GFAP over-expression and accumulation in a transgenic mouse model results in activation of a significant stress response within astrocytes, microglia activation, and eventually decreased neuronal function and synaptic density (Hagemann et al. 2005). The same group provided further evidence that transgenic expression of the most commonly found GFAP mis-sense mutations in human disease (*R76H* and *R236H*) results

44

in typical Rosenthal fiber formation, astrocyte hypertrophy, and increased response to oxidative stress, linking GFAP mutations with Rosenthal fiber formation, oxidative stress, and white matter toxicity (Hagemann et al. 2006). Moreover, increased levels of GFAP expression appeared to significantly accelerate the course of the disease by decreasing the solubility of GFAP aggregates (Hagemann et al. 2006).

Taken together, the manifestation and progression in Alexander disease appears to be a complex process involving mutant GFAP expression and function, formation of Rosenthal fibers, and white matter breakdown that is likely to be mediated by increased stress response. Additional factors, including sex (Cerghet et al. 2006) and activity of other genes are likely to contribute to the manifestation and course of the disease.

VANISHING WHITE MATTER DISEASE

Vanishing white matter (VWM) disease, also known as childhood ataxia with central nervous system hypomyelination (CACH), myelinoapthia centralis diffusa, or Cree leukodystrophy, is an autosomal recessive leukodystrophy (Hanefeld et al. 1993, Schiffmann et al. 1994, van der Knaap et al. 1997). The disease usually manifests after initial normal development between age 2 and 5 years, and is characterized by progressive loss of motor function, spasticity, ataxia, and seizures. Cognitive function remains relatively preserved. The disease is ultimately fatal. As summarized elsewhere (Fogli and Boespflug-Tanguy 2006), clinical symptoms and severity of the disease vary significantly and correlate with age of symptom onset. The classical form, with disease onset in children between 2 and 5 years old, represents the largest group, whereas the most severe phenotype with rapid decline is seen with disease onset before age 2. Interestingly, episodic deterioration may occur after mild head trauma, or following febrile illnesses. Radiographic findings on MRI demonstrate diffuse white matter loss and cystic degeneration (Fig. 3.2).

Oligodendrocyte numbers may be increased in affected patients and may exhibit a foamy cytoplasm. In addition, decreased numbers and abnormal appearing astrocytes are characteristic histological features of the disease (Rodriguez et al. 1999, Wong et al. 2000, Fogli et al. 2002, Van Haren et al. 2004, Dietrich et al. 2005).

The disease has been linked to mutations in each of the genes encoding for the five subunits of the translation factor "eukaryotic initiation factor 2B" (eIF2B) (Leegwater et al. 2001, Fogli et al. 2002, van der Knaap et al. 2002, Fogli and Boespflug-Tanguy 2006), which is required for the formation of the 43S initiation complex and considered a rate-limiting step in mRNA translation (Proud 2005).

About 90% of all mutations identified so far in affected individuals are mis-sense mutations and certain genotype–phenotype correlations have been suggested (Fogli et al. 2004, Fogli and Boespflug-Tanguy 2006). The effects of *EIF2B* mutations probably reflect an incomplete disruption of protein function, as the complete loss of eIF2B function is considered lethal and frame-shift mutations have not been observed in a homozygous state (Fogli and Boespflug-Tanguy 2006).

Analysis of neural cells obtained from an affected individual have revealed initial insights into the cellular dysfunction as a consequence of *EIF2B5* mutations, suggesting that an abnormal astrocyte function underlies VWM leukodystrophy. These studies

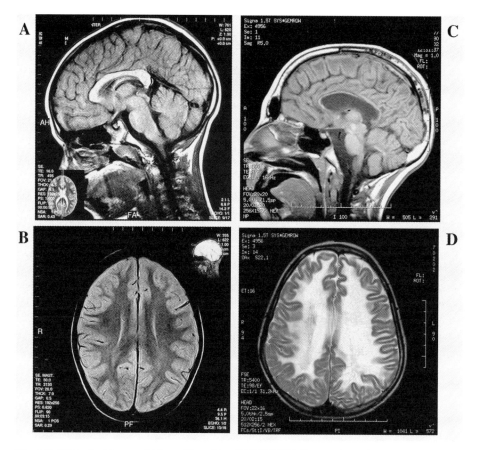

Fig. 3.2. MRI of a 12-year-old boy affected by CACH/VWM disease. Parts **A** (T1/sagittal) and **B** (T2/axial) show the comparable scans of an age-matched healthy individual. Parts **C** (T1/sagittal) and **D** (T2/axial) demonstrate widespread and bi-hemispheric demyelination with evidence of vacuolating leukoencephalopathy.

demonstrated that *EIF2B5* mutations severely compromise generation of GFAP-positive astrocytes. Despite profound myelin disruption and white matter loss in the reported individual, normal appearing oligodendrocytes were readily generated from neural precursor cells. In contrast, astrocyte development was largely abnormal with generation of fewer and dystrophic cell types (Fig. 3.3), and RNAi targeting of EIF2B5 severely compromised induction of GFAP-positive astrocytes from normal human glial progenitors (Dietrich et al. 2005).

Collectively, we demonstrated that disruption of eIF2B5 function by either spontaneous mutation or by RNAi targeting of normal human neural progenitor cells, consistently impaired generation of GFAP-positive astrocytes. This effect could be partially rescued by transient expression of the normal protein in human precursor cells, supporting the assumption that CACH/VWM disease may be primarily caused by astrocyte dysfunction with

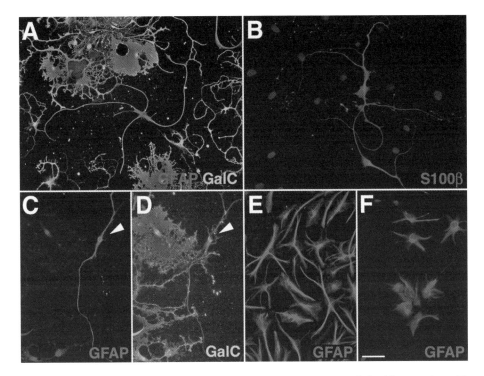

Fig. 3.3. Abnormal astrocytic phenotypes in CACH/VWM disease. Astrocytes derived from a patient with VWM disease show an unusual morphology. Freshly isolated frontal cortex cells have unusually long processes; stained with (**A**) glial fibrillary acidic protein (GFAP) (tetramethylrhodamine isothiocyanate, TRITC), galactosylceramide (GalC) (fluorescein isothiocyanate, FITC), and (**B**) protein S-100b (TRITC). **C, D**: Some GFAP+ cells also co-label with GalC, normally a marker for oligodendrocyte lineage cells. **E**: Normal astrocytes derived from BMP-treated human glial precursor cells, GFAP (TRITC). **F**: Primary human post-natal astrocytes derived from temporal lobe of a 17-year-old patient. Scale bars: **A–D** 75 μm and **E, F** 25 μm. Adopted from Dietrich J. et al. *EIF2B5* mutations compromise GFAP+ astrocyte generation in vanishing white matter leukodystrophy. Nature Medicine 2005; 11(3): 277–283; with permission. (A color version of this figure is available in the Plate section.)

subsequent disruption of myelination (Dietrich et al. 2005). In addition to the paucity of GFAP-positive astrocytes in patients with VWM disease, it remains unclear whether the astrocytes that are found in such patients retain normal functionality and can mount an adequate stress response.

Given the broad function of eIF2B in overall protein biosynthesis, the specificity of the cellular dysfunction within the nervous system with clinical presentation as a leukodystrophy has been surprising, although cellular function may partially be compromised in non-CNS tissues, such as liver, kidney, eyes, and ovaries (Fogli and Boespflug-Tanguy 2006).

It is conceivable that defective or absent astrocytes may explain the gelatinous consistency of affected white matter (van der Knaap et al. 1997, Wong et al. 2000); however, the exact mechanism by which white matter breakdown occurs is unclear.

There has been increasing evidence that a reduction of eIF2B function in patients with CACH/VWM disease alters the cellular stress response (Kantor et al. 2005). This effect may be preferentially harmful to myelin maintenance and oligodendrocytes that are dependent on high rates of protein metabolism and highly vulnerable to oxidative stress (Back et al. 1998).

Taken together, compromised neural precursor cell function and impaired astrocyte maturation, in combination with alterations in the cellular stress response level by impaired eIF2B activity, may result in increased oligodendrocyte vulnerability in particular during periods of augmented energy demand and oxidative stress, such as during febrile illness and head trauma.

MEGALENCEPHALIC LEUKOENCEPHALOPATHY WITH SUBCORTICAL CYSTS

Abnormal astrocyte function has also been postulated in megalencephalic leukoen-cephalopathy with subcortical cysts (MLC), a rare and progressive leukodystrophy characterized by macrocephaly, myelin fiber vacuolization, and formation of subcortical cysts predominantly in temporal, frontal, and parietal distribution (van der Knaap et al. 1995, 1996, Singhal et al. 1996).

The disease has its onset early in childhood and may present with motor impairment, ataxia, and spasticity. Individuals may become wheelchair dependent in their second decade of life. The degree of mental impairment varies and may not even be part of the symptom complex. Other symptoms include seizures, dysphagia, and speech abnormalities. As seen in VWM disease, minor head traumas or infections can significantly accelerate disease progression (Bugiani et al. 2003). MLC is an autosomal recessive disease. The causative gene mutation has been located to chromosome 22qtel (Topcu et al. 2000) affecting the MLC1 protein (Leegwater et al. 2002). MLC1 initially was thought to represent a membrane channel protein localized to distal astrocyte and glia processes in perivascular, subependy-mal, and subpial regions (Boor et al. 2005). MLC1 is also expressed in Bergmann glia and astrocytes located in the olfactory bulb, but lacks expression in oligodendrocytes (Schmitt et al. 2003, Teijido et al. 2004). Strong protein expressions were notable within the membrane domain of adjacent astrocyte processes and at brain-barrier sites, including periventricular ependymal cells, perivascular and subpial regions (Teijido et al. 2004).

MLC shows considerable clinical heterogeneity in symptom presentation and severity. Significant genetic heterogeneity was reported in a series of 18 cases, but without a clear genotype-phenotype correlation (Patrono et al. 2003). Only about 70% of cases demonstrate MRI findings and a clinical picture consistent with MLC, which is why it has been postulated that other genes may be involved in the disease manifestation in approximately 30% of patients (Blattner et al. 2003, Gorospe and Maletkovic 2006).

The exact function of the MLC1 protein is unclear, and the exact mechanisms by which white matter tracts are disrupted secondary to MLC1-associated astrocyte dysfunction remain elusive. An abnormal function of molecule transportation in glia cells has been discussed (Boor et al. 2005). Based on the MLC-1 expression pattern with predisposition to distal astrocytic processes at brain-barrier sites of perivascular, ependymal, and subpial locations, one key mechanism may involve the impaired integrity of the blood–brain barrier with disruption of fluid and electrolyte homeostasis (Sofroniew 2005).

Possible mechanisms of white matter damage secondary to astrocyte dysfunction

As illustrated by three genetically distinct leukodystrophies (Table 3.1), even partial interference with astrocyte function may result in white matter disease. Considering the growing list of cellular functions of astrocytes and their precursor cells in the developing and mature CNS, their disruption at any level may severely compromise oligodendrocyte function and myelin integrity. Impairment of GFAP-positive astrocytes disrupts the organization of a filamentous network in the CNS (Hsiao et al. 2005), offering a possible explanation for the formation of vacuolization and myelin cavitations, as it can be seen in Alexander disease, VMW disease and MLC.

Under physiological conditions, astrocytes act as paracrine regulators of oligodendrocyte and oligodendrocyte precursor survival, partially mediated via platelet-derived growth factor production and leukemia inhibitory factor (Gard et al. 1995).

As discussed earlier, oligodendrocytes and their precursor cells belong to the most vulnerable CNS populations to cytotoxic stress and oxidative damage. For example, glutamate and tumor necrosis factor-α have been shown to be toxic to oligodendroglia (Oka et al. 1993, Mayer and Noble 1994, McDonald et al. 1998a, Miller et al. 2005). Toxicity to astrocytes may propagate damage to oligodendrocytes and their precursors through glutamate release into the extracellular matrix from dying astroglia cells, and the associated lack of glutamate uptake through astrocytes (Wilke et al. 2004). Moreover, it has been demonstrated that increased glutamate concentration in the extracellular space may subsequently activate and reverse the glutamate/cysteine co-transporter in oligodendrocytes leading to overall glutathione depletion, increased oxidative stress, and subsequent oligodendrocyte death (Back et al. 1998). Astrocytes are able to store glycogen, which can be utilized as an energy source by surrounding cells at times of glucose deprivation after metabolism into lactate and subsequent release into the extracellular matrix. Consequently, lack of glycogen storage in astrocytes may render both oligodendrocytes and neurons more vulnerable (Brucklacher et al. 2002).

The formation of "reactive astrocytes," as seen in numerous pathological conditions (Fig. 3.4), is associated with the production of cytokines toxic to oligodendrocytes and precursor cells, such as tumor necrosis factor-α, interferon-γ, and glutamate (Baerwald and Popko 1998, Jurewicz et al. 2005). Progressive white matter damage could play an increasing role in aging, as the ability of astrocytes to become "reactive" appears to be enhanced in the adult brain when compared with the immature brain (Sumi and Hager 1968,

TABLE 3.1
Leukodystrophies with known gene mutations and associated astrocyte pathology

Disease	Gene	Inheritance	Postulated mechanism
Alexander Disease	*GFAP*	Autosomal dominant	Astrocyte dysfunction
VWM/CACH	*EIF2B5*	Autosomal recessive	Astrocyte generation and dysfunction
Megalencephalic leukoencephalopathy with subcortical cysts	*MLC1*	Autosomal recessive	Abnormal membrane function and transport mechanisms in glia cells

CACH, childhood ataxia with central nervous system hypomyelination; VWM, vanishing white matter.

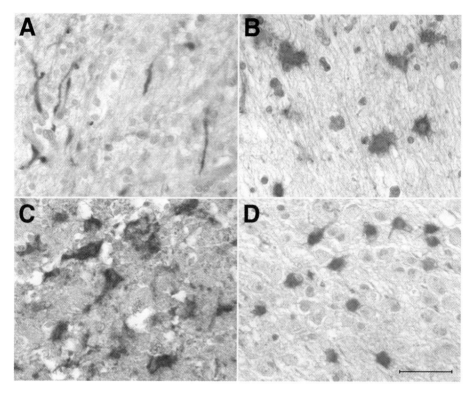

Fig. 3.4. Phenotype of GFAP-positive astrocytes in different neurological conditions. **A**: CACH/VWM disease. **B**: Adrenoleukodystrophy. **C**: Stroke. **D**: Progressive multifocal leukoencephalopathy. Error bar: 50 μm. Adopted from Dietrich J. et al. *EIF2B5* mutations compromise GFAP+ astrocyte generation in vanishing white matter leukodystrophy. Nature Medicine 2005; 11(3): 277–283; with permission. (A color version of this figure is available in the Plate section.)

Berry et al. 1983) and parallels the degree of microglial activation (Balasingam et al. 1994). However, the effects of "reactive astrocytes" on oligodendrocytes are complex and possibly have additional positive effects on surrounding cells, as cytokine-activated glia cells have been shown to produce energy substrates and trophic factors important for neurons and oligodendrocytes, and may even promote remyelination and restoration of homeostasis (Liberto et al. 2004). In support of this view, inhibition of reactive astrocytosis in transgenic models promotes gray and white matter degeneration (Bush et al. 1999, Faulkner et al. 2004).

The vulnerability of glial cells and their precursors depends on their developmental stage (Back et al. 1998, Volpe 2001, Morath and Mayer-Proschel 2002, Andersen 2003, Garcia et al. 2004), raising the question as to whether lineage specificity and clinical disease progression in patients correlate with cellular vulnerability during certain time windows of development. Moreover, a selectively diminished progenitor cell population during development could also explain prolonged effects on delayed myelin disruption later in life (Corbin et al. 1996, Chew et al. 2005).

Considering the evidence currently available, abnormal astrocytes may impair myelin maintenance and generation by different mechanisms, ranging from direct effects on progenitor cell populations and oligodendrocytes to indirect effects, such as increased oxidative stress, cytokine toxicity, and growth factor depletion.

Summary and future perspectives

Astrocytes are the most abundant cell type of the CNS and have diverse functions in the developing and adult brain. Given their enormous complexity and critical role in cellular communication, signaling, protein synthesis, metabolism, and homeostasis, abnormal astrocyte function is likely to play a fundamental role in various neurological diseases, such as white matter diseases. Recent molecular and cell-biological studies and collective evidence from genetically unrelated leukodystrophies (Alexander disease, VWM disease, MLC) have provided evidence that astrocytes play a vital role in myelin function. Moreover, there is increasing evidence that astrocyte dysfunction may be the primary cause of some forms of leukodystrophies. Identification of the exact mechanisms that underlie the pathophysiology of leukodystrophies and other forms of white matter diseases and further study of the cross-talk between astrocytes and oligodendrocytes are areas of ongoing investigation that will allow the identification of new therapeutic targets.

REFERENCES

Abbott NJ, Ronnback L, Hansson E (2006). Astrocyte-endothelial interactions at the blood–brain barrier. Nat Rev Neurosci 7, 41–53.

Alexander WS. (1949) Progressive fibrinoid degeneration of fibrillary astrocytes associated with mental retardation in a hydrocephalic infant. Brain 72, 373–381.

Alfei L, Aita M, Caronti B, et al. (1999) Hyaluronate receptor CD44 is expressed by astrocytes in the adult chicken and in astrocyte cell precursors in early development of the chick spinal cord. Eur J Histochem 43: 29–38.

Allen NJ, Barres BA. (2009) Neuroscience: Glia – more than just brain glue. Nature 457: 675–677.

Aloisi F, Giampaolo A, Russo G, Peschle C, Levi G. (1992) Developmental appearance, antigenic profile, and proliferation of glial cells in the human embryonic spinal cord: an immunocytochemical study using dissociated cultured cells. Glia 5: 171–181.

Altman J, Das GD. (1965) Autoradiographic and histological evidence of postnatal hippocampal neurogenesis in rats. J Comp Neurol 124: 319–335.

Alvarez-Buylla A, Lim DA. (2004) For the long run: maintaining germinal niches in the adult brain. Neuron 41: 683–686.

Amiry-Moghaddam M, Ottersen OP. (2003) The molecular basis of water transport in the brain. Nat Rev Neurosci 4: 991–1001.

Andersen SL. (2003) Trajectories of brain development: point of vulnerability or window of opportunity? Neurosci Biobehav Rev 27: 3–18.

Anderson CM, Swanson RA. (2000) Astrocyte glutamate transport: review of properties, regulation, and physiological functions. Glia 32: 1–14.

Arsenijevic Y, Villemure JG, Brunet JF, et al. (2001). Isolation of multipotent neural precursors residing in the cortex of the adult human brain. Exp Neurol 170: 48–62.

Asher RA, Morgenstern DA, Moon LD, Fawcett JW. (2001) Chondroitin sulphate proteoglycans: inhibitory components of the glial scar. Prog Brain Res 132: 611–619.

Back SA, Gan X, Li Y, Rosenberg PA, Volpe JJ. (1998) Maturation-dependent vulnerability of oligodendrocytes to oxidative stress-induced death caused by glutathione depletion. J Neurosci 18: 6241–6253.

Baerwald KD, Popko B. (1998) Developing and mature oligodendrocytes respond differently to the immune cytokine interferon-gamma. J Neurosci Res 52: 230–239.

Balasingam V, Tejada-Berges T, Wright E, Bouckova R, Yong VW. (1994) Reactive astrogliosis in the neonatal mouse brain and its modulation by cytokines. J Neurosci 14: 846–856.

Barnabe-Heider F, Wasylnka JA, Fernandes KJ, et al. (2005) Evidence that embryonic neurons regulate the onset of cortical gliogenesis via cardiotrophin-1. Neuron 48: 253–265.

Berry M, Maxwell WL, Logan A, et al. (1983) Deposition of scar tissue in the central nervous system. Acta Neurochir Suppl (Wien) 32: 31–53.

Bignami A, Eng LF, Dahl D, Uyeda CT. (1972) Localization of the glial fibrillary acidic protein in astrocytes by immunofluorescence. Brain Res 43: 429–435.

Blattner R., Von Moers A, Leegwater PA, Hanefeld FA, Van Der Knaap MS, Kohler W. (2003) Clinical and genetic heterogeneity in megalencephalic leukoencephalopathy with subcortical cysts (MLC). Neuropediatrics 34: 215–218.

Bonaguidi MA, McGuire T, Hu M, Kan L, Samanta J, Kessler JA. (2005) LIF and BMP signaling generate separate and discrete types of GFAP-expressing cells. Development 132: 5503–5514.

Bonni A, Sun Y, Nadal-Vicens M, et al. (1997) Regulation of gliogenesis in the central nervous system by the JAK-STAT signaling pathway. Science 278: 477–483.

Boor PK, de Groot K, Waisfisz Q, et al. (2005) MLC1: a novel protein in distal astroglial processes. J Neuropathol Exp Neurol 64: 412–419.

Borrett D, Becker LE. (1985) Alexander's disease. A disease of astrocytes. Brain 108(2): 367–385.

Bovolenta P, Liem RK, Mason CA. (1984) Development of cerebellar astroglia: transitions in form and cytoskeletal content. Dev Biol 102: 248–259.

Boyes BE, Kim SU, Lee V, Sung SC. (1986) Immunohistochemical co-localization of S-100b and the glial fibrillary acidic protein in rat brain. Neuroscience 17: 857–865.

Brenner M, Johnson AB, Boespflug-Tanguy O, Rodriguez D, Goldman JE, Messing A. (2001) Mutations in GFAP, encoding glial fibrillary acidic protein, are associated with Alexander disease. Nat Genet 27: 117–120.

Brown AM, Baltan Tekkok S, Ransom BR. (2004) Energy transfer from astrocytes to axons: the role of CNS glycogen. Neurochem Int 45: 529–536.

Brucklacher RM, Vannucci RC, Vannucci SJ. (2002) Hypoxic preconditioning increases brain glycogen and delays energy depletion from hypoxia–ischemia in the immature rat. Dev Neurosci 24: 411–417.

Bugiani M, Moroni I, Bizzi A, et al. (2003) Consciousness disturbances in megalencephalic leukoencephalopathy with subcortical cysts. Neuropediatrics 34: 211–214.

Burrows RC, Lillien L, Levitt, P. (2000) Mechanisms of progenitor maturation are conserved in the striatum and cortex. Dev Neurosci 22: 7–15.

Bush TG, Puvanachandra N, Horner CH, et al. (1999) Leukocyte infiltration, neuronal degeneration, and neurite outgrowth after ablation of scar-forming, reactive astrocytes in adult transgenic mice. Neuron 23: 297–308.

Cajal SR. (1913) Contribucitm al conocimiento de la neuroglia del cerebro humane. Trab Lab Inv Biol (Madrid) 11: 255–315.

Cameron HA, McKay RD. (2001) Adult neurogenesis produces a large pool of new granule cells in the dentate gyrus. J Comp Neurol 435: 406–417.

Cerghet M, Skoff RP, Bessert D, Zhang Z, Mullins C, Ghandour MS. (2006) Proliferation and death of oligodendrocytes and myelin proteins are differentially regulated in male and female rodents. J Neurosci 26: 1439–1447.

Chan-Ling T, Chu Y, Baxter L, Weible Ii, M, Hughes S. (2009) In-vivo characterization of astrocyte precursor cells (APCs) and astrocytes in developing rat retina: differentiation, proliferation, and apoptosis. Glia 57: 39–53.

Chang A, Nishiyama A, Peterson J, Prineas J, Trapp BD. (2000) NG2-positive oligodendrocyte progenitor cells in adult human brain and multiple sclerosis lesions. J Neurosci 20: 6404–6412.

Chew LJ, King WC, Kennedy A, Gallo V. (2005) Interferon-gamma inhibits cell cycle exit in differentiating oligodendrocyte progenitor cells. Glia 52: 127–143.

Chojnacki AK, Mak GK, Weiss S. (2009) Identity crisis for adult periventricular neural stem cells: subventricular zone astrocytes, ependymal cells or both? Nat Rev Neurosci 10: 153–163.

Coles BL, Angenieux B, Inoue T, et al. (2004) Facile isolation and the characterization of human retinal stem cells. Proc Natl Acad Sci USA 101: 15 772–15 777.

Corbin JG, Kelly D, Rath EM, Baerwald KD, Suzuki K, Popko B. (1996) Targeted CNS expression of interferon-gamma in transgenic mice leads to hypomyelination, reactive gliosis, and abnormal cerebellar development. Mol Cell Neurosci 7: 354–370.

Curtis MA, Kam M, Nannmark U, et al. (2007) Human neuroblasts migrate to the olfactory bulb via a lateral ventricular extension. Science 315: 1243–1249.

Dahl D. (1981) The vimentin-GFA protein transition in rat neuroglia cytoskeleton occurs at the time of myelination. J Neurosci Res 6: 741–748.

Davies JE, Huang C, Proschel C, Noble M, Mayer-Proschel M, Davies SJ. (2006) Astrocytes derived from glial-restricted precursors promote spinal cord repair. J Biol 5: 7.

Davies JE, Proschel C, Zhang N, Noble M, Mayer-Proschel M, Davies SJ. (2008) Transplanted astrocytes derived from BMP- or CNTF-treated glial-restricted precursors have opposite effects on recovery and allodynia after spinal cord injury. J Biol 7: 24.

De Keyser J, Mostert JP, Koch MW. (2008) Dysfunctional astrocytes as key players in the pathogenesis of central nervous system disorders. J Neurol Sci 267: 3–16.

Dietrich J, Han R, Yang Y, Mayer-Proschel M, Noble M. (2006) CNS progenitor cells and oligodendrocytes are targets of chemotherapeutic agents in vitro and in vivo. J Biol 5: 22.

Dietrich J, Kempermann G. (2006) Role of endogenous neural stem cells in neurological disease and brain repair. Adv Exp Med Biol 557: 191–220.

Dietrich J, Lacagnina M, Gass D, et al. (2005) EIF2B5 mutations compromise GFAP+ astrocyte generation in vanishing white matter leukodystrophy. Nat Med 11: 277–283.

Dietrich J, Noble M, Mayer-Proschel M. (2002) Characterization of A2B5+ glial precursor cells from cryopreserved human fetal brain progenitor cells. Glia 40: 65–77.

Doetsch F. (2003) The glial identity of neural stem cells. Nat Neurosci 6: 1127–1134.

Doetsch F, Caille I, Lim DA, Garcia-Verdugo JM, Alvarez-Buylla A. (1999) Subventricular zone astrocytes are neural stem cells in the adult mammalian brain. Cell 97: 703–716.

Drager UC, Edwards DL, Barnstable CJ. (1984) Antibodies against filamentous components in discrete cell types of the mouse retina. J Neurosci 4: 2025–2042.

Eng LF. (1985) Glial fibrillary acidic protein (GFAP): the major protein of glial intermediate filaments in differentiated astrocytes. J Neuroimmunol 8: 203–214.

Eriksson PS, Perfilieva E, Bjork-Eriksson T, et al. (1998) Neurogenesis in the adult human hippocampus. Nat Med 4: 1313–1317.

Farina C, Aloisi F, Meinl E. (2007) Astrocytes are active players in cerebral innate immunity. Trends Immunol 28: 138–145.

Faulkner JR., Herrmann JE, Woo MJ, Tansey KE, Doan NB, Sofroniew MV. (2004) Reactive astrocytes protect tissue and preserve function after spinal cord injury. J Neurosci 24: 2143–2155.

Fields RD, Stevens-Graham B. (2002) New insights into neuron–glia communication. Science 298: 556–562.

Fogli A, Boespflug-Tanguy O. (2006) The large spectrum of eIF2B-related diseases. Biochem Soc Trans 34: 22–29.

Fogli A, Dionisi-Vici C, Deodato F, Bartuli A, Boespflug-Tanguy O, Bertini E. (2002) A severe variant of childhood ataxia with central hypomyelination/vanishing white matter leukoencephalopathy related to EIF21B5 mutation. Neurology 59: 1966–1968.

Fogli A, Schiffmann R, Bertini E, et al. (2004) The effect of genotype on the natural history of eIF2B-related leukodystrophies. Neurology 62: 1509–1517.

Fok-Seang J, Miller RH. (1992) Astrocyte precursors in neonatal rat spinal cord cultures. J Neurosci 12: 2751–2764.

Friede RL. (1964) Alexander's Disease. Arch Neurol 11: 414–422.

Fukuda S, Kondo T, Takebayashi H, Taga T. (2004) Negative regulatory effect of an oligodendrocytic bHLH factor OLIG2 on the astrocytic differentiation pathway. Cell Death Differ 11: 196–202.

Gage FH. (2000) Mammalian neural stem cells. Science 287: 1433–1438.

Garcia A, Steiner B, Kronenberg G, Bick-Sander A, Kempermann G. (2004) Age-dependent expression of glucocorticoid- and mineralocorticoid receptors on neural precursor cell populations in the adult murine hippocampus. Aging Cell 3: 363–371.

Gard AL, Burrell MR, Pfeiffer SE, Rudge JS, Williams WC, 2nd. (1995) Astroglial control of oligodendrocyte survival mediated by PDGF and leukemia inhibitory factor-like protein. Development 121: 2187–2197.

Ge W, Martinowich K, Wu X, et al. (2002) Notch signaling promotes astrogliogenesis via direct CSL-mediated glial gene activation. J Neurosci Res 69: 848–860.

Gieselmann V, Franken S, Klein D, et al. (2003) Metachromatic leukodystrophy: consequences of sulphatide accumulation. Acta Paediatr Suppl 92: 74–79; discussion 45.

Goldman JE, Zerlin M, Newman S, Zhang L, Gensert, J. (1997) Fate determination and migration of progenitors in the postnatal mammalian CNS. Dev Neurosci 19: 42–48.

Gomi H, Yokoyama T, Fujimoto K, et al. (1995) Mice devoid of the glial fibrillary acidic protein develop normally and are susceptible to scrapie prions. Neuron 14: 29–41.

Gorospe JR, Maletkovic J. (2006) Alexander disease and megalencephalic leukoencephalopathy with subcortical cysts: leukodystrophies arising from astrocyte dysfunction. Ment Retard Dev Disabil Res Rev 12: 113–122.

Gregori N, Proschel C, Noble M, Mayer-Proschel M. (2002) The tripotential glial-restricted precursor (GRP) cell and glial development in the spinal cord: generation of bipotential oligodendrocyte-type-2 astrocyte progenitor cells and dorsal-ventral differences in GRP cell function. J Neurosci 22: 248–256.

Grinspan JB, Edell E, Carpio DF, et al. (2000) Stage-specific effects of bone morphogenetic proteins on the oligodendrocyte lineage. J Neurobiol 43: 1–17.

Gross RE, Mehler MF, Mabie PC, Zang Z, Santschi L, Kessler JA. (1996) Bone morphogenetic proteins promote astroglial lineage commitment by mammalian subventricular zone progenitor cells. Neuron 17: 595–606.

Hagemann TL, Connor JX, Messing A. (2006) Alexander disease-associated glial fibrillary acidic protein mutations in mice induce Rosenthal fiber formation and a white matter stress response. J Neurosci 26: 11162–11173.

Hagemann TL, Gaeta SA, Smith MA, Johnson DA, Johnson JA, Messing A. (2005) Gene expression analysis in mice with elevated glial fibrillary acidic protein and Rosenthal fibers reveals a stress response followed by glial activation and neuronal dysfunction. Hum Mol Genet 14: 2443–2458.

Hallervorden J. (1961) [The development of the myelin sheath and Rosenthal's fibers.] (in German) Dtsch Z Nervenheilkd 181: 547–580.

Hanefeld F, Holzbach U, Kruse B, Wilichowski E, Christen HJ, Frahm J. (1993) Diffuse white matter disease in three children: an encephalopathy with unique features on magnetic resonance imaging and proton magnetic resonance spectroscopy. Neuropediatrics 24, 244–248.

Hartfuss E, Galli R, Heins N, Gotz M. (2001) Characterization of CNS precursor subtypes and radial glia. Dev Biol 229: 15–30.

Hastings NB, Seth MI., Tanapat P, Rydel TA, Gould E. (2002) Granule neurons generated during development extend divergent axon collaterals to hippocampal area CA3. J Comp Neurol 452: 324–333.

Hatten ME, Liem RK, Shelanski ML, Mason CA. (1991) Astroglia in CNS injury. Glia 4: 233–243.

Head MW, Goldman JE. (2000) Small heat shock proteins, the cytoskeleton, and inclusion body formation. Neuropathol Appl Neurobiol 26: 304–312.

Helmuth L. (2001) Neuroscience. Synchronizing the brain's signals. Science 292: 2233.

Hirato J, Nakazato Y, Sasak A, Hikima A, Shimizu S, Yamanouchi H. (1994) Krabbe's disease with giant lamellar bodies in Purkinje cells. Acta Neuropathol 88: 78–84.

Hitoshi S, Tropepe V, Ekker M, van der Kooy D. (2002) Neural stem cell lineages are regionally specified, but not committed, within distinct compartments of the developing brain. Development 129: 233–244.

Horner PJ, Palmer TD. (2003) New roles for astrocytes: the nightlife of an "astrocyte." La vida loca! Trends Neurosci 26: 597–603.

Hsiao VC, Tian R, Long H, et al. (2005) Alexander-disease mutation of GFAP causes filament disorganization and decreased solubility of GFAP. J Cell Sci 118: 2057–2065.

Hughes SM, Lillien LE, Raff MC, Rohrer H, Sendtner M. (1988) Ciliary neurotrophic factor induces type-2 astrocyte differentiation in culture. Nature 335, 70–73.

Iwaki T, Iwaki A, Tateishi J, Sakaki Y, Goldman JE. (1993) Alpha B-crystallin and 27-kd heat shock protein are regulated by stress conditions in the central nervous system and accumulate in Rosenthal fibers. Am J Pathol 143: 487–495.

Iwaki T, Kume-Iwaki, A, Liem RK, Goldman JE. (1989) Alpha B-crystallin is expressed in non-lenticular tissues and accumulates in Alexander's disease brain. Cell 57: 71–78.

Johe KK, Hazel TG, Muller T, Dugich-Djordjevic MM, McKay RD. (1996) Single factors direct the differentiation of stem cells from the fetal and adult central nervous system. Genes Dev 10: 3129–3140.

Johnson AB. (1996) Alexander disease. In: Handbook of Clinical Neurology M. HW, ed. Amsterdam: Elsevier, pp. 701–710.

Jurewicz A, Matysiak M, Tybor K, Kilianek L, Raine CS, Selmaj K. (2005) Tumour necrosis factor-induced death of adult human oligodendrocytes is mediated by apoptosis inducing factor. Brain 128: 2675–2688.

Kantor L, Harding HP, Ron D, et al. (2005) Heightened stress response in primary fibroblasts expressing mutant eIF2B genes from CACH/VWM leukodystrophy patients. Hum Genet 118: 99–106.

Kimelberg HK. (1995) Receptors on astrocytes – what possible functions? Neurochem Int 26: 27–40.

Kimelberg HK. (2004) The problem of astrocyte identity. Neurochem Int 45: 191–202.

Klein EA, Anzil AP. (1994) Prominent white matter cavitation in an infant with Alexander's disease. Clin Neuropathol 13: 31–38.

Knopman D, Sung JH, Davis D. (1996) Progressive familial leukodystrophy of late onset. Neurology 46: 429–434.

Kuhn HG, Dickinson-Anson H, Gage FH. (1996) Neurogenesis in the dentate gyrus of the adult rat: age-related decrease of neuronal progenitor proliferation. J Neurosci 16: 2027–2033.

Lee JC, Mayer-Proschel M, Rao MS. (2000) Gliogenesis in the central nervous system. Glia 30: 105–121.

Leegwater PA, Boor PK, Yuan BQ, et al. (2002) Identification of novel mutations in MLC1 responsible for megalencephalic leukoencephalopathy with subcortical cysts. Hum Genet 110: 279–283.

Leegwater PA, Vermeulen G, Konst AA, et al. (2001) Subunits of the translation initiation factor eIF2B are mutant in leukoencephalopathy with vanishing white matter. Nat Genet 29: 383–388.

Lehre KP, Levy LM, Ottersen OP, Storm-Mathisen J, Danbolt NC. (1995) Differential expression of two glial glutamate transporters in the rat brain: quantitative and immunocytochemical observations. J Neurosci 15: 1835–1853.

Li R, Messing A, Goldman JE, Brenner M. (2002) GFAP mutations in Alexander disease. Int J Dev Neurosci 20: 259–268.

Li Z, Dong T, Proschel C, and Noble M. (2007) Chemically diverse toxicants converge on Fyn and c-Cbl to disrupt precursor cell function. PLoS Biol 5: e35.

Liberto CM, Albrecht PJ, Herx LM, Yong VW, Levison SW. (2004) Pro-regenerative properties of cytokine-activated astrocytes. J Neurochem 89: 1092–1100.

Lichtman JW, Smith SJ. (2008) Seeing circuits assemble. Neuron 60: 441–448.

Lie DC, Song H, Colamarino SA, Ming GL, Gage FH. (2004) Neurogenesis in the adult brain: new strategies for central nervous system diseases. Annu Rev Pharmacol Toxicol 44: 399–421.

Liedtke W, Edelmann W, Bieri PL, et al. (1996) GFAP is necessary for the integrity of CNS white matter architecture and long-term maintenance of myelination. Neuron 17: 607–615.

Lillien LE, Sendtner M, Rohrer H, Hughes SM, Raff MC. (1988) Type-2 astrocyte development in rat brain cultures is initiated by a CNTF-like protein produced by type-1 astrocytes. Neuron 1: 485–494.

Liu Y, Han SS, Wu Y, et al. (2004) CD44 expression identifies astrocyte-restricted precursor cells. Dev Biol 276: 31–46.

Liu Y, Rao MS. (2004) Glial progenitors in the CNS and possible lineage relationships among them. Biol Cell 96: 279–290.

Liu Y, Wu Y, Lee JC, et al. (2002) Oligodendrocyte and astrocyte development in rodents: an in situ and immunohistological analysis during embryonic development. Glia 40: 25–43.

Lois C, Garcia-Verdugo JM, Alvarez-Buylla A. (1996) Chain migration of neuronal precursors. Science 271: 978–981.

Lubetzki C, Goujet-Zalc C, Demerens C. Danos O, Zalc B. (1992) Clonal segregation of oligodendrocytes and astrocytes during differentiation of glial progenitor cells. Glia 6: 289–300.

Luskin MB. (1993) Restricted proliferation and migration of postnatally generated neurons derived from the forebrain subventricular zone. Neuron 11: 173–189.

Mabie PC, Mehler MF, Marmur R, Papavasiliou A, Song Q, Kessler JA. (1997) Bone morphogenetic proteins induce astroglial differentiation of oligodendroglial–astroglial progenitor cells. J Neurosci 17: 4112–4120.

Marmur R, Mabie PC, Gokhan S, Song Q, Kessler JA, Mehler MF. (1998) Isolation and developmental characterization of cerebral cortical multipotent progenitors. Dev Biol 204: 577–591.

Marshall CA, Suzuki SO, Goldman JE. (2003) Gliogenic and neurogenic progenitors of the subventricular zone: who are they, where did they come from, and where are they going? Glia 43: 52–61.

Mayer M, Noble M. (1994) N-acetyl-L-cysteine is a pluripotent protector against cell death and enhancer of trophic factor-mediated cell survival in vitro. Proc Natl Acad Sci USA 91: 7496–7500.

Mayer-Proschel M, Kalyani AJ, Mujtaba T, Rao MS. (1997) Isolation of lineage-restricted neuronal precursors from multipotent neuroepithelial stem cells. Neuron 19: 773–785.

McCall MA, Gregg RG, Behringer RR, et al. (1996) Targeted deletion in astrocyte intermediate filament (Gfap) alters neuronal physiology. Proc Natl Acad Sci USA 93: 6361–6366.

McDonald JW, Althomsons SP, Hyrc KL, Choi DW, Goldberg MP. (1998a) Oligodendrocytes from forebrain are highly vulnerable to AMPA/kainate receptor-mediated excitotoxicity. Nat Med 4: 291–297.

McDonald JW, Levine JM, Qu Y. (1998b) Multiple classes of the oligodendrocyte lineage are highly vulnerable to excitotoxicity. Neuroreport 9: 2757–2762.

Meaney JA, Balcar VJ, Rothstein JD, Jeffrey PL. (1998) Glutamate transport in cultures from developing avian cerebellum: presence of GLT-1 immunoreactivity in Purkinje neurons. J Neurosci Res 54: 595–603.

Mehler MF, Mabie PC, Zhu G, Gokhan S, Kessler JA. (2000) Developmental changes in progenitor cell responsiveness to bone morphogenetic proteins differentially modulate progressive CNS lineage fate. Dev Neurosci 22: 74–85.

Mennerick S, Dhond RP, Benz A, et al. (1998) Neuronal expression of the glutamate transporter GLT-1 in hippocampal microcultures. J Neurosci 18: 4490–4499.

Messing, A., Goldman, J.E., Johnson, A.B., and Brenner, M. (2001) Alexander disease: new insights from genetics. J Neuropathol Exp Neurol 60, 563–573.

Messing A, Head MW, Galles K, Galbreath EJ, Goldman JE, Brenner M. (1998) Fatal encephalopathy with astrocyte inclusions in GFAP transgenic mice. Am J Pathol 152: 391–398.

Mi H, Barres BA. (1999) Purification and characterization of astrocyte precursor cells in the developing rat optic nerve. J Neurosci 19: 1049–1061.

Mignot C, Boespflug-Tanguy O, Gelot A, Dautigny A, Pham-DinhD, Rodriguez D. (2004) Alexander disease: putative mechanisms of an astrocytic encephalopathy. Cell Mol Life Sci 61: 369–385.

Miller BA, Sun F, Christensen RN, Ferguson AR, Bresnahan JC, Beattie MS. (2005) A sublethal dose of TNFalpha potentiates kainate-induced excitotoxicity in optic nerve oligodendrocytes. Neurochem Res 30: 867–875.

Miller G. (2005) Neuroscience. The dark side of glia. Science 308: 778–781.

Miller RH, Abney ER, David S, et al. (1986) Is reactive gliosis a property of a distinct subpopulation of astrocytes? J Neurosci 6: 22–29.

Miller RH, Raff MC. (1984) Fibrous and protoplasmic astrocytes are biochemically and developmentally distinct. J Neurosci 4: 585–592.

Miller RH, Szigeti V. (1991) Clonal analysis of astrocyte diversity in neonatal rat spinal cord cultures. Development 113: 353–362.

Molne M, Studer L, Tabar V, Ting YT, Eiden MV, McKay RD. (2000) Early cortical precursors do not undergo LIF-mediated astrocytic differentiation. J Neurosci Res 59: 301–311.

Morath DJ, Mayer-Proschel M. (2002) Iron deficiency during embryogenesis and consequences for oligodendrocyte generation in vivo. Dev Neurosci 24: 197–207.

Morrison SJ, Perez SE, Qiao Z, et al. (2000) Transient Notch activation initiates an irreversible switch from neurogenesis to gliogenesis by neural crest stem cells. Cell 101: 499–510.

Nakagaito Y, Yoshida T, Satoh M, Takeuchi M. (1995) Effects of leukemia inhibitory factor on the differentiation of astrocyte progenitor cells from embryonic mouse cerebral hemispheres. Brain Res Dev Brain Res 87: 220–223.

Nakashima K, Takizawa T, Ochiai W, et al. (2001) BMP2-mediated alteration in the developmental pathway of fetal mouse brain cells from neurogenesis to astrocytogenesis. Proc Natl Acad Sci USA 98, 5868–5873.

Nakashima K, Wiese S, Yanagisawa, M, et al. (1999a) Developmental requirement of gp130 signaling in neuronal survival and astrocyte differentiation. J Neurosci 19, 5429–5434.

Nakashima K, Yanagisawa M, Arakawa H, Taga T. (1999b) Astrocyte differentiation mediated by LIF in cooperation with BMP2. FEBS Lett 457: 43–46.

Nedergaard M. (1994) Direct signaling from astrocytes to neurons in cultures of mammalian brain cells. Science 263: 1768–1771.

Nedergaard M, Ransom B, Goldman SA. (2003) New roles for astrocytes: redefining the functional architecture of the brain. Trends Neurosci 26: 523–530.

Newman EA. (2003) New roles for astrocytes: regulation of synaptic transmission. Trends Neurosci 26: 536–542.

Nielsen S, Nagelhus EA, Amiry-Moghaddam M, Bourque C, Agre P, Ottersen OP. (1997) Specialized membrane domains for water transport in glial cells: high-resolution immunogold cytochemistry of aquaporin-4 in rat brain. J Neurosci 17: 171–180.

Nishiyama A, Yang Z, Butt A. (2005) Astrocytes and NG2-glia: what's in a name? J Anat 207: 687–693.

Nishiyama K, Collodi P, Barnes D. (1993) Regulation of glial fibrillary acidic protein in serum-free mouse embryo (SFME) cells by leukemia inhibitory factor and related peptides. Neurosci Lett 163: 114–116.

Noble M, Proschel C, Mayer-Proschel M. (2004) Getting a GR(i)P on oligodendrocyte development. Dev Biol 265: 33–52.

Noble M, Smith J, Power J, Mayer-Proschel M. (2003) Redox state as a central modulator of precursor cell function. Ann N Y Acad Sci 991: 251–271.

Norenberg MD. (1979) Distribution of glutamine synthetase in the rat central nervous system. J Histochem Cytochem 27: 756–762.

Nunes MC, Roy NS, Keyoung HM, et al. (2003) Identification and isolation of multipotential neural progenitor cells from the subcortical white matter of the adult human brain. Nat Med 9: 439–447.

Ohno M, Kohyama J, Namihira M, et al. (2006) Neuropoietin induces neuroepithelial cells to differentiate into astrocytes via activation of STAT3. Cytokine 36: 17–22.

Oka A, Belliveau MJ, Rosenberg PA,Volpe JJ. (1993) Vulnerability of oligodendroglia to glutamate: pharmacology, mechanisms, and prevention. J Neurosci 13: 1441–1453.

Palmer TD, Willhoite AR, Gage FH. (2000) Vascular niche for adult hippocampal neurogenesis. J Comp Neurol 425: 479–494.

Patrono C, Di Giacinto G, Eymard-Pierre E, et al. (2003) Genetic heterogeneity of megalencephalic leukoencephalopathy and subcortical cysts. Neurology 61: 534–537.

Pfeiffer J. (1968) Alexander's disease – really a leucodystrophy? Pathol Eur 3: 305–312.

Pekny M, Leveen P, Pekna M, et al. (1995) Mice lacking glial fibrillary acidic protein display astrocytes devoid of intermediate filaments but develop and reproduce normally. EMBO J 14: 1590–1598.

Pekny M, Pekna M. (2004) Astrocyte intermediate filaments in CNS pathologies and regeneration. J Pathol 204: 428–437.

Porter JT, McCarthy KD. (1997) Astrocytic neurotransmitter receptors in situ and in vivo. Prog Neurobiol 51: 439–455.

Privat A, Rataboul P. (1986) Fibrous and protoplasmic astrocytes. In: Fedoroff S, Vernadakis A, Eds. Astrocytes: Development, Morphology, and Regional Specialization of Astrocytes. Orlando, FL: Academic Press, pp. 105–129.

Proud CG. (2005) eIF2 and the control of cell physiology. Semin Cell Dev Biol 16: 3–12.

Quinones-Hinojosa A, Sanai N, Soriano-Navarro M, et al. (2006) Cellular composition and cytoarchitecture of the adult human subventricular zone: a niche of neural stem cells. J Comp Neurol 494: 415–434.

Raff MC, Abney ER, Miller RH. (1984) Two glial cell lineages diverge prenatally in rat optic nerve. Dev Biol 106: 53–60.

Ransom B, Behar T, Nedergaard, M. (2003) New roles for astrocytes (stars at last). Trends Neurosci 26: 520–522.

Rao MS. (1999) Multipotent and restricted precursors in the central nervous system. Anat Rec 257: 137–148.

Rao MS, Noble M, Mayer-Proschel M. (1998) A tripotential glial precursor cell is present in the developing spinal cord. Proc Natl Acad Sci USA 95: 3996–4001.

Reynolds BA, Weiss S. (1992) Generation of neurons and astrocytes from isolated cells of the adult mammalian central nervous system. Science 255: 1707–1710.

Ridet JL, Malhotra SK, Privat A, Gage FH. (1997) Reactive astrocytes: cellular and molecular cues to biological function. Trends Neurosci 20: 570–577.

Rodriguez D, Gauthier F, Bertini E, et al. (2001) Infantile Alexander disease: spectrum of GFAP mutations and genotype-phenotype correlation. Am J Hum Genet 69: 1134–1140.

Rodriguez D, Gelot A, della Gaspera B, et al. (1999) Increased density of oligodendrocytes in childhood ataxia with diffuse central hypomyelination (CACH) syndrome: neuropathological and biochemical study of two cases. Acta Neuropathol 97: 469–480.

Rothstein JD, Martin L, Levey AI, et al. (1994) Localization of neuronal and glial glutamate transporters. Neuron 13: 713–725.

Sanai N, Tramontin AD, Quinones-Hinojosa A, et al. (2004) Unique astrocyte ribbon in adult human brain contains neural stem cells but lacks chain migration. Nature 427: 740–744.

Schiffmann R, Moller JR, Trapp BD, et al. (1994) Childhood ataxia with diffuse central nervous system hypomyelination. Ann Neurol 35: 331–340.

Schiffmann R, Tedeschi G, Kinkel RP, et al. (1997) Leukodystrophy in patients with ovarian dysgenesis. Ann Neurol 41: 654–661.

Schmitt A, Gofferje V, Weber M, Meyer J, Mossner R, Lesch KP. (2003) The brain-specific protein MLC1 implicated in megalencephalic leukoencephalopathy with subcortical cysts is expressed in glial cells in the murine brain. Glia 44: 283–295.

Schwankhaus JD, Parisi JE, Gulledge WR, Chin L, Currier RD. (1995) Hereditary adult-onset Alexander's disease with palatal myoclonus, spastic paraparesis, and cerebellar ataxia. Neurology 45: 2266–2271.

Seidman KJ, Teng AL, Rosenkopf R, Spilotro P, Weyhenmeyer JA. (1997) Isolation, cloning and characterization of a putative type-1 astrocyte cell line. Brain Res 753: 18–26.

57

Sendtner M, Carroll P, Holtmann B, Hughes RA, Thoenen H. (1994) Ciliary neurotrophic factor. J Neurobiol 25: 1436–1453.

Shen Q, Goderie SK, Jin L, et al. (2004) Endothelial cells stimulate self-renewal and expand neurogenesis of neural stem cells. Science 304: 1338–1340.

Shen Q, Wang Y, Dimos JT, et al. (2006) The timing of cortical neurogenesis is encoded within lineages of individual progenitor cells. Nat Neurosci 9: 743–751.

Shibuki K, Gomi H, Chen L, et al. (1996) Deficient cerebellar long-term depression, impaired eyeblink conditioning, and normal motor coordination in GFAP mutant mice. Neuron 16: 587–599.

Silver J, Miller JH. (2004) Regeneration beyond the glial scar. Nat Rev Neurosci 5: 146–156.

Singhal BS, Gursahani RD, Udani VP, Biniwale AA. (1996) Megalencephalic leukodystrophy in an Asian Indian ethnic group. Pediatr Neurol 14: 291–296.

Sofroniew MV. (2005) Reactive astrocytes in neural repair and protection. Neuroscientist 11: 400–407.

Stockli KA, Lillien LE, Naher-Noe M, et al. (1991) Regional distribution, developmental changes, and cellular localization of CNTF-mRNA and protein in the rat brain. J Cell Biol 115: 447–459.

Sumi SM, Hager H. (1968) Electron microscopic study of the reaction of the newborn rat brain to injury. Acta Neuropathol 10: 324–335.

Sun Y, Nadal-Vicens M, Misono S, et al. (2001) Neurogenin promotes neurogenesis and inhibits glial differentiation by independent mechanisms. Cell 104: 365–376.

Suzuki K. (2003) Globoid cell leukodystrophy (Krabbe's disease): update. J Child Neurol 18: 595–603.

Takano T, Tian GF, Peng W, et al. (2006) Astrocyte-mediated control of cerebral blood flow. Nat Neurosci 9: 260–267.

Tanigaki K, Nogaki F, Takahashi J, Tashiro K, Kurooka H, Honjo T. (2001) Notch1 and Notch3 instructively restrict bFGF-responsive multipotent neural progenitor cells to an astroglial fate. Neuron 29: 45–55.

Tansey FA, Farooq M, Cammer W. (1991) Glutamine synthetase in oligodendrocytes and astrocytes: new biochemical and immunocytochemical evidence. J Neurochem 56: 266–272.

Teijido, O, Martinez A, Pusch M, et al. (2004) Localization and functional analyses of the MLC1 protein involved in megalencephalic leukoencephalopathy with subcortical cysts. Hum Mol Genet 13: 2581–2594.

Temple S. (2001) The development of neural stem cells. Nature 414: 112–117.

Temple S., and Alvarez-Buylla, A. (1999) Stem cells in the adult mammalian central nervous system. Curr Opin Neurobiol 9, 135–141.

Terada S, Ishizu H, Yokota O, et al. (2004) An autopsy case of hereditary diffuse leukoencephalopathy with spheroids, clinically suspected of Alzheimer's disease. Acta Neuropathol 108: 538–545.

Tomokane N, Iwaki T, Tateishi J, Iwaki A, Goldman JE. (1991) Rosenthal fibers share epitopes with alpha B-crystallin, glial fibrillary acidic protein, and ubiquitin, but not with vimentin. Immunoelectron microscopy with colloidal gold. Am J Pathol 138: 875–885.

Topcu M, Gartioux C, Ribierre F, et al. (2000) Vacuoliting megalencephalic leukoencephalopathy with subcortical cysts, mapped to chromosome 22qtel. Am J Hum Genet 66: 733–739.

Tsacopoulos M, Magistretti PJ. (1996) Metabolic coupling between glia and neurons. J Neurosci 16: 877–885.

Ullian EM, Sapperstein SK, Christopherson KS, Barres BA. (2001) Control of synapse number by glia. Science 291: 657–661.

van der Knaap MS, Barth PG, Gabreels FJ, et al. (1997) A new leukoencephalopathy with vanishing white matter. Neurology 48: 845–855.

van der Knaap MS, Barth PG, Stroink H, et al. (1995) Leukoencephalopathy with swelling and a discrepantly mild clinical course in eight children. Ann Neurol 37: 324–334.

van der Knaap MS, Barth PG, Vrensen GF, Valk J. (1996) Histopathology of an infantile-onset spongiform leukoencephalopathy with a discrepantly mild clinical course. Acta Neuropathol 92: 206–212.

van der Knaap MS, Leegwater PA, Konst AA, et al. (2002) Mutations in each of the five subunits of translation initiation factor eIF2B can cause leukoencephalopathy with vanishing white matter. Ann Neurol 51: 264–270.

van der Knaap MS, Naidu S, Breiter SN, et al. (2001) Alexander disease: diagnosis with MR imaging. AJNR Am J Neuroradiol 22: 541–552.

van der Knaap MS, Ramesh V, Schiffmann R, et al. (2006) Alexander disease: ventricular garlands and abnormalities of the medulla and spinal cord. Neurology 66: 494–498.

van der Knaap MS, Salomons GS, Li R, et al. (2005) Unusual variants of Alexander's disease. Ann Neurol 57: 327–338.

Van Haren K, van der Voorn JP, Peterson DR, van der Knaap MS, Powers JM. (2004) The life and death of oligodendrocytes in vanishing white matter disease. J Neuropathol Exp Neurol 63: 618–630.

58

van Praag H, Schinder AF, Christie BR, Toni N, Palmer TD, Gage FH. (2002) Functional neurogenesis in the adult hippocampus. Nature 415: 1030–1034.

Verkman AS, Binder DK, Bloch O, Auguste K, Papadopoulos MC. (2006) Three distinct roles of aquaporin-4 in brain function revealed by knockout mice. Biochim Biophys Acta 1758: 1085–1093.

Viti J, Feathers A, Phillips J, Lillien L. (2003) Epidermal growth factor receptors control competence to interpret leukemia inhibitory factor as an astrocyte inducer in developing cortex. J Neurosci 23: 3385–3393.

Vizuete ML, Venero JL, Vargas C, et al. (1999) Differential upregulation of aquaporin-4 mRNA expression in reactive astrocytes after brain injury: potential role in brain edema. Neurobiol Dis 6: 245–258.

Voigt T. (1989) Development of glial cells in the cerebral wall of ferrets: direct tracing of their transformation from radial glia into astrocytes. J Comp Neurol 289: 74–88.

Volpe JJ. (2001) Neurobiology of periventricular leukomalacia in the premature infant. Pediatr Res 50: 553–562.

Volterra A, Meldolesi J. (2005) Astrocytes, from brain glue to communication elements: the revolution continues. Nat Rev Neurosci 6: 626–640.

Webster H, Astrom KE. (2009) Gliogenesis: historical perspectives, 1839–1985. Adv Anat Embryol Cell Biol 202: 1–109.

Weible MW, 2nd, Chan-Ling T. (2007) Phenotypic characterization of neural stem cells from human fetal spinal cord: synergistic effect of LIF and BMP4 to generate astrocytes. Glia 55: 1156–1168.

Weinstein DE, Shelanski ML, Liem RK. (1991) Suppression by antisense mRNA demonstrates a requirement for the glial fibrillary acidic protein in the formation of stable astrocytic processes in response to neurons. J Cell Biol 112: 1205–1213.

Wilke S, Thomas R, Allcock N, Fern R. (2004) Mechanism of acute ischemic injury of oligodendroglia in early myelinating white matter: the importance of astrocyte injury and glutamate release. J Neuropathol Exp Neurol 63; 872–881.

Wong K, Armstrong RC, Gyure KA, et al. (2000) Foamy cells with oligodendroglial phenotype in childhood ataxia with diffuse central nervous system hypomyelination syndrome. Acta Neuropathol 100: 635–646.

Xu L, Sapolsky RM, Giffard R.G. (2001) Differential sensitivity of murine astrocytes and neurons from different brain regions to injury. Exp Neurol 169: 416–424.

Yanagisawa M, Takizawa T, Ochiai W, Uemura,A, Nakashima K, Taga T. (2001) Fate alteration of neuroepithelial cells from neurogenesis to astrocytogenesis by bone morphogenetic proteins. Neurosci Res 41: 391–396.

Zaheer A, Zhong W, Uc EY, Moser DR, Lim R. (1995) Expression of mRNAs of multiple growth factors and receptors by astrocytes and glioma cells: detection with reverse transcription-polymerase chain reaction. Cell Mol Neurobiol 15: 221–237.

4
MICROGLIA AND LEUKODYSTROPHIES

Patricia Musolino and Florian Eichler

Introduction

Tissue macrophages are found to reside in the central nervous system (CNS), just as they reside in all other tissues in the body. Microglia are the most numerous of brain macrophages and account for about 10% of the non-neuronal cells in brain parenchyma. They are of myeloid lineage, which was conclusively established by the fact that microglia are absent from the CNS of PU.1-null mice but can be readily re-populated by bone marrow transplantation (McKercher et al. 1996, Beers et al. 2006). In healthy brain, microglia have a distinct phenotype induced by molecules expressed on, or secreted by, adjacent neurons and astrocytes. This phenotype is maintained in part by exclusion of serum components by the blood–brain barrier (BBB).

In this chapter we focus upon important aspects of microglial physiology in the context of the leukodystrophies. To this end, we review the role of microglia in health and neurodegeneration. In the leukodystrophies, microglia may be the first sensors of disturbed homeostasis. They are likely to be the first cells to react to aberrant products of lipid metabolism within the CNS. While many questions surrounding microglia in the leukodystrophies remain unanswered, we draw upon the increasing literature regarding microglia in multiple sclerosis and neurodegeneration to frame the context of future studies. Lastly, microglia have been implicated in the mechanism by which bone marrow transplantation salvages the brain of leukodystrophy patients (Priller 2003, Fabriek et al. 2005, Mildner et al. 2007). We must therefore investigate these cells more throroughly if therapies for leukodystrophy patients are to improve in the years to come.

Macrophage populations in the central nervous system

Several different macrophage populations can be distinguished within the CNS. In the adult brain, microglia have a small cell soma, little perinuclear cytoplasm, and numerous branched processes that are covered in fine protrusions. With these fine protrusions, microglia continually palpate and monitor their local microenvironment. Microglia rapidly change their phenotype in response to any disturbance of nervous system homeostasis and are then commonly referred to as "activated" on the basis of changes in their morphology or expression of cell surface antigens (see section on "Defining microglial activation").

In addition to microglia, there are macrophage populations associated with the perivascular space, the circumventricular organs, the choroid plexus, and the meninges (Perry and Gordon 1987, Bechmann et al. 2001, Fabriek et al. 2005). These macrophages have a different phenotype than microglia and express different antigens. These cells are also more overtly phagocytic than microglia, and their expression of major histocompatibility complex (MHC) antigens is more widespread. Such phenotypic differences may arise in part from the fact that, due to their location in the circumventricular organs and choroid plexus, they are exposed to blood and serum proteins, the latter being a possible regulator of microglial phenotype.

Within healthy brain, the homeostasis of immune responses is regulated and adapted to protect neurons and their connections from immune-mediated damage that could compromise survival of the host. This state of "immune privilege" may be radically altered in the diseased brain, allowing for introduction of a population of dendritic cells, the "professional" antigen-presenting cells of the immune system. There has been no convincing demonstration of dendritic cells, either by expression of the relevant surface markers or by characteristic function in the healthy brain parenchyma, although they are present in the meninges and choroid plexus.

Defining microglial activation

Original studies of microglial activation began with the premise that activated microglia emerge from a resting state and undergo morphological transformation from ramified to various activated forms, including ameboid, rod-like, and phagocytic. This view has expanded to include alternate modes of progression from surveillant to effector states, replacing the notion that microglia proceed from resting to activated. In this context, it is instructive to compare microglia with peripheral macrophages.

Both peripheral macrophages and microglia, as members of the family of mononuclear phagocytic cells, can be stimulated by non-self pathogens (stranger signals) or by injured-self components (danger signals). These stimuli activate pattern-recognition receptors such as the Toll-like receptors (TLRs), scavenger receptors, and nucleotide-binding oligomerization domain-containing protein receptors. The goal of this activation is clearance of tissue debris, generation of cues for tissue restoration, and resistance to pathogens. Together these reactions comprise the innate immune response. In turn, this may lead to activation of an adaptive immune response including lymphocyte and antibody functions.

Despite these commonalities, microglia differ decisively from peripheral macrophages in three important respects. (1) Microglia reside behind the BBB, so that serum products represent danger signals indicating a breach of the BBB. Active brain disease in adrenoleukodystrophy is associated with an opening of the BBB, which may in itself lead to microglial activation. (2) Microglia, as brain glial cells, are affected by altered synaptic activity and perturbations of neurotransmitter availability. Responses to acute and chronic injury are in part regulated by selective activation of metabotropic glutamate receptors upon microglia. The impact of altered chemistry in the leukodystrophies upon neurotransmitter receptors remains unknown. (3) Microglia exhibit an actively repressed phenotype, so that removal of constraints that are primarily neuronally derived constitutes a type of danger signal, indicating that neuronal function is impaired. CXCL1 is a membrane-tethered chemokine that is tonically released from CNS neurons and inhibits microglia through its receptor, CX3CR1. If this tonic inhibition is removed, microglial neurotoxicity is unleashed in response to either systemic inflammatory stimuli or damage to resident neurons. This phenomenon may be a consequence of microglia coexisting among fragile, non-renewing neurons. Analogous scenarios may hold true for microglia and their relation to functionally impaired oligodendrocytes and astrocytes.

Microglia in development and repair

Microglia have been assigned an important role in synaptic remodeling. During CNS development, axonal connections with synaptic targets exceed those required and are reduced in a process termed pruning. It is known that in mice lacking specific MHC class I determinants, this process of synaptic pruning is aberrant. Mice lacking complement components C1q or C3 exhibit defects in visual system synaptic refinement, similar to those found in MHC class I–deficient animals.

In normal conditions, microglia will ensure a "silent" clearance of apoptotic neurons and glial cells in the CNS. This process ensures the uptake of cells committed to death before their membrane lyses, thus preventing release of their intracellular content and disruption of tissue homeostasis. Several molecules on the surface of apoptotic cells and cognate receptors have been shown to be involved in the recognition and ingestion of apoptotic cells by macrophages. Among these, phosphatidylserine (PS), a phospholipid normally found in the inner leaflet of the plasma membrane and externalized during the early phase of the apoptotic process, has received great attention since the identification of a specific macrophage receptor (PS-R).

Several lines of evidence, such as the expression of mRNA for the PS-R, indicate that phosphatidylserine externalization is necessary for microglial recognition and phagocytosis of the apoptotic neurons. Recently, Minghetti et al. (2005) demonstrated that chronic stimulation and interaction with phosphatidylserine-expressing apoptotic cells contributed to a progressive downregulation of pro-inflammatory molecule expression and a sustained release of immunoregulatory substances, such as prostaglandin (PG) E2 and transforming growth factor-1, by microglia. Despite its classical pro-inflammatory role on vascular permeability and leukocyte extravasation, PGE2 regulates several immune functions and downregulates the release of interleukin (IL)-1, tumor necrosis factor (TNF)-α and nitric oxide (NO) by activated macrophages and microglia. The enhancement of PGE2 synthesis in microglia interacting with apoptotic neurons expressing membrane phosphatidylserine could contribute to the silent clearance of dying neurons and other non-neuronal cell types.

Thus, while activated microglia responding to apoptotic neurons are turned into a phenotype that releases anti-inflammatory cytokines that prevent further damage, activated microglia lacking this interaction with the PS-R can produce a burst of pro-inflammatory cytokines and oxidative stress.

Brain colonization, self-renewal, and post-lesional recruitment of microglia

In the CNS, two populations of cells derived from bone marrow (BM) execute the functions of resident macrophages: microglial cells and perivascular macrophages. Both belong to the myelomonocytic lineage and are derived from the embryonic hemangioblastic mesoderm. Microglial cells populate the developing neuroectoderm early in embryonic life and represent around 10% of the brain cell population. Later and during the lifespan of the host, a group of undefined BM precursor cells constantly migrates into the CNS and repopulates resident perivascular macrophages and occasionally microglia. Studies tracking BM-transplanted cells expressing galactosidase show that these cells engraft slowly following transplantation, and that 1 year after transplantation 30% of resident microglia are replaced (Kennedy and Abkowitz 1997). Yet, only rarely do donor-derived cells become parenchymal microglia. Possible explanations for this finding are that parenchymal cells can arise from cells other than BM-derived cells or, more likely, that they are of hematopoietic origin but enter the CNS before birth and turn over at an extremely slow rate.

Even though BM-derived cells can enter the brain parenchyma throughout the CNS in normal mice, they seem to be preferentially attracted to regions afflicted by neurodegeneration or neurological insults. This is also true in models where the BBB is not compromised, such as in the case of facial nerve axotomy. Following prion neuroinvasion, another neurodegenerative model without BBB disruption, Priller et al. (2006) found that more than 50% of all brain microglia were replaced by BM-derived cells before clinical disease onset and that in terminally sick mice, microglial density increased three to four fold. These findings suggest that blood monocytes infiltrate the brain and later differentiate into ramified microglia, and that they are able to enter the CNS, even if the BBB is intact, and massively colonize the CNS in particular diseases.

The exact mechanisms involved in these events have yet to be fully characterized. It is likely that stressed or damaged neurons send signals to resident microglia or produce specific chemokines to cause recruitment of BM-derived microglia. A number of proteins can act as endogenous ligands for TLRs expressed on the surface of microglia and then trigger NF-kB signaling, leading to a subtle inflammatory response and subsequent proliferation and chemoattraction of myeloid cells without the need for massive neurodegeneration and BBB breakdown. We speculate that this process takes place to provide survival signals in support of stressed, injured, or infected neurons.

Microglia in the pathogenesis of leukodystrophies

Although the gene and enzymatic defects have been identified in most forms of leukodystrophies described to date, the pathogenesis of CNS destruction and the wide phenotypic variation among patients with the same genotype are still poorly understood. Whereas lipid accumulation correlates with the deficiency of enzymes involved in substrate catabolism in several disorders – such as arylsulfatase A in metachromatic leukodystrophy or galactocerebrosidase in globoid cell leukodystrophy – the mechanism by which adrenoleukodystrophy protein (ALDP), a peroxisomal transporter protein, leads to accumulation of very long chain fatty acids (VLCFAs) in adrenoleukodystrophy (ALD) is less well understood. However, the mere accumulation of substrate in any one of these disorders may not be sufficient cause for progressive demyelination, implying that other elements may be crucial in the pathogenesis of CNS disease.

Using experimental models, the quantity and duration of substrate exposure upon tissue can be examined. Most animal models that show phenotypic resemblance to human leukodystrophies demonstrate microglial activation. This suggests that microglia play a vital role as sensors of aberrant lipids and are critical to early reactivity to abnormal metabolic substrates (Fig. 4.1). Beyond the metabolic substrate, the immune system itself may act as a modifier of disease. This observation is supported by the fact that knockout mice for *ABCD1*, the defective gene in ALD, show increased VLCFA levels but no inflammatory reaction (Kobayashi et al. 1997, Lu et al. 1997). This warrants closer examination of the immune regulatory mechanisms involved in the pathogenesis of a wide range of myelinopathies, particularly the behavior of microglial cells and their immunomodulatory role.

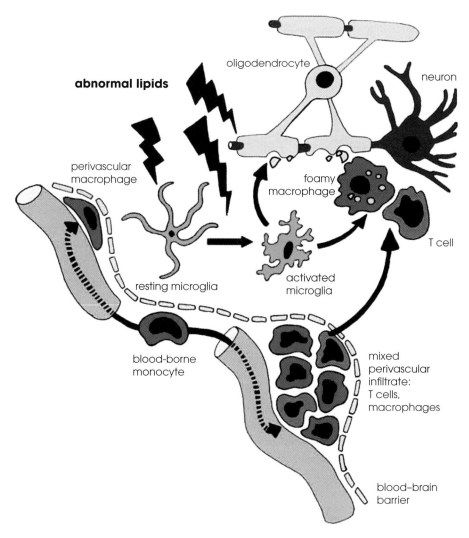

Fig. 4.1. Microglia are critical to early reactivity to abnormal lipids and initiate a cascade of cytokine release, macrophage and lymphocyte recruitment, and demyelination.

The scavenger receptor CD36 is expressed on a wide variety of cells and is thought to play a vital role in the uptake of lipid molecules such as fatty acids (Abumrad et al. 2005, Drover et al. 2008, Goldberg et al. 2008). In brain tissue, the expression of CD36 has been established on both microglia and microvascular endothelial cells. Beyond the innate response CD1, which is a family of surface glycoproteins with the ability to present foreign and self-lipid antigens to unconventional or MHC-unrestricted T cells, has been identified on microglial cells and resident CNS macrophages and may be responsible for the massive lymphocytic inflammation seen in ALD (Ito et al. 2001, Moody et al. 2005).

Environmental factors such as head trauma may also play a role in microglial activation. During BBB disruption, serum constituents such as fibrinogen can activate microglia (Adams et al. 2007). Surface receptors on microglia, such as P2Y12, are known to be sensitive to purinergic signaling and have recently been recognized to play a role in brain trauma (Haynes et al. 2006, Kettenmann 2006). The altered lipid substrate may further modify the response. Below we will review the knowledge accumulated to date about the role of microglia in the pathogenesis of three of the most prevalent and extensively studied leukodystrophies: adrenoleukodystrophy, metachromatic leukodystrophy, and globoid cell leukodystrophy.

Adrenoleukodystrophy

X-linked adrenoleukodystrophy (X-ALD) is a common peroxisomal disease affecting 1 in 15 000 to 1 in 20 000 boys annually (Moser et al. 2001). The principal biochemical abnormality identified in X-ALD patients is the accumulation of unbranched saturated VLCFAs, particularly in the adrenal cortex, testis, and brain, which are constituents of complex lipids (e.g., glycerophospholipids, gangliosides, and cholesterol esters) and proteolipid protein. The gene responsible for ALD resides on chromosome Xq28 and codes for a 84-kDa protein of the peroxisomal membrane, referred to as ALDP, which is an ATP-binding cassette (ABC) half-transporter.

The inflammatory nature of brain demyelination in ALD aligns it with multiple sclerosis, the most common demyelinative disease. Like multiple sclerosis, much of the destruction of myelin in X-ALD appears to be mediated by an immunologic response. The lymphocyte infiltration in X-ALD is comprised mostly of T cells (cytotoxic lymphocytes) and macrophages, tends to occur behind the demyelinating edge, and is implicated in subsequent secondary tract degeneration. This is in contrast to multiple sclerosis, where the inflammatory infiltrates accumulate at the active demyelinating edge, and suggests differential mechanisms of disease pathogenesis.

Demyelination in X-ALD evolves systematically. It is first seen in the splenium or genu of the corpus callosum and then extends symmetrically outward, creating a confluent lesion within the white matter. Demyelination regularly spares the subcortical white matter. Pathological descriptions of the inflammatory lesion of X-ALD demarcate three zones (Schaumburg et al. 1975). The first zone consists of a dense mesh of glial fibrils and scattered astrocytes without any evidence of an active process; here, oligodendroglia, axons, and myelin sheaths are absent. Moving outward, the leading edge consists of two closely aligned zones: one in which many macrophages are present; and the most peripheral edge, where destruction of myelin is apparent but axons are spared.

Expansion of lesion

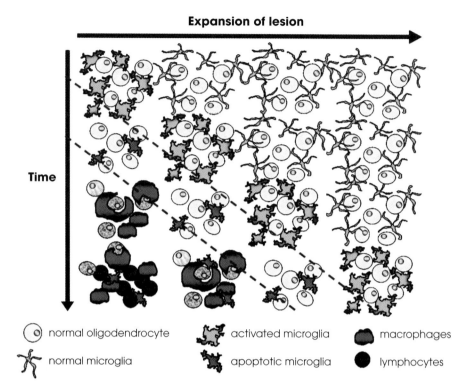

Time

normal oligodendrocyte	activated microglia	macrophages
normal microglia	apoptotic microglia	lymphocytes

Fig. 4.2. Loss of microglia precedes demyelination in cerebral adrenoleukodystrophy. Early microglial activation is followed by microglial apoptosis and subsequent demyelination. Macrophages and lymphocytes are recruited to clear myelin debris.

Recently, we discovered a zone within myelinated white matter that lacks microglia beyond the leading edge of the lesion (Eichler et al. 2008). Given the spatial and temporal evolution of lesions in X-ALD, this observation suggests that loss of microglia precedes demyelination (Fig. 4.2). This region contains factors that are critical to the progression of demyelination in X-ALD. Interestingly, this area of activation is only seen in perilesional myelin, not in unaffected regions of the brain, and corresponds to areas where myelin contains six to seven times higher levels of VLCFAs. It is possible that microglia in this region are unable to degrade VLCFAs, and that those VLCFAs, in turn, may cause microglial activation and apoptosis.

Does VLCFA accumulation cause microglial activation?
VLCFAs, defined as saturated fatty acids greater than 22 carbons in length, are metabolized in peroxisomes, and it is known that lipopolysaccharide-induced cytokines can decrease peroxisomal β-oxidation activity in rat liver and cultured oligodendrocytes. This suggests that the release of cytokines (i.e., TNF-α, IL-1ß) and expression of ICAMs (intercellular adhesion molecules) by activated astrocytes and microglia at the active edge of the

demyelinating lesion in X-ALD affected brain may modulate peroxisomal metabolism of VLCFAs in the actively demyelinating region. In fact, it has been shown that pro-inflammatory cytokines (TNF-α, IL-1ß, and interferon-γ) can downregulate peroxisomal beta-oxidation activity of fatty acids. The resulting excessive production of NO and reactive oxygen species may be a mediator of this impaired peroxisomal function, leading to the accumulation of VLCFAs in glial cells. Many studies have implicated pro-inflammatory cytokines and inducible NO synthase in the pathogenesis of brain disorders, including multiple sclerosis, Alzheimer disease, and ALD, but the signaling pathways remain poorly understood.

How does microglial activation relate to demyelination in adrenoleukodystrophy?
Reactive astrocytes, macrophages, and T lymphocytes are the most prevalent cellular elements in X-ALD lesions. Ito et al. (2001) showed that while active lesions in both ALD and adrenomyeloneuropathy have occasional CD4+ perivascular lymphocytes, the majority of perivascular and infiltrating lymphocytes are CD8+. These CD8+ cytotoxic lymphocytes (CTLs) may be the effectors of cytolytic killing of oligodendrocytes in X-ALD, a process consisting of rapid cytoplasmatic swelling and disruption of cytoplasm and nucleolus. The authors proposed that target cell lysis by CTLs could be initiated by CD1-mediated lipid antigen presentation via in-situ activation of microglia/macrophages and reactive astrocytes and perpetuated by glycolipid-rectricted T lymphocytes that cross the BBB when activated in peripheral tissues. In support of these observations, several studies have demonstrated that the immune response in ALD is neither classical Th1 nor Th2, and that MHC haplotype differences do not explain the striking phenotypic variation in ALD.

More recent evidence suggests that although the oligodendrocyte and axon may be the evident targets in cerebral ALD, the process might not be cell-autonomous, and injury to oligodendrocytes may be enhanced through damage incurred by neighboring microglia via an inflammatory or metabolic imbalance that initiates and accelerates disease progression (Eichler et al. 2008). The prominence of macrophages around blood vessels at the leading edge of the lesion in cerebral X-ALD suggests that these macrophages are blood borne. Hematogenous macrophages play a crucial role in the removal of myelin debris, as evidenced by luxol fast blue inclusions. In addition, a zone lacking microglia has recently been described within non-lesional myelinated white matter, beyond the leading edge of inflammation/demyelination (Eichler et al. 2008) (Fig. 4.3).

Although the mechanisms underlying the apoptosis of perilesional activated microglia are still under debate, this loss of microglia could abrogate the production of neuroprotective factors, including immunoregulatory molecules that prevent the initiation or acceleration of a harmful inflammatory response, for cells at risk of degeneration. Moreover, there is recent evidence that the fine branches of "resting" microglia are highly motile and provide extensive and continuous surveillance of their cellular environment. These moving branches show a rapid chemotactic response to tissue injury and take cues from surrounding astrocytes both in the normal and in the injured brain.

In summary, the degeneration and death of oligodendrocytes in ALD appear to be due at least in part to metabolic and immunologic disturbances suffered by local microglia

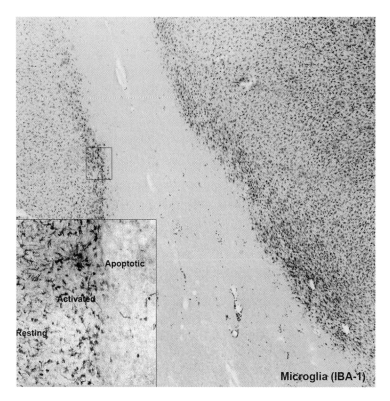

Fig. 4.3. IBA-1 staining showing distribution and morphology of microglia in the cortex and perilesional white matter. Cortical microglia show a normal morphology ("resting"), while microglia within white matter are either ameboid ("activated") or dying ("apoptotic"). The spatial distribution of altered microglial morphology indicates that selective microglial cell loss is an early phenomenon that probably precedes demyelination.

during the early stages of disease. Thereafter, activated microglia may initiate lysis of oligodendrocytes through lipid–antigen presentation to CTLs. The ensuing activation or overactivation of microglia generates a metabolic stress, which in addition to the protein deficiency causes further accumulation of VLCFAs. Thus, these "abnormal" microglia may become vulnerable to increased levels of cytokines present in the media, in particular TNF-α, and undergo apoptosis, further impairing the balance between pro-inflammatory and neuroprotective molecules.

Metachromatic leukodystrophy
Metachromatic leukodystrophy (MLD) is an autosomal recessive lipidosis caused by a deficiency of the lysosomal enzyme arylsulfatase A and is mapped to chromosome 22q13.31 (Gieselmann and von Figura 2000, Gieselmann et al. 2003). The enzymatic defect results in accumulation of its substrate, galactosylceramide I 3-sulfate (sulfatide), a major sphingolipid of myelin. The disease is characterized by myelin degeneration in both the CNS and

peripheral nervous system, associated with the accumulation of sulfatide in glial cells and neurons. Despite the fact that the enzymatic deficiency is systemic, disease manifestations are restricted to the nervous system.

CONSEQUENCES OF SULFATIDE ACCUMULATION AND MICROGLIAL ACTIVATION
The polar head of sulfatide consists of a galactose molecule, which is sulfated in position 3, where arylsulfatase A desulfates it. Due to deficiency of the enzyme, desulfation cannot take place and sulfatide accumulates. Sulfatide is found in the external layer of the plasma membrane, represents 4% to 5% of myelin lipids and is, besides galactosylceramide, the major glycosphingolipid of myelin. Within plasma membranes, sulfatide, together with cholesterol, is restricted to the outer layer of the membrane and forms aggregates that float in the liquid phase of diacylglycerol-based lipids. These floating sphingolipid/cholesterol platforms have been termed lipid rafts (Simons and Ehehalt 2002). These lipid rafts are involved in signal-transduction pathways and may play a role in intracellular trafficking, and sulfatide accumulation within lipid rafts may contribute to neuronal and oligodendrocytic degeneration through changes in intracellular sorting and signal transduction pathways (Simons and Toomre 2000).

Despite the fact that lack of residual arylsulfatase A (ASA) activity always results in severe late-infantile MLD in humans, the phenotype of the ASA-deficient mouse is surprisingly mild (Hess et al. 1996, Gieselmann et al. 2003). Abnormal sulfatide accumulation is seen in the nervous system, kidney, and bile ducts. Within the brain, neuronal sulfatide storage is most prominent in nuclei of the medulla oblongata, pons, and several nuclei of the mid-brain and forebrain. The extent of storage increases with age, and the overall organ distribution largely resembles that found in humans. However, although animals lose 30% of the fibers in the peripheral nervous system by 18 months of age, they do not develop significant demyelination up to 2 years of age.

Ameboid microglial cells in the brains of ASA/ mice are round or ovoid and congested with alcianophilic material, which often obscures the nucleus (Muschol et al. 2002, Molander-Melin et al. 2004, Wittke et al. 2004). On an ultrastructural level, in both ASA/ mice and humans, the storage material within the inclusions displays lamellated and occasionally prismatic and herring-bone patterns. The abnormal composition of the sufatide-loaded lipidic membrane may give rise to antigens as the basis of instability and disruption with release of fragments that, engulfed by microglia, could in turn expand the inflammatory response. However, our understanding of the precise role of microglia in the pathogenesis of MLD is nascent and remains to be explored.

Microglia in globoid cell leukodystrophy (Krabbe disease)
Globoid cell leukodystrophy, also known as Krabbe disease, is an autosomal recessive disorder resulting from a deficiency of the lysosomal enzyme galactocerebrosidase (GALC), mapped to chromosome 14q31 (Wenger et al. 2000). While most patients present within the first 6 months of life ("infantile" or "classic" disease), later-onset patients have been reported, even into adulthood. In its infantile form, Krabbe disease manifests as a rapidly progressive neurological deterioration leading to death within the first two years of life.

Main clinical features include marked irritability, pyramidal tract dysfunction, optic atrophy, sensorineural deafness, and seizures within the first months of life. The neuropathological hallmark is that of large macrophages filled with periodic acid–Schiff positive material (globoid cells).

THE TWITCHER MOUSE, AN ANIMAL MODEL OF KRABBE DISEASE

The twitcher mouse, a mouse in which the *GALC* gene has been knocked out, resembles the human counterpart in its main histopathological findings (Kobayashi et al. 1986, Wu et al. 2000). Demyelination in twitcher mice commences in orderly fashion and the nerve-fiber tracts that myelinated earlier start demyelinating first. In the cerebellar white matter and brainstem, demyelination and increased numbers of macrophages are recognized earlier (postnatal day 20) than in the cerebral white matter (postnatal day 25). With progression of demyelination, the number of astrocytes and microglia/macrophages increase and MHC class II-expressing cells appear within areas of demyelination. IL-6 and TNF-α–positive reactive astrocytes are increased in the brain of the twitcher mice with respect to controls, and in more advanced demyelination TNF-α–positive macrophages can be found in the cerebral white matter, the pons, and the medulla. Moreover, T lymphocytes immunoreactive for leukocyte common antigen and CD3 were found increased around the vessel in white matter. These data suggest that inflammatory-immunological mechanisms may be involved in the myelin breakdown and glial pathology of globoid cell leukodystrophy, as reported in the twitcher mouse.

MICROGLIA IN THE PATHOGENESIS OF KRABBE DISEASE

Signs of inflammation have been described in immunohistological studies of human Krabbe disease. The deficient enzyme, galactocerebrosidase, leads to an accumulation of its substrates galactosylceramide and psychosine. Mononuclear phagocytic cells engulf and remove galatosylceramide, and globoid cells are present early in the disease. It is unclear whether psychosine is also removed by phagocytes. More importantly, psychosine appears to be cytotoxic to oligodendrocytes. In human autopsy cases, ramified microglia, immunoreactive for ferritin and HLA-DR-α, can be seen scattered in the white matter, with some also immunoreactive for TNF-α.

Among other proinflammatory cytokines, microglia produce NO and prostaglandins (PGs). In the twitcher mouse, activated brain microglia express hematopoetic PGD synthase (HPGDS), the enzyme responsible for production of PGD2 (Mohri et al. 2006). Further, activated astrocytes express the DP1 receptor for PGD2 in the brain of these mice. Mohri et al. postulate that the molecular events leading to neuroinflammation in the twitcher mouse brain first involve apoptosis of oligodendrocytes, activation of microglia by myelin debris, and synthesis of PGD2 in activated microglia. PGD2 in turn stimulates both DP1 and DP2 receptors on neighboring astrocytes in a paracrine manner and upregulates the expression of DP1, a Gs-coupled receptor that increases intracellular cAMP levels leading to hypertrophy of these cells. Engagement of DP2, a Gi-coupled receptor, also increases glial fibrillary acidic protein expression, presumably through elevation of intracellular calcium levels. Both genetic and pharmacological inhibition of HPGDS have been shown to suppress astrogliosis and demyelination in the twitcher mouse, indicating a key role of the pro-inflammatory prostaglandins within microglia.

In order to determine the source of the inflammatory infiltrate, Wu et al. (2000) tracked hematopoietic cells labeled with rhodamine isothiocynate and found that these cells migrate to the lesion parenchyma after PND 30. The majority of BM-derived cells emerge in the spinal cord and brainstem at PND 30 and are found in the cerebrum at PND 32, gradually increasing in number and expressing MHC class II. However, at PND 45, despite the presence of macrophages and demyelination, these double-labeled cells are no longer detected in the CNS parenchyma. The authors hypothesize that in the early stage of demyelination, local microglial cells are activated to become ameboid microglia/ macrophages engaging in phagocytic activity, and hematogenous cells are only called in when the need for phagocytic activity extends beyond the capacity of local microglia. Expression of these hematogenous cells appears to reach a plateau between PND 30 and 40 and rapidly decreases thereafter. Thus, the most likely scenario is that activated resident microglia and astroglia secret various cytokines to recruit hematogenous cells from the circulation. The finding of increased expression of MCP-1 mRNA during the critical time period supports this hypothesis.

The role of microglia in transplantation
Allogenic bone marrow transplantation (BMT) is an effective therapeutic approach in ALD, MLD, and Krabbe disease, significantly delaying disease onset and progression in early symptomatic patients (Krivit et al. 1999a, b, Peters et al. 2004). However, the efficacy of and optimal circumstances for BMT remain an issue of great concern in the clinical arena for management of leukodystrophy patients. While many questions remain regarding the degree of risk associated with immunsuppression, and the morbidity of the procedure itself, there appears to be consensus over the role of microglia in the process, a better understanding of which may aid in the development of safer, more effective therapies (Eglitis and Mezey 1997, Wehner et al. 2003, Priller 2003, Djukic et al. 2006, Ransohoff 2007).

With the advent of green fluorescent protein (GFP) technology, it has become possible to track engrafted cells in the CNS. GFP is a fluorophore with high fluorescence yield, resistance to photobleaching, and no endogenous counterpart in mammals. Several studies have shown that following transplantation of GFP-expressing BM cells into myeloablated adult mice, perivascular spaces become rapidly populated by donor-derived monocytes/ macrophages (Priller et al. 2001, Vallieres and Sawchenko 2003). The number of donor-derived microglia increases over time. When adult male BM cells are transplanted into non-irradiated female PU.1-deficient neonatal mice, all microglia in the recipient mice are donor-derived and Y-chromosome positive. After irradiation and transplant, marrow-derived cells can be detected in the mouse brain as early as 3 days post-procedure, and the number of marrow-derived cells continues to increase for several weeks. These marrow-derived cells ultimately become widely distributed throughout the brain, including in the cortex, hippocampus, thalamus, brainstem, and cerebellum. El Khoury and Luster (2008) have shown that by 6 months post-irradiation and BMT, approximately 60% of CD11b+ cells (i.e., microglia/mononuclear phagocytes) in the brain of transplanted mice are donor derived.

In humans, autopsy data demonstrating donor-derived parenchymal microglia following transplantation are sparse (Schonberger et al. 2007). BM-transplanted cells are thought to re-populate microglia in perivascular and leptomeningeal sites. They engraft slowly following transplantation, with 30% replacement at 1 year. Hence, timing and the rapid search for a matched donor remain vital to successful BMT in leukodystrophy patients.

Partial correction of enzymatic activity in lysosomal storage diseases likely occurs through delivery of missing enzymes by BM-derived migrated monocytic cells, a phenomenon known as cross-correction. It has been shown that BM-derived monocytes/ macrophages can cross the BBB and become perivascular macrophages and microglia. The secretion of lysosomal enzymes from hematopoietic donor cells and their recapture by surrounding diseased brain cells has long been proposed to be the corrective mechanism. However, recent analysis has shown that lysosomal enzymes secreted by human macrophages or a mouse microglial cell line cannot be endocytosed by brain cells owing to the failure to efficiently equip newly synthesized lysosomal enzymes with the M6P recognition marker (Muschol et al. 2002). These data suggest that mechanisms other than the proposed M6P-dependent secretion/recapture of lysosomal enzymes might be responsible for therapeutic effects of BMT in the brain.

In X-ALD, the gene mutation results in a defective protein. Unlike lysosomal enzymes, this protein cannot be secreted. Nevertheless, BMT performed in the early stages of X-ALD is highly effective. This supports the notion that microglia in X-ALD play a vital role, and their correction alone may suffice to halt progression of the devastating inflammatory demyelination.

Concluding remarks

Microglia play various roles in the leukodystrophies. On the one hand, they provide trophic support to surrounding neurons and glia and perform the necessary function of removal of debris. The loss of microglia may in some diseases, such as X-ALD, initiate the cascade of demyelination. On the other hand, microglia may aggravate the disease process by secretion of pro-inflammatory substances such as prostaglandins, as seen in Krabbe disease. A closer phenotypic characterization of microglia is required to understand the balance of microglial functions needed to maintain health within the nervous system. As cells of myeloid origin, microglia are vital to the efficacy of transplantation procedures in the leukodystrophies, and in the future microglia may represent vehicles for gene delivery in these monogenic disorders.

REFERENCES

Abumrad NA, Ajmal M, Pothakos K, Robinson JK. (2005) CD36 expression and brain function: does CD36 deficiency impact learning ability? Prostaglandins Other Lipid Mediat 77: 77–83.
Adams RA, Bauer J, Flick MJ, et al. (2007) The fibrin-derived gamma377–395 peptide inhibits microglia activation and suppresses relapsing paralysis in central nervous system autoimmune disease. J Exp Med 204: 571–582.
Bechmann I, Priller J, Kovac A, et al. (2001) Immune surveillance of mouse brain perivascular spaces by blood-borne macrophages. Eur J Neurosci 14: 1651–1658.
Beers DR, Henkel JS, Xiao Q, et al. (2006) Wild-type microglia extend survival in PU.1 knockout mice with familial amyotrophic lateral sclerosis. Proc Natl Acad Sci USA 103: 16 021–16 026.

Djukic M, Mildner A, Schmidt H, et al. (2006) Circulating monocytes engraft in the brain, differentiate into microglia and contribute to the pathology following meningitis in mice. Brain 129: 2394–2403.

Drover VA, Nguyen DV, Bastie CC, et al. (2008) CD36 mediates both cellular uptake of very long chain fatty acids and their intestinal absorption in mice. J Biol Chem 283: 13 108–13 115.

Eglitis MA, Mezey E. (1997) Hematopoietic cells differentiate into both microglia and macroglia in the brains of adult mice. Proc Natl Acad Sci USA 94: 4080–4085.

Eichler FS, Ren JQ, Cossoy M, et al. (2008) Is microglial apoptosis an early pathogenic change in cerebral X-linked adrenoleukodystrophy? Ann Neurol 63: 729–742.

El Khoury J, Luster AD. (2008) Mechanisms of microglia accumulation in Alzheimer's disease: therapeutic implications. Trends Pharmacol Sci 29: 626–632.

Fabriek BO, van Haastert ES, Galea I, et al. (2005) CD163-positive perivascular macrophages in the human CNS express molecules for antigen recognition and presentation. Glia 51: 297–305.

Gieselmann V, Franken S, Klein D, et al. (2003) Metachromatic leukodystrophy: consequences of sulphatide accumulation. Acta Paediatr Suppl 92: 74–79; discussion 45.

Gieselmann V, von Figura K. (2000) Metachromatic Leukodystrophy. New York: McGraw Hill.

Goldberg IG, Eckel RH Abumrad NA. (2008) Regulation of fatty acid uptake into tissues: lipoprotein lipase- and CD36-mediated pathways. J Lipid Res Suppl 50: 86–90.

Haynes SE, Hollopeter G, Yang G, et al. (2006) The P2Y12 receptor regulates microglial activation by extracellular nucleotides. Nat Neurosci 9: 1512–1519.

Hess B, Saftig P, Hartmann D, et al. (1996) Phenotype of arylsulfatase A-deficient mice: relationship to human metachromatic leukodystrophy. Proc Natl Acad Sci USA 93: 14 821–14 826.

Ito M, Blumberg BM, Mock DJ, et al. (2001) Potential environmental and host participants in the early white matter lesion of adreno-leukodystrophy: morphologic evidence for CD8 cytotoxic T cells, cytolysis of oligodendrocytes, and CD1-mediated lipid antigen presentation. J Neuropathol Exp Neurol 60: 1004–1019.

Kennedy DW, Abkowitz JL. (1997) Kinetics of central nervous system microglial and macrophage engraftment: analysis using a transgenic bone marrow transplantation model. Blood 90: 986–993.

Kettenmann H. (2006) Triggering the brain's pathology sensor. Nat Neurosci 9: 1463–1464.

Kobayashi S, Chiu FC, Katayama M, Sacchi RS, Suzuki K, Suzuki K. (1986) Expression of glial fibrillary acidic protein in the CNS and PNS of murine globoid cell leukodystrophy, the twitcher. Am J Pathol 125: 227–243.

Kobayashi T, Shinnoh N, Kondo A, Yamada T. (1997) Adrenoleukodystrophy protein-deficient mice represent abnormality of very long chain fatty acid metabolism. Biochem Biophys Res Commun 232: 631–636.

Krivit W, Aubourg P, Shapiro E, Peters C. (1999a) Bone marrow transplantation for globoid cell leukodystrophy, adrenoleukodystrophy, metachromatic leukodystrophy, and Hurler syndrome. Curr Opin Hematol 6: 377–382.

Krivit W, Peters C, Shapiro EG. (1999b) Bone marrow transplantation as effective treatment of central nervous system disease in globoid cell leukodystrophy, metachromatic leukodystrophy, adrenoleukodystrophy, mannosidosis, fucosidosis, aspartylglucosaminuria, Hurler, Maroteaux-Lamy, and Sly syndromes, and Gaucher disease type III. Curr Opin Neurol 12: 167–176.

Lu JF, Lawler AM, Watkins PA, et al. (1997) A mouse model for X-linked adrenoleukodystrophy. Proc Natl Acad Sci USA 94: 9366–9371.

McKercher SR, Torbett BE, Anderson KL, et al. (1996) Targeted disruption of the PU.1 gene results in multiple hematopoietic abnormalities. Embo J 15: 5647–5658.

Mildner A, Schmidt H, Nitsche M, et al. (2007) Microglia in the adult brain arise from Ly-6ChiCCR2+ monocytes only under defined host conditions. Nat Neurosci 10: 1544–1553.

Minghetti L, Ajmone-Cat MA, De Berardinis MA, De Simone R. (2005) Microglial activation in chronic neurodegenerative diseases: roles of apoptotic neurons and chronic stimulation. Brain Res Rev 48: 251–256.

Mohri I, Taniike M, Taniguchi H, et al. (2006) Prostaglandin D2-mediated microglia/astrocyte interaction enhances astrogliosis and demyelination in twitcher. J Neurosci 26: 4383–4393.

Molander-Melin M, Pernber Z, Franken S, Gieselmann V, Mansson JE, Fredman P. (2004) Accumulation of sulfatide in neuronal and glial cells of arylsulfatase A deficient mice. J Neurocytol 33: 417–427.

Moody, DB Zajonc DM, Wilson IA. (2005) Anatomy of CD1-lipid antigen complexes. Nat Rev Immunol 5: 387–399.

Moser H, Smith K, Watkins P, Powers J, Moser A. (2001) X-linked adrenoleukodystrophy. In: Scriver C, Beaudet A, Sly W, Valle D, Eds. The Metabolic and Molecular Bases of Inherited Disease, 8th edn. New York: McGraw Hill, pp. 3257–3301.

Muschol N, Matzner U, Tiede S, Gieselmann V, Ullrich K, Braulke T. (2002) Secretion of phosphomannosyl-deficient arylsulphatase A and cathepsin D from isolated human macrophages. Biochem J 368: 845–853.

Perry VH, Gordon S. (1987) Modulation of CD4 antigen on macrophages and microglia in rat brain. J Exp Med 166: 1138–1143.

Peters C, Charnas LR, Tan Y, et al. (2004) Cerebral X-linked adrenoleukodystrophy: the international hematopoietic cell transplantation experience from 1982 to 1999. Blood 104: 881–888.

Priller J. (2003) Robert Feulgen Prize Lecture. Grenzganger: adult bone marrow cells populate the brain. Histochem Cell Biol 120: 85–91.

Priller J, Flugel A, Wehner T, et al. (2001) Targeting gene-modified hematopoietic cells to the central nervous system: use of green fluorescent protein uncovers microglial engraftment. Nat Med 7: 1356–1361.

Priller J, Prinz M, Heikenwalder M, et al. (2006) Early and rapid engraftment of bone marrow-derived microglia in scrapie. J Neurosci 26: 11 753–11 762.

Ransohoff RM. (2007) Microgliosis: the questions shape the answers. Nat Neurosci 10: 1507–1509.

Schaumburg HH, Powers JM, Raine CS, Suzuki K, Richardson EP, Jr. (1975) Adrenoleukodystrophy. A clinical and pathological study of 17 cases. Arch Neurol 32: 577–591.

Schonberger S, Roerig P, Schneider DT, Reifenberger G, Gobel U, Gartner J. (2007) Genotype and protein expression after bone marrow transplantation for adrenoleukodystrophy. Arch Neurol 64: 651–657.

Simons K, Ehehalt R. (2002) Cholesterol, lipid rafts, and disease. J Clin Invest 110 597–603.

Simons K, Toomre D. (2000) Lipid rafts and signal transduction. Nat Rev Mol Cell Biol 1: 31–39.

Vallieres L, Sawchenko PE. (2003) Bone marrow-derived cells that populate the adult mouse brain preserve their hematopoietic identity. J Neurosci 23: 5197–5207.

Wehner T, Bontert M, Eyupoglu I, et al. (2003) Bone marrow-derived cells expressing green fluorescent protein under the control of the glial fibrillary acidic protein promoter do not differentiate into astrocytes in vitro and in vivo. J Neurosci 23: 5004–5011.

Wenger D, Suzuki K, Suzuki YS. (2000) Galactosylceramide Lipidosis: Globoid Cell Leukodystrophy (Krabbe Disease). New York: McGraw Hill.

Wittke D, Hartmann D, Gieselmann V, Lullmann-Rauch R. (2004) Lysosomal sulfatide storage in the brain of arylsulfatase A-deficient mice: cellular alterations and topographic distribution. Acta Neuropathol (Berl) 108: 261–271.

Wu YP, Matsuda J, Kubota A, Suzuki K, Suzuki K. (2000) Infiltration of hematogenous lineage cells into the demyelinating central nervous system of twitcher mice. J Neuropathol Exp Neurol 59: 628–639.

5
X-LINKED ADRENOLEUKODYSTROPHY

Gerald V. Raymond

Introduction

X-linked adrenoleukodystrophy (X-ALD) is a peroxisomal disorder characterized by adrenal insufficiency and neurological manifestations which are extraordinarily variable and complex. X-ALD is due to a defect in the *ABCD1* gene located on chromosome Xq28, which alters peroxisomal beta-oxidation, resulting in elevated levels of very long chain fatty acids (VLCFAs). As will be discussed, these unique saturated fatty acids play a central role in the diagnosis, treatment, and potential pathogenesis of ALD. Among the many peroxisomal disorders that have been associated with myelin destruction, X-ALD is the most common. Whether X-ALD shares a common path of injury with the other peroxisomal disorders is not certain.

X-ALD has been recognized from early in the twentieth century when it was first described as an inflammatory demyelination associated with adrenal insufficiency (Moser et al. 2005a). It was later recognized to have an X-linked pattern of inheritance, but the major steps to unraveling the disorder came with the discovery of inclusions in the adrenal gland followed by the finding of an elevation of saturated VLCFAs. This in turn led to the development of an assay, which could be performed on a variety of tissues including plasma (Moser et al. 1999) and allowed the simple screening of extended family members. The view that X-ALD was rare, affecting boys with a severe, progressive disorder was quickly dispatched when it became apparent that the manifestations could be highly variable, even within a family. The frequency of the disorder has been estimated to be 1 in 17 000 similar to that of phenylketonuria. All ethnic groups are affected equally. With this increasing understanding, prevention and therapies are now being developed.

Biochemical and molecular basis

The characteristic diagnostic abnormality in all affected males is the elevation of VLCFAs. These are saturated fatty acids with chain lengths greater than 22 carbons. This, however, is not specific to X-ALD but is, rather, a finding in all disorders that affect peroxisomal beta-oxidation.

The peroxisome is an organelle found in nearly all eukaryotic cells. Within this compartment, a variety of catabolic and anabolic activities occur including the metabolism of VLCFAs. Similar, but distinct from the mitochondrial fatty-acid oxidation pathways, the peroxisomal beta-oxidation pathway consists of four enzymatic steps. Before the substrates can enter this pathway the acyl residues require activation by transfer of coenzyme A (CoA). For VLCFAs entering the L-specific beta-oxidation pathway, lignoceryl-CoA ligase (also referred to as lignoceryl-CoA synthetase) is the activating enzyme. Deficiency of this enzyme was initially implicated as the basis of the VLCFA accumulation in X-ALD, but is now known not to be the cause.

The genetic basis for X-ALD is mutations of the *ABCD1* gene. The gene, located at Xq28, encodes a protein belonging to a large family, the ATPase Binding Cassette proteins (Mosser et al. 1993). Other peroxisomal proteins with homology to ABCD1 have been described: (1) ALDR or ALD-related protein; (2) PMP70, peroxisomal membrane protein 70 kDa; and (3) PMP70-related protein. All of these proteins are located within the peroxisomal membrane and contain the ATP-binding cassette motif. Experimental data indicates that these proteins form homodimers and heterodimers (Valle and Gartner 1993) and it has been hypothesized that they are involved in the transport of substrates or other protein complexes across the membrane.

The gene occupies approximately 26 kb of genomic DNA, is composed of 10 exons, and encodes an mRNA of 4.3 kb with a predicted protein (ALDP) of 745 amino acids. (Sarde et al. 1994) There have now been nearly 1000 mutations identified in patients with X-ALD. The mutations are archived at the X-linked Adrenoleukodystrophy Database (www.x-ald.nl). Alterations are found throughout the coding regions and over half of the mutations identified are private mutations. The nature of the mutations includes mis-sense, nonsense, frame-shift, amino acid insertion/deletions, and one or more exons deleted. Three-quarters of the genetic alterations result in failure to produce a protein. About 93% of index cases have inherited the *ABCD1* mutation from one parent; at most, 7% of individuals with X-ALD have de-novo mutations.

Sequence analysis of genomic DNA is made difficult because of the presence of *ABCD1* paralogs on four autosomes. At a point in evolution, a 9.7-kb DNA segment encompassing exons 7 though 10 of the *ABCD1* gene was duplicated from the X-chromosome to four of the autosomes (2p11; 10p11; 16p11; 22q11). Because of this very high homology between the pseudogenes and the *ABCD1* gene, care should be taken when mutation analysis using genomic DNA is performed. In 1999, a genomic DNA-based test for X-ALD was developed and serves as the basis of molecular DNA diagnosis and the utility of this testing is discussed in the section on diagnosis (Boehm et al. 1999).

Clinical features

While VLCFAs accumulate in all tissues of the body, the clinical features of X-ALD are normally restricted to the adrenal cortex and nervous system, and the disease that results is highly variable in age of onset and manifestations. This has resulted in the description of several differing phenotypes (see Table 5.1). The frequency listed in the table has been ascertained by attempts to identify all individuals in their respective populations.

CHILDHOOD CEREBRAL ADRENOLEUKODYSTROPHY

The childhood cerebral form is the most well recognized of the presentations and for many years was the only form of the condition recognized. The clinical characteristics have been presented in several large series. This group is generally restricted to boys who develop clinically apparent disease by 10 to 13 years of age. Initial birth and development are

TABLE 5.1
Clinical presentation of adrenoleukodystrophy in males

Phenotype	Description	Estimated relative frequency
Childhood cerebral (CCER)	Onset at 3–10 years of age. Progressive behavioral, cognitive and neurologic deficit, often leading to total disability or death within 2 years. Inflammatory demyelination	31–35%
Adolescent	Onset age 11–18 years. Similar to CCER, but slower progression	4–7%
Adrenomyeloneuropathy (AMN)	Onset 28 ± 9 years, progressive over decades. Involves spinal cord mainly as a distal axonopathy	40–46%
Adult cerebral	Dementia and behavioral disturbances without preceding AMN. White matter inflammatory response present. Progression parallels that of childhood cerebral form	2–5%
Addison-only	Primary adrenal insufficiency without apparent neurologic involvement. Onset common before 7.5 years	Varies with age. Up to 50% in childhood
Asymptomatic	Biochemical and gene abnormality without demonstrable adrenal or neurologic deficit	Diminishes with age

unremarkable. The mean age at onset is generally between 4 and 10 years with peak incidence at 7 ± 1.7 years.

Manifestations in an affected boy are usually subtle changes in behavior or cognition. These initial difficulties are most often only picked up in a school setting and labeled as attentional issues (attention deficit hyperactivity disorder, ADHD), learning issues, or adjustment disorders. Slow to progress at first, other neurological findings then become apparent with a more rapid accumulation of findings. A seizure may be the first neurological manifestation and virtually all boys develop seizures during the course of the illness.

Initial diagnosis is often made by neuroimaging. Computed tomographic and magnetic resonance imaging (MRI) abnormalities are well described, with the MRI being more definitive. The MRI demonstrates bilateral symmetric hyperintense lesions on T2-weighted and FLAIR (fluid-attenuated inversion recovery) imaging (see Fig. 5.1) with concordant hypointensity on the T1-weighted images. This pattern is primarily posterior in 85% of affected individuals with the majority of the remainder being frontal. Occasionally, one may see in affected boys a distinct unilateral involvement which may be confused with a primary neoplasm. A hallmark of X-ALD is the appearance after the administration of contrast with a hyperintense garland at the leading edge of the lesion.

Other distinctive features include the involvement of the corpus callosum – in the posterior pattern, the splenium is the initial involvement and nearly always affected in this pattern. In the frontal involvement, the genu of the corpus callosum is involved. The other noted feature is the striking fiber track involvement – for example, involvement of the corticospinaltract may be traced from the brain through the mid-brain down into the medulla.

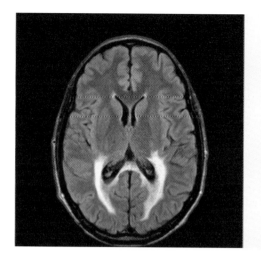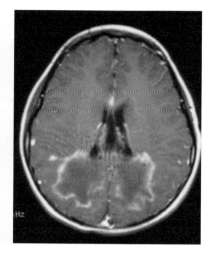

Fig. 5.1. T2-weighted MRI in adrenoleukodystrophy. Note the hyperintensity of the posterior white matter with involvement of the splenium of the corpus callosum and symmetrical parieto-occipital disease.

Progression of the condition is characterized by the advancement of the lesion from affected to unaffected tissue. The alterations in MRI appearance have correlated closely with the changes seen in pathological material.

Once clinically apparent, the disease progresses rapidly. There is development of cortical blindness, loss of auditory processing, dementia, and spastic quadriplegia. The motor involvement includes the inability to walk, use the arms, and oromotor abilities. The loss of ability to chew and swallow may be relatively early in the progression and may require enteral feeding with a gastrostomy tube. The time from first symptom to this is as short as 6 to 12 months. Death often occurs in the initial years, but with the institution of enteral feeding, the condition may plateau and we are aware of individuals alive 5 to 10 years after initial presentation.

ADRENOMYELONEUROPATHY

Adrenomyeloneuropathy (AMN) is by definition an adult disorder affecting the long tracts of the spinal cord and the peripheral nerves as a primary axonopathy. It may be the most common neurological manifestation of this genetic disorder affecting approximately 65% of at-risk males, and is certainly underdiagnosed. Affected men usually present in their twenties to thirties with a slowly progressive spastic paraparesis, distal sensory loss, and bladder and bowel involvement. Unlike the childhood cerebral form of the condition, progression is slow.

In examining the long-term outcome of men with AMN, van Geel et al. (2001) reported a subset of 60 patients with AMN without cerebral involvement using a modification of the Rankin scale. This six-point scale was used retrospectively to study changes in disability during follow-up and ranged from 0 with no symptoms through a score of 5 indicating severe disability. Symptoms of myelopathy began at a mean age of 28.2 ± 8.1 years. At the first visit, 9.1 ± 8.2 years after the onset of symptoms, the mean of the modified Rankin score was 1.7 ± 0.9. At last admission, 16.2 ± 8.9 years after the onset of myelopathy, the mean score had increased to 2.9 ± 1.1 (95% CI of the difference, 0.8 to 1.6) indicating a progression from minor disability through a moderate one that was now significantly affecting their lives. Many individuals eventually require the use of bilateral canes or a wheelchair.

Standard imaging of the spinal cord demonstrates typically only atrophy of the cord (Snyder et al. 1991, Kumar et al. 1995). Recent techniques in imaging using diffusion fiber tracking and magnetization transfer weighted imaging have allowed improved visualization of tract involvement and correlation with disease (Dubey et al. 2005a b, Fatemi et al. 2005, Smith et al. 2009).

Cerebral findings on MRI have been reported in 40% of individuals in one series (Kumar et al. 1995). This was certainly complicated by referral bias. In a different series, van Geel et al. (2001) found the development occurrence of cerebral disease of 19% in individuals followed up for a period of 10 years. Cerebral disease when it occurs may progress as rapidly as in the childhood form (van Geel et al. 2001).

Adolescent and adult cerebral diseases are occasionally listed as a separate presentation. These individuals have minimal findings of spinal cord disease, but have cerebral disease similar to the childhood form. A spinocerebellar presentation has also been reported and appears to be a variation on cerebral AMN.

PRIMARY ADRENAL INSUFFICIENCY

Primary adrenal insufficiency or Addison disease may occur at any age in affected males and does not correlate with neurological involvement. Affected individuals manifest a deficiency of glucocorticoid and mineralocorticoids with an elevation in the pituitary hormone ACTH. With the rise in ACTH, hyperpigmentation may occur. X-ALD is esti- mated to be the cause of adrenal insufficiency in approximately 35% of patients with idiopathic Addison disease, and over 70% of individuals with X-ALD will develop evidence of adrenal insufficiency (Dubey et al. 2005c). This group is reported to make up 8% to 14% of patients with X-ALD. It is important to emphasize that while adrenal disease may occur in childhood, it is presumed that many affected individuals will develop neurological manifestations in adulthood and the incidence of this subgroup diminishes with age.

Affected males may present with adrenal crisis characterized by hypotension with hypoglycemia secondary to influenza, varicella, or other mild infection. Adrenal crisis is potentially lethal and there are reports of cerebral edema and death as the initial presentation in a tragic number of boys – the diagnosis of adrenal insufficiency and X-ALD made only at postmortem (Stephenson et al. 2000). In addition, there are a number of individuals who have had repeated presentations to emergency facilities with dehydration following minor illnesses before the diagnosis of adrenal insufficiency is considered. A more chronic presen- tation has also been seen with general decline in health and cognition. These individuals, who do not have cerebral demyelination on initial presentation, may gradually improve with treatment.

The age at onset of adrenal insufficiency is highly variable, but in one series approx- imately 80% of 49 asymptomatic boys with X-ALD, identified by plasma VLCFA screening of at-risk relatives, already had biochemical evidence of clinically silent adrenal insufficiency at the time of their diagnosis (Dubey et al. 2005c). It is important to emphasize in this series that two boys already had evidence of early adrenal failure at 6 months of age. However, we are not aware of clinically evident adrenal insufficiency occurring in the first years of life. It is not certain at what point a biochemical abnormality can cross over to clinical manifestations.

We recommend the monitoring of cortisol and ACTH levels in males identified with X-ALD. The latter is very important because cortisol levels alone lack appropriate sensitivity. ACTH stimulation tests may have a role in the decision as to when to begin treatment in certain situations. There is no need for imaging of the adrenal glands or testing for autoantibodies. The time that steroid replacement therapy should be initiated involves clinical judgment, but it is important to emphasize that once begun, treatment is life long and should not be discontinued.

ASYMPTOMATIC INDIVIDUALS

These are tested individuals who have an elevation in VLCFAs, but do not have adrenal or neurological manifestations. Similar to the "Addison-only" (see Table 5.1), prevalence of this group shrinks with age and monitoring. All affected newborn males would fall into this group, but by the end of the first decade, over one-third of untreated boys would have developed childhood cerebral disease.

HETEROZYGOTES

Carrier females are asymptomatic in childhood, but may develop myelopathic and neuro-pathic changes in their adult years. In the past it was generally stated that only a minority of carriers was affected, but this has been determined to be a significant underestimation; in the experience of our group at the Kennedy Krieger Insitute, the recognition of symptoms is mainly a function of the evaluation and appreciation of what is related to carrier status. Many women (>50%) will develop spasticity affecting walking, painful dysesthesias, and bladder involvement. It is rare, however, for women to develop adrenal insufficiency or cerebral involvement and we do not recommend the routine monitoring of brain MRIs or adrenal function.

Diagnosis

The plasma VLCFA assay is the recommended diagnostic procedure in males (Moser et al. 1999). Plasma VLCFA levels are increased on the day of birth in infants with X-ALD. The assay provides a rapid distinction between X-ALD and all other conditions that it can mimic. It is particularly important that the assay be performed in all males with idiopathic Addison disease and in men with progressive paraparesis. The early symptoms of childhood cerebral X-ALD are difficult to distinguish from the much more frequent ADHD. Although it is not practical to screen all boys with ADHD for X-ALD, the assay should be performed when there are unusual or progressive features. It is important to screen at-risk family members of known patients with X-ALD including as many members of the extended family as practical. In this way, asymptomatic males may be identified and appropriately counseled and potentially treated. This reaching out to individuals potentially at risk remains a delicate and ethical dilemma for which there are presently no definitive answers (Minkoff and Ecker 2008).

Plasma VLCFA levels may be increased in women who are heterozygous for X-ALD, but false-negative test results can occur. DNA-based diagnosis in carriers is reliable and is recommended as the diagnostic assay in women (Boehm et al. 1999). After the DNA mutation in the kindred has been defined, heterozygotes can be identified accurately and rapidly by determining whether the specific mutation is present in at-risk women.

Levels of VLCFAs are increased in cultured amniocytes and chorionic villus cells, permitting prenatal identification of affected male fetuses. Appropriate quality assurance measures need to be undertaken to monitor for maternal contamination. The use of DNA testing is also possible when the familial mutation is known.

Animal models

Mouse models of X-ALD have been produced by targeted inactivation of the *ABCD1* gene (Forss-Petter et al. 1997, Kobayashi et al. 1997, Lu et al. 1997). VLCFA levels in brain and adrenals are increased as in the human disease, but the animals appear to develop normally. The inflammatory brain disease observed in patients with the cerebral phenotypes has never been observed in the mouse model. It has been shown that the animals develop an AMN-like syndrome at the advanced age of 18 to 24 months (Pujol et al. 2002).

Pathogenesis

The understanding of the pathogenesis of the various neurological manifestations of X-ALD is incomplete, but certain features are known. The principal two manifestations of disease are a non-inflammatory axonal disorder of peripheral nerves and spinal cord tracts versus inflammatory disease affecting the cerebral white matter.

We hypothesize that the axonopathy seen in AMN is the primary lesion in X-ALD. Males who survive to adulthood will develop evidence of AMN. However, for unknown reasons, 50% of males succumb to inflammatory brain disease in childhood or adolescence before AMN manifests. This percentage does not include the ongoing loss of affected men to cerebral disease, which is often under-reported.

There are several lines of evidence for this hypothesis. The X-ALD (ALDP-/-) mouse models (Forss-Petter et al. 1997, Kobayashi et al. 1997, Lu et al. 1997) develop AMN-like lesions (Pujol et al. 2002). Postmortem studies in humans also provide evidence that distal dying-back axonopathy is the primary pathology in AMN, with loss of myelin secondary to it (Powers et al. 2000, 2001). Neuroimaging studies show an axonopathy by both diffusion tensor imaging and spectroscopy (Dubey et al. 2005a, b). The reduction of *N*-acetylaspartic acid, a high level of which is often the first abnormality demonstrated in boys with inflammatory cerebral X-ALD (Eichler et al. 2002), also indicates that axonopathy is an early feature in this phenotype.

It is likely that this primary lesion is secondary to the accumulation and excess of VLCFAs in tissues. This is based on several points of evidence albeit circumstantial – VLCFAs are the principal biochemical abnormality and their excess is greatest in the affected tissues. The excess co-localizes with brain inflammatory lesions (Paintlia et al. 2003) and appears to be most severe in cerebral disease (Asheuer et al. 2005). VLCFAs have been demonstrated to be cytotoxic to adrenal cells (Powers et al. 1980) and to impair a variety of membrane functions (Knazek et al. 1983,Whitcomb et al. 1988, Ho et al. 1995).

The greater length of the aliphatic chain causes VLCFAs to be insoluble and therefore their accumulation alters physiological properties of various cellular functions. For instance, while albumin has six or more high-affinity binding sites for fatty acids with 12 to 18 carbon chain length, it has only a single low-affinity binding site for C26:0 (Ho et al. 1995, Choi et al. 2002). Microcalometric studies have shown that inclusion of the VLCFA C26:0 into a model disrupts membrane structure (Ho et al. 1995). We hypothesize that these membrane abnormalities contribute to the pathogenesis of the axonopathy in AMN and other aspects of X-ALD. The excess of VLCFAs in myelin constituents, such as proteolipids (Bizzozero et al. 1991), cerebrosides, and sphingomyelin (Theda et al. 1992) may impair the stability of the myelin sheath. As noted below, the VLCFA excess also probably contributes to the pathogenesis and rapid progress of the inflammatory phenotype.

The onset of cerebral inflammation is most likely due to a "second-hit," superimposed on the axonal pathology and perhaps myelin instability that is postulated to be present in all males with X-ALD. Approximately one-half of males appear vulnerable to this secondary event. For unknown reasons the other half appear not vulnerable or only mildly so; some have escaped it even until the ninth decade, with pure AMN as the only neurological manifestation.

The cerebral inflammatory phenotype is an aggressive, unrelenting inflammatory demyelinative process associated with the accumulation of CD8 cytotoxic lymphocytes, lysis of oligodendrocytes, and reactive astrocytes and loss of axons (Ito et al. 2001). Expression of pro-inflammatory cytokines, such as tumor necrosis factor-α, interleukins 1, 2, 6, 12, γ-interferon, and chemokines are also increased (Powers et al. 1992, Paintlia et al. 2003, Powers et al. 2005). The role of the microglia in this process has recently come under investigation (Eichler et al. 2008) with evidence that apoptosis of these cells is a notable step in the pathogenesis of the immune response.

The widely variant phenotypes of X-ALD listed in Table 5.1 often co-occur in the same family. Indeed it is more common for the phenotypes in a kindred to be diverse than identical (Moser et al. 1992). No consistent correlation between phenotype and the nature of the mutation or X-ALD expression has been documented. The action of a modifier gene has been postulated (Smith et al. 1991, 1999) and investigation continues.

Therapy in adrenoleukodystrophy
It is important to understand at the outset that there is presently no complete curative therapy for X-ALD.

SYMPTOMATIC THERAPY FOR AFFECTED INDIVIDUALS
Men with AMN and symptomatic women carriers will often benefit from physiotherapy and agents that address spasticity, neuropathic pain, and bladder issues. Boys and men with cerebral disease will require monitoring of nutrition and when appropriate a gastrostomy

tube. Their function may deteriorate quickly and there are often severe and painful muscle spasms associated with progression. This will require antispasticity medications and analgesia. Families will often benefit from palliative care services.

ADRENAL REPLACEMENT

Adrenal hormone therapy is mandatory and life-saving for patients with adrenal insufficiency. Individuals and their families should receive proper instruction and management of adrenal replacement, requirements for medical alert bracelets, and the recognition and rapid treatment of impending crisis. Treatment of individuals with adrenal insufficiency requires monitoring of proper dosage and growth since both undertreatment and overtreatment may affect growth and wellbeing. Adrenal replacement does not alter neurologic progression.

HEMATOPOIETIC STEM CELL TRANSPLANT

Hematopoietic stem cell or bone marrow transplants can be useful for patients with MRI and clinical evidence of mild cerebral involvement (Aubourg et al. 1990, Shapiro et al. 2000, Peters et al. 2004), though its use is limited by several factors. It is recommended only for boys or adolescents who have evidence of active inflammatory cerebral demyelination that is still in its early stages. When the neurological involvement is advanced, the quality of life outcome has been poor and the procedure may accelerate disease progression. Because of its risk the procedure is not recommended for young patients who have no evidence of cerebral involvement.

DIETARY RESTRICTION AND INHIBITION OF ENDOGENOUS SYNTHESIS OF VLCFAs

The demonstration that the abnormal accumulation of VLCFAs is the principal biochemical abnormality in X-ALD led to the introduction of dietary therapy aimed to reduce VLCFA levels. The first attempt at dietary therapy involved the stringent reduction of VLCFA intake. A diet which reduced the intake of saturated VLCFAs to less than 3 mg a day compared with the 12 to 40 mg a day that is customary in United States diets (Van Duyn et al. 1984) was administered for 1 year to six patients with X-ALD (Brown et al. 1982). Plasma C26:0 levels remained unaltered and there was no effect on clinical progression.

Rizzo et al. (1984) introduced a different strategy in which the aim was to diminish the synthesis of saturated VLCFAs. They demonstrated that the addition of monounsaturated oleic acid (C18:1) reduced the levels and the rate of synthesis of saturated VLCFAs in cultured skin fibroblasts of X-ALD patients. Rizzo et al. then administered glyceryl trioleate oil to X-ALD patients and showed that this reduced plasma VLCFA levels by 50% after 3 months (Rizzo et al. 1987). No definitive effect on clinical course was demonstrated.

LORENZO OIL THERAPY

Based on these initial findings that monounsaturated fatty acid therapy led to inhibition of the endogenous production of long chain fatty acids, it was then determined that erucic acid (C22:1) offered additional efficacy. This led to the development of a 4:1 mixture of glyceryl trioleate and glyceryl trierucate, subsequently named Lorenzo Oil. The administration of this mixture normalizes plasma C26:0 levels within 4 weeks (Rizzo et al. 1989, Moser et al. 1991). This result led to a series of clinical trials, which are summarized briefly in the following paragraphs.

Studies in boys with symptomatic cerebral X-ALD demonstrated that although Lorenzo oil drastically reduced plasma levels of VLCFAs, it had no effect on neurological progression of the disease in patients already advanced in this severest manifestation of X-ALD (Moser et al. 2005b).

Limited studies in AMN have not produced a definitive answer. Cappa et al. (1994) reported that CNS demyelination occurred in only 2 out of 11 asymptomatic patients treated with Lorenzo oil; another study found that symptoms of spasticity improved in one adult AMN patient treated with the oil (Asano et al. 1994) A study by van Geel et al. (1999) examined 22 Lorenzo oil–treated X-ALD patients with a range of phenotypes, including asymptomatic (median age 25 years), AMN (median age 44 years), and symptomatic heterozygotes (median age 52 years). Four out of the six neurologically asymptomatic patients with X-ALD remained free of neurological involvement during the study period, though disease in other patients with neurological involvement generally progressed. Aubourg et al. (1993) found that while 5 oil-treated symptomatic X-ALD heterozygotes did not show clinical deterioration during the duration of the study, 9 of the 14 oil-treated male AMN patients did deteriorate, although there was improvement in certain measured parameters. It should be noted, however, that several of the AMN patients included in this work had cerebral lesions at the time of entry into the study, and thus would be classified with the AMN-cerebral phenotype, and not "pure" AMN.

All of these studies were uncontrolled; the number of individuals examined was small with a wide range of ages, disability, and phenotypes; and limited information is provided on compliance and effective reduction of VLCFAs. However in spite of the poor design of the clinical evaluation, the lack of clear improvement led to the presumption that Lorenzo oil was ineffective in all forms of X-ALD.

This opinion was initially bolstered by studies of postmortem tissue of Lorenzo oil–treated patients in which it was not possible to demonstrate erucic acid in sampled tissues. This led to the question as to whether the oil had crossed the blood–brain barrier (Poulos et al. 1994). It has since been shown that labeled erucic acid does enter the brain in rodents (Golovko and Murphy 2006) and, as will be discussed, other studies have demonstrated the possibility of a clinical effect.

The previously cited clinical studies do highlight the difficulties that have been encountered in determining the potential efficacy of Lorenzo oil. In summary, it is clear that Lorenzo oil effectively lowers VLCFAs, but that this is not sufficient to repair injury already present or arrest the most devastating manifestations of the disease. More recently a larger cohort has suggested that Lorenzo oil does have a clinical effect in certain circumstances, namely as a preventive of neurological damage in asymptomatic patients (Moser et al. 2003, 2005b)

RESULTS OF LORENZO OIL STUDY IN ASYMPTOMATIC BOYS

Moser et al. (2005b) performed a prospective trial examining the reduction of plasma VLCFAs and clinical outcome. This study examined the hypothesis that there is an association

84

between the decrease in C26:0 levels and two measures of clinical outcome: the time to development of neurological and/or MRI abnormalities in boys with X-ALD in whom the therapy was initiated when both their neurological exam and MRI were normal. The study population was 89 asymptomatic boys with X-ALD who were enrolled between 1989 and 2002. The boys had a mean age at entry of 4.75 years and the mean follow-up was 6.9 ± 2.7 years (range 6 to 15). All boys were offered dietary therapy with Lorenzo oil. At the time of analysis, 12 patients were lost to follow-up and 14 boys received hematopoietic stem cell transplantation.

Sixty-six (74%) of the patients remained free of neurological involvement. Twenty-one (24%) developed MRI abnormalities and 8 patients (9%) developed both neurological and MRI abnormalities. All MRI abnormalities preceded neurological abnormalities. In 9 patients whose MRIs became abnormal, neurological status continued to be normal. All patients with neurological abnormalities had the childhood cerebral phenotype.

There was a significant association between reductions of plasma C26:0 levels and clinical outcome. The time-weighted average of C26:0 levels since study entry was a significant predictor ($p = 0.01$; hazard ratio = 21.56) of the time to neurological progression. A statistically significant risk of progression was seen in boys with elevated VLCFAs. Boys who developed a neurological abnormality had significantly higher weighted average C26:0 levels than those who did not have an abnormality, suggesting that a decrease in C26:0 level induced by Lorenzo oil protected against inflammatory cerebral disease.

It was also demonstrated that erucic acid levels were a measure of the extent to which Lorenzo oil was consumed and absorbed. The observed correlation suggests that compliance with oil intake is a significant factor in the reduction of the plasma C26:0 levels with the degree of fat reduction being a second factor. There was no correlation between the reduction of C26:0 level and the nature of the *ABCD1* mutation or the phenotypic pattern of affected relatives.

This was the first follow-up study to examine the preventative effect in asymptomatic boys and suggests that long-term reduction of C26:0 levels reduces the risk of developing brain MRI abnormalities. It is important to emphasize that the most recent year of C26:0 measurements did not show this significant association, suggesting that long-term elevation of the plasma C26:0 is more deleterious and that, for benefit, reduced levels may need to be in place for longer than 1 year.

On the basis of this data, we hypothesize that lowering plasma C26:0 levels lowers the risk of childhood cerebral X-ALD, but the prevention is not absolute. The mechanism of the preventative effect is incompletely understood owing to our inability to measure C26:0 levels in vivo.

OTHER POTENTIAL THERAPIES FOR ADRENOLEUKODYSTROPHY

A variety of other potential therapies for X-ALD have been suggested.

4-Phenylbutyrate has been of interest because of the studies of Kemp and colleagues (Kemp et al. 1998; Wei et al. 2000), which showed that 4-phenylbutyrate increases the capacity of cultured skin fibroblasts of X-ALD patients to metabolize VLCFAs, resulting in the normalization of VLCFA levels in these cultures. But the mechanism of action is not yet clear. One finding is that 4-phenylbutyrate increased the expression of ALDR, which can substitute at least in part for the action of ALDP (Netik et al. 1999). However, preliminary studies at the Kennedy Krieger Institute, where 4-phenylbutyrate was administered orally to 6 AMN patients at a dose of 9 to 13 g/kg per day for two, 6-week periods found that VLCFA levels in plasma, white blood cells, and red blood cells remained unchanged. Furthermore, there was no change in the VLCFA oxidation or ALDR expression in white blood cells (Smith, KD, unpublished observations).

Lovastatin has been administered because of its favorable effect on VLCFA metabolism in X-ALD fibroblasts combined with its anti-inflammatory action (Stanislaus et al. 1999, Kwak et al. 2000). One group has reported that lovastatin is able to lower VLCFA levels in X-ALD patients (Pai et al. 2000). However, it did not alter VLCFA levels in the X-ALD mouse model (Cartier et al. 2000) and additional studies have given equivocal biochemical results.

Hematopoietic stem cell transplantation has been used in X-ALD treatment and offers a clear benefit for selected patients with early cerebral disease. It is limited in application due to the narrow window of opportunity, donor availability, and significant morbidity. Other immunosuppressive treatments have shown little or no benefit, most likely because patients already had significant neurological symptoms at the time treatment was initiated. High-dose cyclophosphamide therapy is encouraging in a number of autoimmune diseases including multiple sclerosis, and it has the distinct and unique property of being immunoablative but not myeloablative (Drachman and Brodsky 2005). Recently developed immunosuppressive agents that mitigate the cerebral inflammatory response in multiple sclerosis may represent an important opportunity for the cerebral forms of X-ALD (Farrell et al. 2005, Linsen et al. 2005, Cavaletti 2006, Neuhauser et al. 2006). They could be especially promising if administered to those patients with early cerebral disease or possibly in asymptomatic individuals. As the pathogenesis of this disease becomes better understood, a number of the currently available immunotherapies may become potential candidates for evaluation in X-ALD.

A gene therapy approach using autologous transplantation has recently been undertaken. Initial results of this promising new avenue are preliminary but hopeful.

Expanded screening for asymptomatic individuals

Because of the ability to prevent and treat many of the features of X-ALD, it has been the goal to diagnose all at-risk individuals at an earlier stage. The ideal opportunity to perform this would be when boys are asymptomatic prior to adrenal or neurological involvement. Because of the early age of adrenal insufficiency, we have focused on using the newborn screening methodology and have recently developed a method that uses tandem mass spectroscopy and the blood spots of newborns. We have demonstrated that examining a phosphatidyl choline fraction allows the determination of affected individuals (Hubbard et al. 2006). Pilot studies in populations of newborns have recently been initiated.

The improved understanding of the breadth of X-ALD has occurred over a relatively short period of time. While there is still much to learn, improved diagnostics and institution of earlier preventative therapies, including potentially the use of gene therapy, offer hope that the most severe manifestations of the disease may be avoided (Raymond et al. 2007).

REFERENCES

Asano J, Suzuki Y, Yajima S, et al. (1994) Effects of erucic-acid therapy on Japanese patients with X-linked adrenoleukodystrophy. Brain Dev 16(6): 454–458.

Asheuer M, Bieche I, Laurendeau I, et al. (2005) Decreased expression of ABCD4 and BG1 genes early in the pathogenesis of X-linked adrenoleukodystrophy. Hum Mol Genet 14 (10): 1293–1303.

Aubourg P, Adamsbaum C, Lavallardrousseau MC, et al. (1993) A 2-year trial of oleic and erucic acids (Lorenzo Oil) as treatment for adrenomyeloneuropathy. N Engl J Med 329(11): 745–752.

Aubourg P, Blanche S, Jambaque I, et al. (1990) Reversal of early neurologic and neuroradiological manifestations of X-linked adrenoleukodystrophy by bone-marrow transplantation. N Engl J Med 322 (26): 1860–1866.

Bizzozero OA, Zuniga G, Lees MB. (1991) Fatty-acid composition of human myelin proteolipid protein in peroxisomal disorders. J Neurochem 56(3): 872–878.

Boehm CD, Cutting GR, Lachtermacher MB, Moser HW, Chong SS. (1999) Accurate DNA-based diagnostic and carrier testing for X-linked adrenoleukodystrophy. Mol Genet Metab 66(2): 128–136.

Brown FR, Vanduyn MAS, Moser AB, et al. (1982) Adrenoleukodystrophy – effects of dietary restriction of very long-chain fatty-acids and of administration of carnitine and clofibrate on clinical status and plasma fatty-acids. Johns Hopkins Med J 151(4): 164–172.

Cappa M, Cambiaso P, Delbalzo P. (1994) Adrenoleukodystrophy: clinical and therapeutic updating. In: Bhatt HR, James VHT, Besser GM, eds. Advances in Thomas Addison's Disease. Bristol, UK: Journal of Endocrinology, pp. 171–180.

Cartier N, Guidoux S, Rocchiccioli F, Aubourg P. (2000) Simvastatin does not normalize very long chain fatty acids in adrenoleukodystrophy mice. FEBS Lett 478(3), 205–208.

Cavaletti G. (2006) Current status and future prospective of immunointervention in multiple sclerosis. Curr Med Chem 13(19): 2329–2343.

Choi JK, Ho J, Curry S, Qin DH, Bittman R, Hamilton JA. (2002) Interactions of very long-chain saturated fatty acids with serum albumin. J Lipid Res 43(7): 1000–1010.

Drachman DB, Brodsky RA. (2005) High-dose therapy for autoimmune neurologic diseases. Curr Opin Oncol 17(2): 83–88.

Dubey P, Fatemi A, Barker PB, et al. (2005a) Spectroscopic evidence of cerebral axonopathy in patients with pure adrenomyeloneuropathy. Neurology, 64(2): 304–310.

Dubey P, Fatemi A, Huang H, et al. (2005b) Diffusion tensor-based imaging reveals occult abnormalities in adrenomyeloneuropathy. Ann Neurol 58(5): 758–766.

Dubey P, Raymond GV, Moser AB, Kharkar S, Bezman L, Moser HW. (2005c) Adrenal insufficiency in asymptomatic adrenoleukodystrophy patients identified by very long-chain fatty acid screening. J Pediatr 146(4): 528–532.

Eichler FS, Barker PB, Cox C, et al. (2002) Proton MR spectroscopic imaging predicts lesion progression on MRI in X-linked adrenoleukodystrophy. Neurology 58(6): 901–907.

Eichler FS, Ren JQ, Cossoy M, et al. (2008) Is microglial apoptosis an early pathogenic change in cerebral X-linked adrenoleukodystrophy? Ann Neurol 63(6): 729–742.

Farrell R, Heaney D, Giovannoni G. (2005) Emerging therapies in multiple sclerosis. Expert Opin Emerg Drugs 10(4): 797–816.

Fatemi A, Smith SA, Dubey P, et al. (2005) Magnetization transfer MRI demonstrates spinal cord abnormalities in adrenomyeloneuropathy. Neurology 64(10): 1739–1745.

Forss-Petter S, Werner H, Berger J, et al. (1997) Targeted inactivation of the X-linked adrenoleukodystrophy gene in mice. J Neurosci Res 50(5): 829–843.

Golovko MY, Murphy EJ. (2006) Uptake and metabolism of plasma-derived erucic acid by rat brain. J Lipid Res 47(6): 1289–1297.

Ho JK, Moser H, Kishimoto Y, Hamilton JA. (1995a) Interactions of a very long-chain fatty-acid with model membranes and serum-albumin – implications for the pathogenesis of adrenoleukodystrophy. J Clin Invest 96(3): 1455–1463.

Hubbard WC, Moser AB, Tortorelli S, Liu A, Jones D, Moser H. (2006) Combined liquid chromatography-tandem mass spectrometry as an analytical method for high throughput screening for X-linked adrenoleukodystrophy and other peroxisomal disorders: preliminary findings. Mol Genet Metab 89(1–2): 185–187.

Ito M, Blumberg BM, Mock DJ, et al. (2001) Potential environmental and host participants in the early white matter lesion of adreno-leukodystrophy: morphologic evidence for CD8 cytotoxic T cells, cytolysis of oligodendrocytes, and CD1-mediated lipid antigen presentation. J Neuropathol Exp Neurol 60(10): 1004–1019.

Kemp S, Wei HM, Lu JF, et al. (1998) Gene redundancy and pharmacological gene therapy: implications for X-linked adrenoleukodystrophy. Nat Med 4(11): 1261–1268.

Knazek RA, Rizzo WB, Schulman JD, Dave JR. (1983) Membrane microviscosity is increased in the erythrocytes of patients with adrenoleukodystrophy and adrenomyeloneuropathy. J Clin Invest 72(1): 245–248.

Kobayashi T, Shinnoh N, Kondo A, Yamada T. (1997) Adrenoleukodystrophy protein-deficient mice represent abnormality of very long chain fatty acid metabolism. Biochem Biophys Res Commun 232(3): 631–636.

Kumar AJ, Kohler W, Kruse B, et al. (1995) MR findings in adult-onset adrenoleukodystrophy. AJNR Am J Neuroradiol 16(6): 1227–1237.

Kwak B, Mulhaupt F, Myit S, Mach F. (2000) Statins as a newly recognized type of immunomodulator. Nat Med 6(12): 1399–1402.

Linsen L, Somers V, Stinissen P. (2005) Immunoregulation of autoimmunity by natural killer T cells. Hum Immunol 66(12): 1193–1202.

Lu JF, Lawler AM, Watkins PA, et al. (1997) A mouse model for X-linked adrenoleukodystrophy. Proc Natl Acad Sci USA 94(17): 9366–9371.

Minkoff H, Ecker J. (2008) Genetic testing and breach of patient confidentiality: law, ethics, and pragmatics. Am J Obstet Gynecol 198(5): 498e1-e4–504.

Moser AB, Kreiter N, Bezman L, et al. (1999) Plasma very long chain fatty acids in 3000 peroxisome disease patients and 29 000 controls. Ann Neurol 45(1): 100–110.

Moser HW, Aubourg P, Cornblath DR, Borel J, Wu Y-W, Bergin A, Naidu S. (1991) Therapy for X-linked adrenoleukodystrophy. In: Desnick RJ, Ed. Treatment of Genetic Disease. New York: Churchill Livingstone, pp. 111–129.

Moser HW, Moser AB, Smith KD, et al. (1992) Adrenoleukodystrophy – phenotypic variability and implications for therapy. J Inherit Metab Dis 15(4): 645–664.

Moser HW, Raymond GV, Dubey P. (2005a) Adrenoleukodystrophy: new approaches to a neurodegenerative disease. JAMA 294(24): 3131–3134.

Moser HW, Raymond GV, Koehler W, et al. (2003) Evaluation of the preventive effect of glyceryl trioleate–trierucate ("Lorenzo's oil") therapy in X-linked adrenoleukodystrophy: results of two concurrent trials. Adv Exp Med Biol 544: 369–387.

Moser HW, Raymond GV, Lu SE, et al. (2005b) Follow-up of 89 asymptomatic patients with adrenoleukodystrophy treated with Lorenzo's oil. Arch Neurol 62(7): 1073–1080.

Mosser J, Douar AM, Sarde CO, et al. (1993) Putative X-linked adrenoleukodystrophy gene shares unexpected homology with ABC transporters. Nature 361(6414): 726–730.

Netik A, Forss-Petter S, Holzinger A, Molzer B, Unterrainer G, Berger J. (1999) Adrenoleukodystrophy-related protein can compensate functionally for adrenoleukodystrophy protein deficiency (X-ALD): implications for therapy. Hum Mol Genet 8(5): 907–913.

Neuhaus O, Kieseier BC, Hartung HP. (2006) Mitoxantrone in multiple sclerosis. Adv Neurol 98: 293–302.

Pai GS, Khan M, Barbosa E, et al. (2000) Lovastatin therapy for X-linked adrenoleukodystrophy: clinical and biochemical observations on 12 patients. Mol. Genet. Metab 69(4): 312–322.

Paintlia AS, Gilg AG, Khan M, Singh AK, Barbosa E, Singh I. (2003) Correlation of very long chain fatty acid accumulation and inflammatory disease progression in childhood X-ALD: implications for potential therapies. Neurobiol Dis 14(3), 425–439.

Peters C, Charnas LR, Tan Y, et al. (2004) Cerebral X-linked adrenoleukodystrophy: the international hematopoietic cell transplantation experience from 1982 to 1999. Blood 104(3): 881–888.

Poulos A, Gibson R, Sharp P, Beckman K, Grattan-Smith P. (1994) Very long chain fatty acids in X-linked adrenoleukodystrophy brain after treatment with Lorenzo's oil. Ann Neurol 36(5): 741–746.

Powers JM, DeCiero DP, Cox C, Richfield EK, Ito M, Boser AB, Moser HW. (2001) The dorsal root ganglia in adrenomyeloneuropathy: Neuronal atrophy and abnormal mitochondria. J Neuropathol Exp Neurol 60(5): 493–501.

Powers JM, DeCiero DP, Ito M, Moser AB, Moser HW. (2000) Adrenomyeloneuropathy: a neuropathologic review featuring its noninflammatory myelopathy. J Neuropathol Exp Neurol 59(2): 89–102.

Powers JM, Liu Y, Moser AB, Moser HW. (1992) The inflammatory myelinopathy of adrenoleukodystrophy – cells, effector molecules, and pathogenetic implications. J Neuropathol Exp Neurol 51(6): 630–643.

Powers JM, Pei ZT., Heinzer AK, et al. (2005) Adreno-leukodystrophy: oxidative stress of mice and men. J Neuropathol Exp Neurol 64(12): 1067–1079.

Powers JM, Schaumburg HH, Johnson AB, Raine CS. (1980) A correlative study of the adrenal-cortex in adreno-leukodystrophy – evidence for a fatal intoxication with very long-chain saturated fatty-acids. Invest Cell Pathol 3(4): 353–376.

Pujol A, Hindelang C, Callizot N, Bartsch U, Schachner M, Mandel JL. (2002) Late onset neurological phenotype of the X-ALD gene inactivation in mice: a mouse model for adrenomyeloneuropathy. Hum Mol Genet 11(5): 499–505.

Raymond GV, Jones RO, Moser AB. (2007) Newborn screening for adrenoleukodystrophy: implications for therapy. Mol Diagn Ther 11(6): 381–384.

Rizzo WB, Avigan J, Chemk J, Schulman JD. (1984) Adrenoleukodystrophy – very long-chain fatty-acid metabolism in fibroblasts. Neurology 34(2): 163–169.

Rizzo, WB, Leshner RT, Odone A, et al. (1989) Dietary erucic acid therapy for X-linked adrenoleukodystrophy. Neurology 39(11): 1415–1422.

Rizzo WB, Phillips MW, Dammann AL, et al. (1987) Adrenoleukodystrophy – dietary oleic-acid lowers hexacosanoate levels. Ann Neurol 21(3): 232–239.

Sarde CO, Mosser J, Kioschis P, et al. (1994) Genomic organization of the adrenoleukodystrophy gene. Genomics 22(1), 13–20.

Shapiro E, Krivit W, Lockman L, et al. (2000) Long-term effect of bone-marrow transplantation for childhood-onset cerebral X-linked adrenoleukodystrophy. Lancet 356(9231): 713–718.

Smith KD, KempS, Braiterman LT, et al. (1999) X-linked adrenoleukodystrophy: genes, mutations, and phenotypes. Neurochem Res 24(4): 521–535.

Smith KD, Sack G, Beaty T, et al. (1991) A genetic-basis for the multiple phenotypes of X-linked adrenoleukodystrophy. Am J Hum Genet 49(4): 165.

Smith SA, Golay X, Fatemi A, et al. (2009) Quantitative magnetization transfer characteristics of the human cervical spinal cord in vivo: application to adrenomyeloneuropathy. Magn Reson Med 61(1): 22–27.

Snyder R.D, King JN, Keck GM, Orrison WW (1991) MR imaging of the spinal cord in 23 subjects with ALD–AMN complex. AJNR Am J Neuroradiol. 12(6): 1095–1098.

Stanislaus R, Pahan K, Singh AK Singh I. (1999) Amelioration of experimental allergic encephalomyelitis in Lewis rats by lovastatin. Neurosci Lett 269(2): 71–74.

Stephenson DJ, Bezman L, Raymond GV. (2000) Acute presentation of childhood adrenoleukodystrophy. Neuropediatrics 31(6), 293–297.

Theda C, Moser AB, Powers JM, Moser HW. (1992) Phospholipids in X-linked adrenoleukodystrophy white matter: fatty acid abnormalities before the onset of demyelination. J Neurol Sci 110(1–2): 195–204.

Valle D, Gartner J. (1993) Human genetics. Penetrating the peroxisome. Nature 361(6414): 682–683.

Van Duyn MA, Moser AE, Brown FR, III, Sacktor N, Liu A, Moser HW. (1984) The design of a diet restricted in saturated very long-chain fatty acids: therapeutic application in adrenoleukodystrophy. Am J Clin Nutr 40(2): 277–284.

van Geel BM, Assies J, Haverkort EB, et al. (1999) Progression of abnormalities in adrenomyeloneuropathy and neurologically asymptomatic X-linked adrenoleukodystrophy despite treatment with "Lorenzo's oil". J Neurol Neurosurg Psychiatry 67(3): 290–299.

van Geel BM, Bezman L, Loes DJ, Moser HW, Raymond GV. (2001) Evolution of phenotypes in adult male patients with X-linked adrenoleukodystrophy. Ann Neurol 49(2): 186–194.

Wei H, Kemp S, McGuinness MC, Moser AB, Smith KD. (2000) Pharmacological induction of peroxisomes in peroxisome biogenesis disorders. Ann Neurol 47(3): 286–296.

Whitcomb RW, Linehan WM, Knazek RA. (1988) Effects of long-chain, saturated fatty-acids on membrane microviscosity and adrenocorticotropin responsiveness of human adrenocortical-cells in vitro. J Clin Invest 81(1): 185–188.

6
KRABBE DISEASE (GLOBOID CELL LEUKODYSTROPHY)

David A. Wenger

Introduction

Krabbe disease, or globoid cell leukodystrophy (GLD), is an autosomal recessive disorder affecting the white matter of the central and peripheral nervous systems. In the USA and Europe, Krabbe disease occurs in about 1 in 100 000 births. The initial report of infants with diffuse brain-sclerosis or diffuse gliosis clearly described patients we now recognize as having Krabbe disease (Krabbe 1916). K. Krabbe described five patients who had onset of symptoms at about 5 months of age. Findings included rigidity of musculature, violent tonic spasms, nystagmus, periodic elevations in temperature, progressive paresis, and early death. He noted the destruction of the white matter of the cerebellum and degeneration of the spinal nerve tracts with replacement by dense fibrillar glia. In 1924 the term "globoid" was first used to describe these abnormal scavenger cells, which are characteristic for this disorder (Collier and Greenfield 1924). Excellent clinical and genetic studies on 32 Swedish patients by Hagberg et al. (1970) provided the basis for the clinical delineation of the infantile form of this disorder. Late-onset forms of Krabbe disease are recognized and they can be accurately diagnosed – if the disease is considered and an appropriate sample is sent to an experienced laboratory.

Early research suggested that these scavenger/storage cells might contain a glycolipid similar to that stored in Gaucher disease. This was confirmed by chemical analysis and production of globoid cells by intracerebral injection of galactosylceramide into brains of experimental animals (Austin et al. 1961). A major breakthrough came in 1970 when it was reported that tissue samples from patients with Krabbe disease could not degrade galactosylceramide due to the deficiency of galactocerebrosidase (GALC) activity (Suzuki and Suzuki 1970). Galactosylceramide and sulfatide (3-sulfo-galactosylceramide) are the two major glycosphingolipids of myelin. They are biosynthesized during active myelination, and the correct ratio of these lipids is necessary for stable, healthy myelin. Galactosylceramide also is produced during the lysosomal degradation of sulfatide when the sulfate is removed by the action of another lysosomal enzyme, arylsulfatase A. The pathways for the biosynthesis of galactosylceramide and the production of galactosylceramide from sulfatide and its degradation to ceramide and galactose are shown in Figure 6.1. As will be discussed, another substrate of GALC, psychosine (galactosylsphingosine), may be the actual pathological agent that initiates the demyelination seen in this disease.

The diagnosis of individuals suspected of having Krabbe disease can be made by measuring GALC activity in leukocytes isolated from whole blood or fibroblasts grown

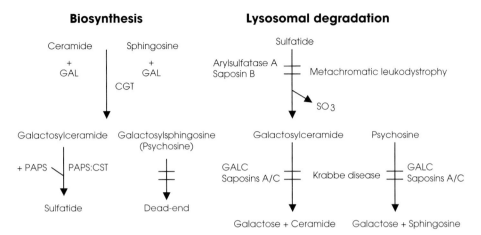

Biosynthesis

Ceramide Sphingosine
+   +
GAL   GAL
   CGT

Galactosylceramide Galactosylsphingosine
      (Psychosine)

+ PAPS PAPS:CST

Sulfatide   Dead-end

Lysosomal degradation

Sulfatide

Arylsulfatase A
Saposin B Metachromatic leukodystrophy

SO_3

Galactosylceramide Psychosine

GALC   GALC
Saposins A/C Krabbe disease Saposins A/C

Galactose + Ceramide Galactose + Sphingosine

Fig. 6.1. Pathways for the biosynthesis of galactosylceramide, psychosine, and sulfatide and their lysosomal degradation showing the required enzymes and sphingolipid activator proteins (saposins). The location of the defects in metachromatic leukodystrophy and Krabbe disease are shown. CGT, ceramide : galactosyltransferase; CST, cerebroside : sulfotransferase; GAL, galactose; GALC, galactocerebrosidase; PAPS, $3'$-phosphoadenosine $5'$-phosphosulfate.

from a skin biopsy. While it is highly probable that late-onset patients have some residual GALC activity allowing some breakdown of galactosylceramide and psychosine, it is not possible to accurately measure this low level of activity in the samples received for diagnostic testing. In August 2006 screening of newborns for Krabbe disease was initiated in New York state. This was done to identify patients needing immediate evaluation and treatment before symptoms become obvious.

In 1993 GALC was first purified, and GALC cDNA was cloned (Chen and Wenger 1993, Chen et al. 1993). This led to the cloning of the gene and the identification of disease-causing and polymorphic mutations (Luzi et al. 1995, reviewed in Wenger et al. 2000, 2001). Identification of the disease-causing mutation(s) in a patient improved carrier testing for other family members. While genotype–phenotype correlations are not perfect, they do help in predicting an infantile versus a later onset of disease if the mutations have been previously identified in a significant number of clinically described patients. In addition, GLD has been identified in a number of animal species, and the mutations in their respective *GALC* genes have been identified (reviewed in Suzuki and Suzuki 1985, Wenger 2000).

Treatment options at this time are limited. Symptomatic infants have a rapid course and little can be done other than supportive care. A number of neonates predicted to become affected because of a previously affected sibling have received umbilical cord hematopoietic stem cell (HSC) transplants within a month of life (Escolar et al. 2005). With newborn screening, additional asymptomatic infants are being identified within a few weeks of life and some have received HSC transplants. A limited number of late-onset patients have received HSC transplants; however, the results have been mixed with significant morbidity and mortality (Krivit et al. 1998). Clearly much more needs to be done before effective therapy for a majority of the patients is a reality.

Clinical features

This laboratory has diagnosed nearly 600 patients with Krabbe disease since 1973, and 85 to 90% of them present before 6 months of age and most die before 15 months of age. Hagberg et al. (1970) described three stages in the progression of the most common infantile form of the disease. Stage I is characterized by general irritability, stiffness of limbs, arrest of mental and motor development, and episodes of temperature elevation without infection. During the stage II phase, the patients are opisthotonic and have myoclonic-like jerks of the arms and legs, hypertonic seizures, continued bouts of fever, and regression of any achieved abilities. By stage III, the patients are severely decerebrate with no voluntary movements. They are hypotonic and cachectic, and they die of respiratory infections or cerebral hyperpyrexia. The average age at onset was 4 months, and the average age at death was 13 months. These averages have not changed much in the past 40 years.

Samples from individuals of any age with neurological symptoms are tested for GALC activity in this laboratory. With this liberal testing policy, a significant number of late infantile, juvenile, and adult cases are diagnosed. Presenting symptoms in the later-onset patients can include vision problems, cerebellar ataxia, spastic hemiparesis, burning paresthesia, peripheral neuropathy, and dementia (reviewed in Lyon et al. 1991). While some individuals remain stable for long periods of time, others show a steady decline in intellect, and develop seizures, severe dysarthria, and blindness leading to a vegetative state and death. The diagnosis of later-onset patients, including siblings with the same *GALC* genotype, raises additional concerns related to predicting the clinical course and the need for therapeutic intervention. This will be illustrated by the following case vignette describing two sisters with late-onset Krabbe disease.

CASE VIGNETTE 1.

The elder sister, currently 45 years of age, was considered normal until about 25 years of age when she suffered the onset of lower extremity paresis with episodes of tripping and clumsiness on walking. Magnetic resonance imaging (MRI) done at this time showed symmetrical white matter lesions affecting the posterior limb of the internal capsules, thalmi, corona radiate, centrum semiovale, and subependymal white matter (especially about the occipital horns). She had leg cord lengthening performed but continued to experience spastic paresis with clumsy gait and difficulty on rising from a squatting or sitting position. There is no obvious intellectual impairment. She is married and is the mother of a daughter born in October 2003. Her sister, who is 1.5 years younger, was considered normal until 4 to 5 years of age when she developed progressive weakness in all extremities. She experienced rapid mental deterioration and onset of seizures. She is currently wheelchair bound and significantly intellectually disabled. Electromyography studies done when the younger sister was 37 years of age showed severe sensorimotor peripheral polyneuropathy with axonal and demyelinating features including median motor distal latency prolongation, median motor conduction velocity-slowing, and prolongation of the median F-response. Similar studies performed at the same time in the older sister showed that the abnormalities were far less severe than in the more symptomatic younger sister. These sisters have the same low GALC activity and the same mutations in the *GALC* gene. Clearly other factors, genetic and/or environmental, play a role in disease onset and progression in the later-onset forms of Krabbe disease.

While it is true that siblings of infantile patients will present in a similar way, it is not true for more distant relatives. Another vignette illustrates the difficulty in predicting the phenotype in patients who have a more distant genetic relationship.

CASE VIGNETTE 2.

Seven years after the diagnosis of a child with symptoms of classic infantile Krabbe disease, including hypotonia, poor head control, gastroesophageal reflux, irritability and loss of milestones at 6 months of age, we were told about a 16-year-old first cousin with progressive spastic paraparesis. Early milestones were normal; however, at 2 years of age it was noted that she fell frequently. As she got older she complained of pain in the right hip and knee and sensation of pins and needles in her right thigh. While she has retained cognitive function in high school, her grades have dropped due to her fatigue and pain level. No neurodiagnostic testing provided an explanation for her symptoms. However, testing of a blood sample confirmed the diagnosis of Krabbe disease. The fathers of both patients are brothers and share a common severe mutation (the common 30-kb deletion). The mother of the infantile patient is a carrier of a severe mutation, and the mother of the later-onset patient is a carrier of a mild mutation resulting in the child with a later onset and milder clinical course.

It is clear that siblings of patients with infantile Krabbe disease will have a similar onset and clinical course; however, it is obvious from the above vignettes that this is not true for individuals, even siblings, with a later-onset form of Krabbe disease. Also, one cannot predict the clinical course in more distant affected family members who may have other mutations brought in from unrelated partners. The author knows of seven additional families with the same *GALC* genotype as the sisters described in case vignette 1 and, although they all have a later-onset form of Krabbe disease, the age at onset and clinical course vary greatly. Interestingly, it is also noted in a number of published papers (Crome et al. 1973, Malone et al. 1975, Goebel et al. 1990, Tada et al. 1992, McGuinness et al. 1996) and in clinical notes attached to samples that we received, that the onset of symptoms in many of these later-onset patients is preceded by an environmental insult such as serious infection or blow to the head. This could indicate that the low, but not zero, GALC activity in these individuals is not adequate for normal remodeling in areas needing remyelination after a demyelinating event.

Diagnostic evaluation

Any of the signs or symptoms given above might lead the physician to request testing for a number of lysosomal disorders that result in neurological abnormalities. In this laboratory, testing for Krabbe disease is usually included in this screen. Patients with Krabbe disease of all ages will have a severe deficiency in GALC activity measured in leukocytes isolated from whole blood and in cultured skin fibroblasts. There is no reproducible difference in residual GALC activity between the infantile and late-onset patients in the tissues used for diagnosis. Obviously, late-onset patients must have some small, but significant, amount of GALC activity in the peripheral and central nervous systems to explain their milder disease, however it cannot be reliably measured. In infantile patients the cerebrospinal fluid protein is usually markedly elevated (>150 mg/dl). It can be greatly elevated even before symptoms are recognized. It is less elevated in late-onset patients. Other signs indicating the need for testing include decreased nerve conduction velocities, magnetic resonance images showing decreased myelination in the brainstem and cerebellum, and computed tomography showing lucencies in the white matter. Some of the late-onset patients diagnosed with Krabbe disease were initially thought to have metachromatic leukodystrophy or adrenoleukodystrophy, especially if male. It should be noted that the initial diagnosis of a new patient is *not* made by mutation analysis. After the diagnosis is made, there may be an indication for mutation analysis to assist in carrier testing for family members and for prenatal diagnosis. However, as will be discussed later, mutation analysis may prove helpful in predicting the clinical subtype once a confirmatory test is made in a presymptomatic individual following newborn screening.

While more than 99% of the patients diagnosed with Krabbe disease have mutations in the *GALC* gene, there have been a few cases of a neurological disorder resembling Krabbe disease, which is caused by mutations in a heat-stable protein called saposin A (Spiegel et al. 2005). This low-molecular-weight protein, and possibly a related protein called saposin C, is required for the in situ lysosomal hydrolysis of galactosylceramide by GALC (see Fig. 6.1). Saposins A and C and two other saposins, B and D, are produced by proteolytic hydrolysis from the same precursor protein encoded for by one gene (Dewji et al. 1987). In fact, a form of metachromatic leukodystrophy can be caused by mutations in saposin B (Rafi et al. 1990). The first reported patient with saposin A deficiency had low GALC activity when measured in leukocytes but the activity was not low compared to normal when measured in cultured skin fibroblasts. It should be emphasized that patients with saposin A deficiency are very rare. While such patients may cause some confusion in diagnosis, never has this author *not* found mutations in the *GALC* gene in over 300 patients who were diagnosed with Krabbe disease because of low GALC activity measured in leukocytes and were subjected to limited or complete mutation analysis.

In general, measurement of GALC activity zero to 5% of our normal mean will suffice to make the diagnosis of Krabbe disease. The "normal" range is quite wide due to a number of factors, including the condition of the sample received for testing and, most importantly, the presence of polymorphic changes in the "normal" allele (Wenger et al. 2000, 2001). While these mutations, which cause amino acid changes, do have a significant effect on the GALC activity measured in vitro, inheriting multiple copies of these polymorphisms on both copies of the GALC gene does not result in Krabbe disease. Such low values can be found in healthy individuals, including obligate carriers of Krabbe disease, and in individuals with neurological disease. The presence of multiple copies of these polymorphisms has resulted in the identification of a significant number of "positive" infants in the New York state newborn screening program (discussed later). These infants usually can be distinguished using the conventional assay to measure GALC activity that has been in use since 1970. Using that assay, together with sequence analysis of the *GALC* gene to look for disease-causing and polymorphic mutations, a fairly reliable prediction of the possibility of disease and onset can be provided to the family.

Carrier testing for Krabbe disease by measurement of GALC activity in leukocytes or cultured skin fibroblasts in the general population is not reliable. It may be possible to predict carrier status in siblings of an affected individual if values from the obligate heterozygous parents are available. As discussed above, the wide range of GALC activities found in the carrier and "control" populations is due to the presence of polymorphic mutations in the *GALC* gene that have significant effects on the GALC activity measured in vitro. Knowing the disease-causing mutation(s) in a family will increase the accuracy of carrier testing for close relatives. Obviously, it will not help to determine the carrier status in those individuals who marry into that family.

Prenatal diagnosis for at-risk couples can be done using a chorionic villi sample or cultured amniocytes by measuring GALC activity or by mutation analysis, if the mutations are known. It is ideal to have the GALC values from the parents before attempting prenatal diagnosis in case one of the parents has low (15–20% of normal) GALC activity due to the presence of polymorphisms on the "normal" allele. Affected fetuses will have zero to 5% of normal GALC activity. Knowing the mutations in a patient with Krabbe disease opens up the possibility of pre-implantation genetic diagnosis using one of several sampling techniques currently under development.

Pathological findings

INFANTILE PATIENTS

In the brain the white matter is firm, reduced in volume, and is of whitish-gray appearance with dilated ventricles. There is a moderate reduction in the cortical thickness in gray matter. The major histopathological changes are extensive demyelination, gliosis, and presence of unique macrophages, the so-called globoid cells, in the white matter. The fornix, hippocampus, mamillothalamic tract, and the nerve fiber bundles in the basal centrum semiovale and the cerebellar white matter are significantly involved. In the spinal cord, the pyramidal tracts are more severely affected than the dorsal columns. In the areas of demyelination, the oligodendroglial cell population is severely diminished and globoid cells are often clustered around blood vessels. Many, but not all, of the globoid cells are multinucleated. They have prominent pseudopods, moderately electron-dense granular cytoplasm containing prominent rough endoplasmic reticulum, many free ribosomes, abundant fine filaments of approximately 9 to 10 nm, and scattered or clustered abnormal cytoplasmic inclusions. The inclusions have moderately electron-dense straight or curved hollow tubular profiles in longitudinal sections and appear irregularly crystalloid in cross-sections. Scattered globoid cells with typical inclusions have been found in the spinal cord in fetuses of 20 to 23 weeks of gestation.

The peripheral nerves tend to be firm and abnormally thick and white on gross inspection. The major pathological features are marked endoneurial fibrosis, proliferation of fibroblasts, demyelination, and infiltration or perivascular aggregation of histiocytes/macrophages containing periodic acid–Schiff positive materials. Thinly myelinated fibers suggestive of remyelination may be present. Axonal degeneration of varying degrees has been reported. Ultrastructurally, inclusions similar to those in globoid cells in the brain are found in the cytoplasm of histiocytes/macrophages, as well as in the Schwann cells.

LATER-ONSET PATIENTS

Despite the increasing diagnosis of late-onset cases in recent years, only limited information on their neuropathology has been reported. In late infantile and juvenile cases, neuropathological changes are similar to those in typical infantile patients. Two identical twin females developed symptoms of weakness and ataxia at about 18 years of age. A brother with similar symptoms died of what was called, probably incorrectly, adrenoleukodystrophy. The young women were diagnosed with Krabbe disease. Both received allogeneic bone marrow transplants and both died of severe graft-versus-host disease within two months of the transplant. Neuropathological changes included degeneration of the fronto-parietal white matter and corticospinal tract. The fronto-parietal lesion consisted of multiple necrotic foci with calcified deposits and active degeneration of the surrounding white matter with globoid cell infiltration. Globoid cell infiltration was noted in the optic radiations. In a 73-year-old woman, the oldest reported case of Krabbe disease, sural nerve biopsy revealed a mild loss of myelinated fibers with disproportionately thin myelin sheaths, and Schwann cells contained needle-like inclusions (Kolodny et al. 1991).

Biochemical findings

Almost all patients with Krabbe disease have a deficiency of GALC activity. This enzyme has specificity toward galactosylceramide, psychosine (galactosylsphingosine), monogalactosyldiglyceride, and lactosylceramide under specific assay conditions. The metabolism of the first two substrates is important to understanding the pathology of this disorder. Globoid cells have been shown to be composed of high concentrations of galactosylceramide, and they can be produced experimentally by injecting this lipid into brain (Austin et al. 1961). However, the pathogenic lipid may be psychosine, which has been demonstrated to inhibit some key enzymes such as protein kinase C, to disrupt peroxisomal functioning, to activate phospholipase A2, and to induce apoptotic death in many cell types including oligodendrocytes and Schwann cells (Hannun and Bell 1987, Jatana et al. 2002, Zaka and Wenger 2004, Khan et al. 2005, Giri et al. 2006, Formichi et al. 2007). Psychosine causes apoptotic death in vitro in all types of cells when taken up from the culture media. While psychosine is a minor component of normal brain, its level increases 10- to 20-fold in white matter of brain and peripheral nerves of humans and animal models with GALC deficiency. GALC is the only enzyme capable of hydrolyzing psychosine. Psychosine is synthesized during active myelination by the enzymatic transfer of galactose to sphingosine catalyzed by ceramide : galactosyltransferase (see Fig. 6.1). In people with sufficient GALC activity psychosine is degraded, but in tissues of patients with Krabbe disease it accumulates.

GALC is synthesized in all tissues of the body, although there is little substrate to hydrolyze in most tissues. The role of so-called sphingolipid activator proteins (saposins, SAPs) in stimulating GALC activity has also been investigated. In 1982 it was demonstrated that SAP-2 or saposin C could stimulate GALC activity in the presence of acidic lipids, including sulfatide and phosphatidylserine (Wenger et al. 1982). The prosaposin gene has been cloned, and it has been shown to encode four saposins, which are produced by proteolytic hydrolysis. A mouse model with a point mutation in the saposin A region of prosaposin was generated and these mice have pathological features resembling a late-onset, chronic form of GLD (Matsuda et al. 2001). The human counterpart to the mouse model was recently described (Spiegel et al. 2005). Therefore, this rare form of a Krabbe-like neurodegenerative disease may be considered if other diagnostic options have been ruled out. Also, there may be a role for the expression of saposins A and C in explaining the clinical variability observed in patients with late-onset Krabbe disease.

Molecular genetics
This laboratory mapped the gene for Krabbe disease to human chromosome 14 by linkage analysis and to the region 14q31 by in-situ hybridization using a probe from the cDNA sequence. Once the GALC protein was purified, the amino acid sequence information was used to clone the cDNA and gene (Chen and Wenger 1993, Chen et al. 1993, Luzi et al. 1995). The cDNA is about 3.8 kb in length including 47 bp 5' to the initiation start site, 2007 bp of open reading frame (coding for 669 amino acids) and 1741 bp of 3' untranslated sequence. The first 78 nucleotides of the open reading frame code for the 26 amino acid leader peptide. The remaining 643 amino acids plus glycosylation of 5 or 6 of the potential sites would constitute the 80 kDa precursor species. The 80 kDa precursor is processed into the 50 to 53 kDa and 30 kDa mature forms by the action of a protease(s), probably localized in lysosomes. The human *GALC* gene is nearly 58 kb in length and contains 17 exons and 16 introns. Other than the first and last exons, the exons are relatively small, ranging from 39 to 181 bp. The introns range in size from 247 bp for intron 2 to about 12 kb for intron 10.

With the available sequence information from the GALC cDNA and gene, mutation analysis of patients with all types of GLD is possible. About 100 mutations, including disease-causing and polymorphisms, have been identified, and a majority have been reported in several recent reviews (Wenger et al. 2000, 2001). The most commonly identified disease-causing mutations are listed in Table 6.1. Of course, knowing the mutation(s) may help to predict the clinical subtype of asymptomatic individuals identified by newborn screening and would improve carrier testing in the immediate family members. We currently test all newly diagnosed patients for the most common mutation found in 40 to 50% of the disease-causing alleles in patients with Krabbe disease who have European ancestry (Rafi et al. 1995). It is a large deletion involving nearly 30 kb of the gene starting within intron 10 and proceeding past the 3' end of the gene. While this severe mutation probably originated in

TABLE 6.1
Most common mutations found in patients with globoid cell leukodystrophy[a]

Designation	Nucleotide change	Effect	Polymorphic background[b]	Comments
635del + ins	del 25 nts + ins 3 nts	del 5 aa + ins 2 aa	?	Infantile Japanese and Koreans
G809A	GGC>GAC	p.G270D	1637C	Results in a later-onset form of GLD when hom or het
502T/del	30 kb deletion	short mRNA	502T	About 40–50% of mutant alleles
1424delA	ATAAGG>ATAGG	FS, PS	1637C	T1873C on same allele
C1538T	ACG>ATG	p.T513M	694A	Infantile
1544A	CGC>CAC	p.R515H	?	Infantile Japanese
G1582A	GAT>AAT	p.D528N	1637C	Infantile Israeli Arab
A1652C	TAC>TCC	p.Y551S	1637C	Infantile
T1748G	ATT>AGT	p.I583S		Infantile Israeli Druze
T1853C	TTA>TCA	p.L618S	1637C	Adult Japanese

[a] All of these mutations have been found homozygous in patients from unrelated parents and/or heterozygous in other unrelated patients.
[b] The polymorphisms examined include c.C502T (p.R168C), c.G694A (p.D224N), and c.T1637C (p.I546T), with the most common nucleotide given first.

Key: hom = homozygous; het = heterozygous; FS = frame-shift; PS = premature stop; del = deletion; ins = insertion; aa = amino acid; c. = change in the cDNA, nucleotide number; p. = change in the protein, codon number; ? = not reported.

Sweden, it has spread throughout Europe, and is also found in patients from India and Mexico. Of the mutations identified in our laboratory and reported by others, some have only been found in one family. However, some mutations do occur in a significant number of patients in certain geographic areas (e.g., Middle East or Japan). Many patients with a late-onset form of Krabbe disease have one copy of the c.G809A (p.G270A) mutation. This mis-sense mutation must result in the production of a small amount of active enzyme that causes a delay in the onset of the disease. This has never been proven because it is difficult to accurately measure very low levels of this enzyme in available tissue samples. This laboratory has identified seven families, including the sisters described above in case vignette 1 and the milder patient in case vignette 2, who have this mutation on one allele and the 30 kb deletion on the other. The age at onset and clinical course of the affected individuals with this genotype are significantly different between and within families. Other patients are compound heterozygotes having different mutations in the two copies of the *GALC* gene. This makes genotype–phenotype correlations difficult. It is interesting that most disease-causing mutations occur together with additional polymorphic changes in the same copy of the *GALC* gene. In addition, the presence of polymorphic mutations in the "normal" allele explains the wide range of GALC values measured in controls and carriers of Krabbe disease.

Newborn screening

Currently, almost all individuals with Krabbe disease are diagnosed after symptoms become apparent. Even when key symptoms, such as irritability, stiffness, fisting, and arching are noted by the parents or caregivers, there may be a significant delay in sending a sample to the correct laboratory for testing. By this time, the options for treatment are very limited. Prior to the newborn screening initiated in New York state, there were newborns who were determined at birth to be affected with Krabbe disease because they had affected siblings, and the parents elected not to have prenatal testing, or had prenatal testing and elected not to terminate a fetus predicted to be affected with Krabbe disease. Some of these children underwent umbilical cord HSC transplantation within a few weeks of the birth (Escolar et al. 2005). While this did not result in a "cure," these transplanted newborns are living longer than their untreated siblings with infantile Krabbe disease (see later).

Newborn screening was initiated in August 2006 in New York state. This was based on the information that treating infantile patients before symptoms were apparent prolonged life and resulted in retention of cognitive function, and the ability to do screening using dried blood spots using an automated method involving tandem mass spectrometry (Li et al. 2004). New York state has about 250 000 births per year, and these newborns are tested for more than 50 conditions.

Briefly, the screening test for Krabbe disease is performed as follows. The 3 mm dried blood punch is hydrated and reacted overnight with a special GALC substrate using specific conditions. After reaction, the mixture is extracted, and the products of the reaction are subjected to tandem mass spectroscopy. Hydrolyzed substrate is visualized on the printout, and the results for each day can be compared. Those samples that fall below a given percentage (now 20% of the daily mean) are repeated with new punches, and if the average of three punches is below 12%, gene sequencing is performed. If disease-causing mutations are found, the family is notified to come in for genetic counseling and for collection of additional samples. DNA is prepared for identification matching, and a sample of heparinized blood is sent to the author's laboratory for measurement of GALC activity using the conventional assay method.

What are the possible reasons for finding low GALC activity in the newborn screening test? The individual will, in fact, be affected with Krabbe disease (when symptoms will begin is a big issue). The individual is a carrier of Krabbe disease with an activity-lowering polymorphism in the "normal" allele. The individual has activity-lowering polymorphisms on both "normal" alleles. The sample was collected or sent in a less than ideal condition. The newborn has a low white blood cell count.

By August 2008 over 500 000 newborns had been screened for Krabbe disease. Six were found to be at high risk because the level of GALC activity in the conventional assay was within the range of values measured in individuals confirmed to have Krabbe disease *and* mutation analysis identified previously known disease-causing mutations or unreported significant mutations (mis-sense, stop codons, insertions or deletions, splice junction errors, etc) in both alleles. While it may be possible to predict an infantile onset if both mutations are severe and previously reported, the situation is more difficult when mild mutations are detected, or when a combination of mutant alleles never seen before is found. As those asymptomatic newborns who are predicted to have rapid onset need immediate neurodiagnostic evaluation and possibly umbilical cord HSC transplantation within the first few weeks of life, the other individuals with low GALC activity create a dilemma. Since the onset of symptoms in later-onset patients varies greatly, there may not be need for any treatment for many years or maybe never. A protocol has been devised to evaluate newborns who are considered high risk. This includes neurological evaluation every month for the first year, neurodiagnostic studies including MRI, lumbar puncture, nerve conduction studies, brainstem auditory evoked responses and visual evoked responses every 3 months, and neuropsychological evaluation annually. Newborns who have lower than normal, but above the affected range, GALC activity (usually caused by the presence of a disease-causing mutation together with enzyme-lowering polymorphisms or polymorphisms on both alleles) are evaluated less frequently for the first two years of life. Parents of all infants with lower than normal GALC activity are given a list of symptoms to watch for and a physician contact. As this is the first lysosomal storage disease to have newborn screening, there is much that can be learned, and issues have arisen that were not considered when the program was initiated.

Studies in animal models

There are well-characterized animal models of GLD available for study. Several reviews describing these models, including their clinical and pathological features, molecular defects, and potential use as models to attempt therapeutic trials, have been published (Suzuki and Suzuki 1985, Wenger 2000). In addition to these naturally occurring models, a new transgenic mouse has been developed (Luzi et al. 2001). As has been demonstrated in human Krabbe disease, the animal models have increased psychosine in nervous tissues, and, in addition, mice have a large increase in galactosylceramide in kidney. Treatment of affected mice by bone marrow transplantation (BMT) has resulted in a prolonged lifespan (Yeager et al. 1984, Ichioka et al. 1987, Luzi et al. 2005). Some mice lived over one year while untreated mice live no longer than 60 days. In our studies there were significant elevations in the GALC activity in lung, liver, heart, kidney, spleen, brain, and peripheral nervous system (Luzi et al. 2005). This rise in enzymatic activity was accompanied by a decrease in the levels of psychosine in brain to near-normal levels in long-lived mice. Histologically there was disappearance of characteristic globoid cells and an infiltration of donor-derived macrophages, which resulted in some remyelination in the central nervous system and the sciatic nerves. Eventually the mice succumb after hind leg weakness hinders eating and movement. This could indicate that therapeutic levels of GALC activity are not getting to the peripheral nervous system, and this appears to mimic the situation in human patients who are treated early by umbilical cord HSC transplantation. Although the lifespan was greatly lengthened by the treatment, all of the affected mice died from neurological complications.

As a prelude to gene therapy trials in animal models, it was demonstrated that cultured oligodendrocytes from twitcher mice could be made to have a normal phenotype when GALC activity was supplied via viral transduction or uptake from transduced neighboring cells (Luddi et al. 2001). The mouse models of GLD have been used for a number of experimental therapy trials including viral gene therapy utilizing adeno-associated virus, adenovirus, and lentivirus containing the GALC cDNA injected directly into the ventricles and the brain cortex (Shen et al. 2001, DeGaspari et al. 2004, Meng et al. 2005, Lin et al. 2005, Rafi et al. 2005, Dolcetta et al. 2006). The treated mice show expression of the gene and some improvement in pathology; however, there is only a small increase in lifespan of these mice. Combining BMT and viral gene therapy into the brain did show synergy in one study (Lin et al. 2007). Neural stem cells have also been injected into the brain with limited success (Croitoru-Lamoury et al. 2006, Pellegatta et al. 2006). However, when oligodendrocytes from twitcher mice were transplanted into the spinal cord of another myelin-deficient mouse model, they myelinated normally once they received GALC activity from the non-twitcher cells (Kondo et al. 2005). Enzyme replacement therapy (ERT) has been tried but it resulted in only a minor extension of the lifespan of affected mice (Lee et al. 2007). As this disease does involve an inflammatory component, a number of non-steroidal anti-inflammatory agents were given alone and together with BMT. Alone, some drugs prolonged the lives of affected mice to about 80 days, however it was difficult to see a synergistic effect when combined with BMT (unpublished data).

Cairn and West Highland white terriers with GLD have been known for many years, and a breeding colony has been established at the University of Pennsylvania School of Veterinary Medicine. This larger animal model has some advantages over the mouse models, which could bridge the gap toward human trials once effective therapies are developed. We have used magnetization transfer imaging to evaluate these dogs (McGowen et al. 2000). As with the mice, bone marrow transplantation in the dog model slows the progression of the disease. A colony of rhesus monkeys that have a mutation in the *GALC* gene is available at the Tulane Primate Research Center. Affected monkeys can be identified in utero using chorionic villi sampling or immediately after birth, and treatment can be instituted. Although only a limited number of affected monkeys will be available, they could be utilized as a final step before human trials to investigate safety and effectiveness of new therapies.

Therapy

At this time the only treatment available for asymptomatic individuals is HSC transplantation. With the use of umbilical cord transplantation, finding a suitable donor is not the problem it was when a compatible bone marrow donor was needed. Transplantation in infantile patients who already have significant neurological symptoms is a procedure with significant morbidity and mortality for the patient and serious emotional consequences for the parents, and has not resulted in improvement in the recipient. Transplantation in late-onset patients who have only mild symptoms and a slower progression has been of benefit to some, but others have not done well following transplantation (Krivit et al. 1998). Some have stabilized and improved, while others have died of complications of the transplantation. The long-term prognosis is not known. The irritability so common in infantile patients has been shown to respond to low-dose morphine (Stewart et al. 2001).

Umbilical cord HSC transplantation of asymptomatic newborns identified at birth because of family history or by newborn screening in New York state has been performed in at least 20 individuals. There is clear evidence that such transplantation in asymptomatic infantile patients slows the clinical course of the disease, and the treated individuals do not follow the clinical course and early death of affected, untreated siblings (Escolar et al. 2005). These newborns received umbilical cord blood from unrelated donors following myeloablative chemotherapy.

Comparing the outcomes of transplanting in asymptomatic and symptomatic individuals, there was little difference regarding engraftment but there were significant differences in survival and neurological functioning. The infants receiving HSC transplantation before symptoms were obvious showed continued myelination and gains in developmental skills. There was a mild beneficial effect on nerve conduction velocity if the transplantation was performed early (Siddiqi et al. 2006). Most had near normal cognitive skills but most had mild-to-moderate delays in expressive language and mild-to-severe delays in gross motor function. Symptomatic infants who had HSC transplantation showed minimal neurological improvement. Recently, an infant identified in the New York state newborn screening program who received an umbilical cord transplantation within the first month of life died of complications from the transplant. Therefore these procedures are not without a significant risk for morbidity and mortality.

Two juvenile-onset patients have done considerably well following BMT. A now 31-year-old woman with onset of symptoms at 5 years of age was given a BMT from her homozygous normal brother. Twenty-six years after transplantation, the patient is stably engrafted, maintaining normal leukocyte GALC activity. Her elevated cerebrospinal fluid protein concentration decreased to normal, her school performance was normal, and she no longer experiences tremors or ataxia. There is an improvement in all of her neuropsychological test results. The other patient, an 8-year-old boy at the time, was determined to be affected with GLD by enzyme studies using leukocytes. He is one of three affected siblings. He received a BMT from his unaffected sister. Ten years after transplantation he is in excellent health and has a donor level of leukocyte GALC activity. There has been a drop in cerebrospinal fluid protein from 125 mg/dl to normal, a rise in his IQ, and an improvement in his MRI.

Although it is too early to reach a conclusion regarding the role of HSC transplantation in Krabbe disease, it should be considered in presymptomatic infantile cases and in mildly affected juvenile and late-onset cases if a suitable donor is available. In-utero BMT has been tried with little success.

Conclusions

At this time Krabbe disease can be readily diagnosed prenatally and postnatally by measuring GALC activity in available tissue samples. The cloning of the *GALC* gene and identification of mutations has led to improved carrier assessment in some families. Although the finding of certain well-characterized mutations in a newly identified patient does help with phenotype prediction, no clear genotype–phenotype correlation can be assigned to novel mutations identified in such patients. In fact, there is considerable clinical variability in late-onset patients with the identical genotype. No completely satisfactory treatment is available; however, HSC transplantation in presymptomatic infantile patients and very mildly affected late-onset patients shows clear beneficial effects. This approach, as well as any treatments developed in the future, will require early diagnosis of affected individuals.

Very recent developments in the isolation and characterization of neural and embryonic stem cells, and the generation of hybrid viral vectors that can infect neural cells with genes of interest, open the way to studies in animal models of GLD. Potentially, stem cells can be transduced to produce high levels of GALC activity, and once injected could spread throughout the brain and supply either GALC activity to viable oligodendrocytes or repopulate large areas of the brain with donor oligodendrocytes that have sufficient GALC activity. While any treatment option should include a method for supplying GALC activity to myelinating oligodendrocytes and Schwann cells or replacing the myelinating cells, a role for anti-apoptotic cytokines and growth factors may have to be considered in future protocols. A combination of therapies may be needed to obtain a more satisfactory outcome. Clearly, the rapid progression of the disease in most patients and the need to supply GALC activity throughout the central and peripheral nervous systems present significant challenges for the treatment.

Acknowledgments
The author thanks the many co-workers who have helped with the research and the diagnosis of patients with this disorder, and the families with Krabbe disease who provided samples and support for our research. This research was supported in part by a grant from the National Institutes of Health (DK 38795).

REFERENCES

Austin J, Lehfeldt D, Maxwell W. (1961) Experimental "globoid bodies" in white matter and chemical analysis in Krabbe's disease. J Neuropathol Exp Neurol 20: 284–285.

Chen YQ, Wenger DA. (1993) Galactocerebrosidase from human urine: purification and partial characterization. Biochim Biophys Acta 1170: 53–61.

Chen YQ, Rafi MA, de Gala G, Wenger DA. (1993) Cloning and expression of cDNA encoding human galactocerebrosidase, the enzyme deficient in globoid cell leukodystrophy. Hum Mol Genet 2: 1841–1845.

Collier J, Greenfield J. (1924) The encephalitis periaxialis of Schilder: a clinical and pathological study, with an account of two cases, one of which was diagnosed during life. Brain 47: 489–519.

Croitoru-Lamoury J, Williams KR, Lamoury FM, et al. (2006) Neural transplantation of human MSC and NT2 cells in the twitcher mouse model. Cytotherapy 8: 445–458.

Crome L, Hanefield F, Patrick D, Wilson J. (1973) Late onset globoid cell leukodystrophy. Brain 96: 841–848.

DeGasperi R, Friedrich VL, Perez GM, et al. (2004) Transgenic rescue of Krabbe disease in the twitcher mouse. Gene Ther 11: 1188–1194.

Dewji NN, Wenger DA, O'Brien JS. (1987) Nucleotide sequence of cloned cDNA for human sphingolipid activator protein 1 precursor. Proc Natl Acad Sci USA 84: 8652–8656.

Dolcetta D, Perani L, Givogri MI, et al. (2006) Design and optimization of lentiviral vectors for transfer of GALC expression in twitcher brain. J Gene Med 8: 962–971.

Escolar ML, Poe MD, Provenzale JM, et al. (2005) Transplantation of umbilical-cord blood in babies with infantile Krabbe's disease. New Engl J Med 352: 2069–2081.

Formichi P, Radi E, Battisti C, et al. (2007) Psychosine-induced apoptosis and cytokine activation in immune peripheral cells of Krabbe patients. J Cell Physiol 212: 737–743.

Giri S, Khan M, Rattan R, Singh I, Singh AK. (2006) Krabbe disease: psychosine-mediated activation of phospholipase A2 in oligodendrocyte cell death. Lipid Res 47: 1478–1492.

Goebel HH, Harzer K, Ernst JP, Bohl J, Klein H. (1990) Late-onset globoid cell leukodystrophy: Unusual ultrastructural pathology and subtotal β-galactocerebrosidase deficiency. J Child Neurol 5: 299–309.

Hagberg B, Kollberg H, Sourander P, Akesson HO. (1970) Infantile globoid cell leucodystrophy (Krabbe's disease): A clinical and genetic study of 32 Swedish cases 1953–1967. Neuropaediatrie 1: 74–88.

Hannun, YA, Bell RM. (1987) Lysosphingolipids inhibit protein kinase C: implication for the sphingolipidoses. Science 235: 670–674.

Ichioka T, Kishimoto Y, Brennan S, Santos GW, Yeager AM. (1987) Hematopoietic cell transplantation in murine globoid cell leukodystrophy (the twitcher mouse): effects on levels of galactosylceramidase, psychosine, and galactocerebrosides. Proc Natl Acad Sci USA 84: 4259–4263.

Jatana M, Giri, S, Singh, AK. (2002) Apoptotic positive cells in Krabbe brain and induction of apoptosis in rat C6 glial cells by psychosine. Neurosci Lett 330: 183–187.

Khan M, Haq E, Giri S, Singh I, Singh AK. (2005) Peroxisomal participation in psychosine-mediated toxicity: implications for Krabbe's disease. J Neurosci Res 80: 845–854.

Kolodny EH, Raghavan S, Krivit W. (1991) Late-onset Krabbe disease (globoid cell leukodystrophy): clinical and biochemical features in 15 patients. Dev Neurosci 13: 232–239.

Kondo Y, Wenger DA, Duncan I. (2005) Galactocerebrosidase-deficient oligodendrocytes maintain stable central myelin by exogenous replacement of the missing enzyme in mice. Proc Natl Acad Sci USA 102: 18 670–18 675.

Krabbe K. (1916) A new familial, infantile form of diffuse brain sclerosis. Brain 39: 74–114.

Krivit W, Shapiro EG, Peters C, et al. (1998) Hematopoietic stem-cell transplantation in globoid-cell leukodystrophy. New Engl J Med 338: 1119–1126.

Lee WC, Tsoi YK, Troendle FJ, et al. (2007) Single-dose intracerebroventricular administration of galactocerebrosidase improves survival in a mouse model of globoid cell leukodystrophy. FASEB J 21: 2520–2527.

Li Y, Scott CR, Chamoles NA, Ghavami A, Pinto BM, Turecek F, Gelb MH. (2004) Direct multiplex assay of lysosomal enzymes in dried blood spots for newborn screening. Clin Chem 50: 1785–1796.

Lin D, Fantz CR, Levy B, et al. (2005) AAV2/5 vector expressing galactocerebrosidase ameliorates CNS disease in the murine model of globoid-cell leukodystrophy more efficiency than AAV2. Mol Ther 12: 422–430.

Lin D, Donsante A, Macauley S, Levy B, Vogler C, Sands MS. (2007) Central nervous system-directed AAV2/5-mediated gene therapy synergizes with bone marrow transplantation in the murine model of globoid-cell leukodystrophy. Mol Ther 15: 44–52.

Luddi A, Volterrani M, Strazza M, et al. (2001) Retrovirus-mediated gene transfer and galactocerebrosidase uptake into twitcher glial cells results in appropriate localization and phenotype correction. Neurobiol Dis 8: 600–610.

Luzi P, Rafi MA, Wenger DA. (1995) Structure and organization of the human galactocerebrosidase (GALC) gene. Genomics 26: 407–409.

Luzi P, Rafi MA, Zaka M, Curtis M, Vanier MT, Wenger DA. (2001) Generation of a mouse with low galactocerebrosidase activity by gene targeting: a new model of globoid cell leukodystrophy (Krabbe disease). Molec Genet Metab 73: 221–223.

Luzi P, Rafi MA, Zaka M, Rao HZ, Curtis M, Vanier MT, Wenger DA. (2005) Biochemical and pathological evaluation of long-lived mice with globoid cell leukodystrophy after bone marrow transplantation. Mol Genet Metab 86: 150–159.

Lyon G, Hagberg B, Evrard Ph, Allaire C, Pavone L, Vanier M. (1991) Symptomatology of late onset Krabbe's leukodystrophy: the European experience. Dev Neurosci 13: 240–244.

Malone MJ, Szöke MC, Looney GL. (1975) Globoid leukodystrophy I. Clinical and enzymatic studies. Arch Neurol 32: 606–612.

Matsuda J, Vanier MT, Saito Y, Tohyama J, Suzuki K, Suzuki K. (2001) A mutation in the saposin A domain of the sphingolipid activator protein (prosaposin) gene results in a late-onset, chronic form of globoid cell leukodystrophy in the mouse. Hum Mol Genet 10: 1191–1199.

McGowan JC, Haskins H, Wenger DA, Vite C. (2000) Investigating demyelination in the brain in a canine model of globoid cell leukodystrophy (Krabbe disease) using magnetization transfer contrast: preliminary results. J Comput Assisted Tomography 24: 316–321.

McGuinness OE, Winrow AP, Smyth DPL. (1996) Krabbe's leukodystrophy precipitated by influenza A infection. Dev Med Child Neurol 38: 460–462.

Meng X-L, Shen J-S, Watabe K, Ohashi T, Eto Y. (2005) GALC transduction leads to morphological improvement of the twitcher oligodendrocytes in vivo. Mol Genet Metab 84: 332–343.

Pellegatta S, Tunici P, Poliani PL, et al. (2006) The therapeutic potential of neural stem/progenitor cells in murine globoid cell leukodystrophy is conditioned by macrophage/microglial activation. Neurobiol Dis 21: 314–323.

Rafi MA, Zhang X-L, DeGala G, Wenger DA. (1990) Detection of a point mutation in sphingolipid activator protein-1 mRNA in patients with a variant form of metachromatic leukodystrophy. Biochem Biophys Res Commun 166: 1017–1023.

Rafi MA, Luzi P, Chen YQ, Wenger DA. (1995) A large deletion together with a point mutation in the GALC gene is a common mutant allele in patients with infantile Krabbe disease. Hum Mol Genet 4: 1285–1289.

Rafi MA, Rao HZ, Passini MA, et al. (2005) AAV-mediated expression of galactocerebrosidase in brain results in attenuated symptoms and extended life span in murine models of globoid cell leukodystrophy. Mol Ther 11: 734–744.

Shen JS, Watabe K, Ohashi T, Eto Y. (2001) Intraventricular administration of recombinant adenovirus to neonatal twitcher mouse leads to clinicopathological improvements. Gene Ther 8: 1081–1087.

Siddiqi ZA, Sanders DB, Massey JM. (2006) Peripheral neuropathy in Krabbe disease. Effect of hematopoietic stem cell transplantation. Neurology 67: 268–272.

Spiegel R, Bach G, Sury V, et al. (2005) A mutation in the saposin A coding region of the prosaposin gene in an infant presenting as Krabbe disease: first report of saposin A deficiency in humans. Mol Genet Metab 84: 160–166.

Stewart WA, Gordon KE, Camfield PR, Wood EP, Dooley JM. (2001) Irritability in Krabbe's disease: dramatic response to low-dose morphine. Pediatr Neurol 25: 344–345.

Suzuki K, Suzuki Y. (1970) Globoid cell leucodystrophy (Krabbe's disease): Deficiency of galactocerebroside β-galactosidase. Proc Natl Acad Sci USA 66: 302–309.

Suzuki K, Suzuki K. (1985) Genetic galactosylceramidase deficiency (globoid cell leukodystrophy, Krabbe disease) in different mammalian species. Neurochem Pathol 3: 53–68.

Tada K, Taniike M, Ono J, Tsukamoto H, Inui K, Okada S. (1992) Serial magnetic resonance imaging studies in a case of late onset globoid cell leukodystrophy. Neuropediatrics 23: 306–309.

Wenger PA, Sattler M, Roth S. (1982) A protein activator of galactosylceramide β-galactosidase. Biochim Biophys Acta 712: 639–649.

Wenger DA. (2000) Murine, canine and non-human primate models of Krabbe disease. Molec Med Today 6: 449–451.

Wenger DA, Rafi MA, Luzi P, Datto J, Costantino-Ceccarini E. (2000) Krabbe disease: genetic aspects and progress toward therapy. Mol Genet Metab 70: 1–9.

Wenger DA, Suzuki K, Suzuki Y, Suzuki K. (2001) Galactosylceramide Lipidosis. Globoid cell leukodystrophy (Krabbe disease). In: Scriver CR, Beaudet AL, Sly WS, Valle D, Eds. The Metabolic and Molecular Bases of Inherited Disease, 8th edn. New York: McGraw-Hill, pp. 3669–3694.

Yeager AM, Brennan S, Tiffany C, Moser HW, Santos GW. (1984) Prolonged survival and remyelination after hematopoietic cell transplantation in the twitcher mouse. Science 225: 1053–1054.

Zaka P, Wenger DA. (2004) Psychosine-induced apoptosis in a mouse oligodendrocyte progenitor cell line is mediated by caspase activation. Neurosci Lett 358: 205–209.

105

7
ALEXANDER DISEASE

Daniel Flint and Michael Brenner

Introduction

Alexander disease, eponymously named after the pathologist who first described the disorder in 1949 (Alexander 1949), is a rarely reported but often fatal genetic neurodegenerative disorder. Its rarity is a consequence of most of the identified causative mutations being dominant, fully penetrant, and resulting in death before reproductive age. Thus, in most reported cases Alexander disease is not transmitted, but arises at the low frequency of de-novo mutations, which is of the order of 1 in 100 000 (Drake et al. 1998). However, the disease has engendered interest that is disproportionate to its frequency. This is in part due to the striking clinical features that characterize the most typical cases – a large head, seizures, and magnetic resonance imaging (MRI) findings of massive bilateral frontal-lobe myelin deficits. Also contributing to interest has been the remarkable pathological hallmark of the disorder – the widespread and abundant presence in astrocytes of protein aggregates, called Rosenthal fibers. Interest has been heightened by the discovery that nearly all cases of Alexander disease are due to mutations in the gene encoding the intermediate filament protein, glial fibrillary acidic protein (GFAP), which is commonly used as an astrocyte marker. This discovery established Alexander disease as the first known genetic disorder of astrocytes, a central nervous system (CNS) cell type whose star has been rapidly rising as burgeoning numbers of regulatory functions are assigned to them. The availability of *GFAP* mutations as a diagnostic has led to better appreciation of the range of presentations that Alexander disease can display. In particular, there has been a substantial increase in reporting of adult onset and familial cases, leading to the possibility that the disorder may not be so rare after all. One consequence of these more recent reports is that it is no longer appropriate to classify Alexander disease purely as a leukodystrophy, since several of these later-onset cases do not reveal any white matter abnormalities. Instead, given that the primary genetic defect is in the astrocytic protein GFAP, the disease might more accurately be classified as an astrogliopathy. There has also been a shift in focus on the primary disease pathology from the myelin defects in the frontal lobes to atrophy in the brainstem, cerebellum, and spinal cord. This chapter presents a brief overview of the major features of Alexander disease, but primarily focuses on these most recent findings, especially those since 2007. It thus updates a recent book chapter by Brenner et al. (2009), which provides a comprehensive review of the literature into early 2007, including a tabulation of all cases for which *GFAP* gene analysis was used as a diagnostic. Other reviews also address aspects of the disease that are not covered here in depth, such as a historical perspective, detailed discussions of the *GFAP* mutations, individual characteristics of affected patients, and exploration of disease mechanisms using animal and cell culture models (e.g., Li et al. 2002, Jacob et al. 2003, Messing and Goldman 2004, Gorospe and Maletkovic 2006, Wippold et al. 2006, Quinlan et al. 2007, Pareyson et al. 2008).

Clinical presentation

Until recently, Alexander disease was clinically fairly well defined. Onset was generally before the age of 2 years with a presentation of psychomotor developmental delay (failure to meet physical and mental milestones), seizures, and megalencephaly. Patients also often displayed ataxia, spasticity, and bulbar and pseudobulbar signs, such as vomiting and difficulty with eating or speaking; and MRI often revealed bilateral white matter anomalies in the frontal lobes. The only other disorder with a highly similar presentation was Canavan disease, and this could be differentially diagnosed by a urinary test for *N*-acetyl aspartate. Although this typical infantile form remains the most frequently encountered, much more variable presentations for the disease, including forms with onset as late as the seventh decade of life, have been revealed by the unexpected presence of Rosenthal fibers in biopsy and autopsy material from patients thought to have other disorders, and the recent availability of *GFAP* gene sequencing for diagnosis.

The clinical presentation of the adult form, generally defined as having an onset at 13 years or later, is quite different from the infantile: psychomotor developmental delay, macrocephaly, and seizures are seldom seen; instead, bulbar/pseudobulbar signs are almost always present, and ataxia and spasticity are common (Tables 7.1 and 7.2). A myriad of additional symptoms has been observed with varying frequency in adult cases, including palatal myoclonus, nystagmus, sleep apnea, scoliosis, autonomic dysfunction (constipation, hyper- or hypothermia), and precocious or delayed sexual maturity (for a detailed list and references see Pareyson et al. 2008, Brenner et al. 2009). Palatal myoclonus is sufficiently common in adult-onset cases to recommend that individuals with this sign be tested for Alexander disease (see Balbi et al. 2008, Howard et al. 2008).

The adult form was classified as Alexander disease on the basis of the abundant presence of the Rosenthal fibers that typified the infantile form. However, given their very different clinical presentations, there was debate about whether they had different causes. This possibility was partially dispelled by finding patients with features of both, leading to a continuum of presentations between the two. This is particularly true for the juvenile onset cases, defined as having an onset between 2 and 13 years. The debate was settled by the finding that *GFAP* mutations account for most cases of all forms of the disease.

In addition to the highly variable clinical presentations of the juvenile and adult forms, there can be considerable ambiguity as to what is considered their age at onset. In this review and most commonly, the age at onset is taken as the age at which medical treatment was first sought for problems clearly due to the disease. However, in many instances there were much earlier clinical signs that in retrospect were likely caused by the disorder. An example is a patient classified as having adult onset because the hospital admission that led to his diagnosis was at age 20, but who had two seizures at age 2. Did these seizures have a different cause, or was onset actually at age 2? Reflecting this uncertainty, one account of

TABLE 7.1
Characteristics of Alexander disease patients recently tested for *GFAP* mutations

Exon	Mutation	Reference[2]	Reported as patient no.	Age at onset	Age last report or at death (†)	Type	Sex
1	R70Q*	Caroli	12	35 y	40 y	Adt	F
1	R70W	Caroli	13	43 y	44 y	Adt	F
1	M73K*	Caroli	1	7 mo	9 y	Inf	M
1	M73T	Vazquez		Birth	2 mo	Inf	–
1	M74T*	Ohnari		51 y	53 y	Adt	M
1	N77S	Caroli	2	6 mo	11 y	Inf	F
1	R79C	Caroli	3	4 mo	10 y	Inf	M
1	R79C	Caroli	4	5 mo	4 y	Inf	M
1	R79C	Caroli	5	9 mo	19 y†	Inf	M
1	R79C	Mignot		14 mo	3 y	Inf	F
1	R79P*	Caroli	6	5 y	19 y	Juv	F
1	Y83H	Ye[3]	1	<1 y	7 y	Inf	M
1	R88C	Ye[3]	2	2 y	8 y	Juv	F
1	R88C	Ye[3]	3	4 y	8 y	Juv	M
1	R88C	Caroli	7	1 y	11 y	Inf	M
1	D128N*	Pareyson	10	62 y	64 y	Adt	M
3	E205K*	Pareyson	5	NA	30 y	Asm	M
3	E205K	Pareyson	8	54 y	58 y	Adt	M
4	L231H*	Delnooz		50 y	61 y	Adt	M
4	R239H	Caroli	8	4 mo	7 y	Inf	F
4	R239P	Caroli	9	10 mo	5 y†	Inf	M
4	Y257C*	Howard	58	59 y	59 y	Adt	M
	A267P*	Hinttala		10 y	35 y†	Juv	M
6	R330G* & E332K*	Balbi	II.4	57 y	61 y	Adt	M
			II.2	53 y	63 y	Adt	F
			II.3	NA	64 y	Asm	F
			III.5	28 y	32 y	Adt	M
6	E332K*	Pareyson	7	57 y	61 y	Adt	M
6	L359P*	Romano;	Proband	19 y	29 y	Adt	M
		Pareyson	Mother	NA	52 y	Asm	F
6	A364V*	Hartmann	2	4 mo	73 mo	Inf	M
6	Y366C*	Hartmann	1	4 mo	43 mo	Inf	F
6	E373K	Matej		5 mo	12 y†	Inf	–
7	R376W*	Hirayama	Proband	29 y	33 y	Adt	F
			Son	4 y	4 y	Juv	M
8	S393I*	Salmaggi	Proband	33 y	35 y	Adt	F
			Son	2 y	6 y	Juv	M
8	S398Y*	Pareyson	9	NA	52 y	Asm	F
8	R416W	Caroli	10	13 y	27 y	Adt	M
8	D417fs*,[1]	Murakami		10 mo	13 mo	Inf	M
	None	Huttner		32 y	32 y†	Adt	M
	None	Pareyson	11	43 y	45 y	Adt	M

This table presents the characteristics of Alexander disease cases tested for the presence of *GFAP* mutations that were published from 2007 into early 2009. Additional details about many of these cases are described in the "Recent cases" section of the text. Previously published cases are described in Table 24.1 of Brenner et al. (2009). Familial cases are shown as multiple entries for a given reference.

Key: Macro = macrocephaly; Spas = spasticity, Bul/psb =bulbar or pseudobulbar signs, Atx = ataxia. Dev dly = mental or physical developmental delay or regression; Inf = infantile; Juv = juvenile; Adt = adult; Asm = asymptomatic (but carries the indicated mutation); – = not reported, NA = not applicable. If symptoms were not explicitly reported, they were scored in the table as follows: macrocephaly and seizures are listed as absent, under the assumption that they would have been reported if present; spasticity, bulbar/pseudobulbar signs, and ataxia are listed as not reported, except that an unsteady gait was assumed to reflect ataxia; developmental delay or regression was listed as unreported for infantile patients and as negative for older patients.

Macro	Seizure	Spas	Bul/psb	Atx	Dev dly	MRI[4]	Comments
o	No	No	Yes	Yes	No	CDF	Also has D157N SNP
o	No	No	Yes	No	No		
o	Yes	Yes	No	No	Yes	ABCD	
es	No	–	No	–	–	ABCDE	
o	No	Yes	Yes	No	No	DF	no WM lesions
es	Yes	Yes	No	No	Yes	ABCD	
es	No	Yes	No	Yes	Yes	ABCD	
es	Yes	Yes	No	Yes	Yes	ABCD	
o	Yes	Yes	Yes	Yes	Yes	ABCD	
es	No	No	No	Yes	Yes	ABCE	
o	Yes	No	No	No	No	ABCD	
es	No	No	No	No	Yes	4 of A–E	
es	Yes	No	Yes	No	No	4 of A–E	
es	Yes	Yes	Yes	No	No	4 of A–E	
es	No	Yes	NA	NA	Yes	ABCD	
Jo	No	Yes	No	No	No	DF	lower limb weakness
Jo	No	No	No	No	No	ABDEF	
Jo	No	Yes	No	Yes	No	DF	lower limb weakness
Jo	No	No	Yes	Yes	No	DF	Sister who died at 64 y almost certainly also affected
es	Yes	Yes	Yes	No	Yes		
es	Yes	Yes	No	No	Yes		
Jo	No	No	Yes	Yes	No	ABD	
Jo	No	Yes	Yes	Yes	No	BCDF	
Jo	No	Yes	Yes	Yes	No	BCDEF	Proband
Jo	No	No	Yes	Yes	No	BD	Sister
Jo	No	No	No	No	No	BDF	Sister
Jo	No		No	No	No	BDE	Son; only symptom is facial & arm pain
Jo	No	No	Yes	Yes	No	DF	
Jo	No[4]	Yes	Yes	No	No	BDEF	
Jo	No	No	No	No	No	–	
Jo	Yes	No	Yes	Yes	Yes	AB	
Yes	Yes	No	Yes	Yes	Yes	ABCE	Abnormal muscle tone & spontaneous movements
No	Yes	Yes	No	No	Yes	–	
No	No	Yes	Yes	Yes	No	D	Both had deep cerebral WM abnormalities
No	Yes	No	No	No	No	–	abnormalities
No	No	Yes	Yes	No	No	BCDF	
No	Yes	No	No	Yes	No	normal	
No	No	No	No	No	No	BDEF	
No	No	No	Yes	Yes	No	ADEF	
No	No	No	No	No	Yes	ABC	
No	Yes	Yes	Yes	Yes	No	BCDF	
No	No	Yes	Yes	Yes	No	BDF	Has D157N SNP

*Mutation is novel.

1 A single base deletion results in a 14 amino acid frame-shift starting at residue 417.

2 First author is listed; all dates are either 2007, 2008, or 2009.

3 Partial data previously reported in abstract form (Wu et al 2006; Brenner et al 2009).

4 MRI findings use the notation of Caroli et al. (2007) based on the criteria set by van der Knaap et al. (2001, 2006): (A) white matter abnormalities with frontal predominance, (B) periventricular rim, (C) basal ganglia and thalami abnormalities, (D) brainstem abnormalities, (E) contrast enhancement, (F) spinal cord abnormalities.

TABLE 7.2
Summary of characteristics for Alexander disease patients with GFAP mutations

Clinical sign	Number Displaying Clinical Sign (yes/total = %)[1]								
	Infantile			Juvenile			Adult		
	Male	Female	Total	Male	Female	Total	Male	Female	Total
Numbers of patients	50	39	91/149 = 61%	24	10	34/149 = 23%	13	10	24/149 = 16%
Macrocephaly	33/50 = 66%	25/39 = 64%	59/91 = 65%	8/24 = 33%	1/10 = 10%	9/34 = 26%	0/13 = 0%	0/10 = 0%	0/24 = 0%
Seizure	39/49 = 80%	29/39 = 74%	69/90 = 77%	11/24 = 46%	3/10 = 30%	14/34 = 41%	0/13 = 0%	0/10 = 0%	0/24 = 0%
Spasticity	20/37 = 54%	16/27 = 59%	37/65 = 57%	11/24 = 46%	2/10 = 20%	13/34 = 38%	7/13 = 54%	4/10 = 40%	11/24 = 46%
Bulbar and/or pseudobulbar	22/38 = 58%	14/26 = 54%	36/66 = 55%	21/24 = 88%	8/10 = 80%	29/34 = 85%	11/13 = 85%	10/10 = 100%	22/24 = 92%
Ataxia	10/21 = 48%	11/18 = 61%	21/40 = 53%	10/21 = 48%	3/8 = 38%	13/29 = 45%	9/13 = 69%	7/10 = 70%	17/24 = 71%
Developmental delay or regression	41/47 = 87%	33/36 = 92%	75/84 = 89%	13/24 = 54%	2/10 = 20%	15/34 = 44%	1/13 = 8%	0/10 = 0%	1/24 = 4%

Data shown are from Table 7.1 of this chapter combined with Table 24.2 of Brenner et al. (2009). For familial cases, entries are for the proband. Asymptomatic patients are not included. Totals vary because of incomplete reporting.

[1] Totals (%) for "Numbers of patients" are the percentage of all cases with *GFAP* mutations that fall within that onset form. All other values are for the % of patients within the given onset category that display the indicated clinical sign.

this patient includes seizures as part of his clinical description (Romano et al. 2007), whereas another does not (Caroli et al. 2007).

Although in a few instances Alexander disease may have a fluctuating course, at least in its early stages (Pareyson et al. 2008), it is nearly always progressive, with most cases eventually leading to death. The rate of progression tends to be faster the earlier the onset. The mean lifespan for infantile patients is about 4 years after presentation, juvenile patients survive about 8 years after presentation and adult-onset patients (based on 4 patients) 14 years (Pareyson et al. 2008, Brenner et al. 2009). However, these numbers are generalizations; some infantile-onset patients have survived for over 20 years, whereas a recently reported adult-onset patient died just 2 months after presentation (Huttner et al. 2007). Nor does death always result; several studies of familial cases have identified individuals carrying the same *GFAP* mutation as an affected family member, yet who display no or very mild clinical signs (Okamoto et al. 2002, Shiihara et al. 2002, Stumpf et al. 2003, Balbi et al. 2008, Pareyson et al. 2008). Interestingly, in four of these five families the asymptomatic member was female. This is consistent with the data presented in Table 7.2, which indicate that males are more likely than females to be diagnosed for each of the three forms of Alexander disease. This difference reaches statistical significance for the juvenile form ($p = 0.016$) and for total cases ($p = 0.02$). In the transitional juvenile form the symptoms of males tend to be more like the infantile cases and those of females more like adult cases, although the numbers are too low for the differences to reach statistical significance ($p = 0.06$ for the sex difference in developmental delay).

MRI characteristics

A major diagnostic advance was the specification of a set of five MRI criteria common to many cases of infantile and juvenile Alexander disease (van der Knaap et al. 2001). These were (1) extensive cerebral white matter anomalies in signal intensity with a frontal predominance, (2) increased signal from the periventricular rim in T1-weighted images and a decreased signal on T2-weighting, (3) anomalous signals from the brainstem or thalamus, (4) brainstem abnormalities, and (5) increased signal with contrast (Fig. 7.1A). The presence of four of these criteria was proposed as sufficient for an accurate diagnosis. Generally, these MRI features do not change much over a period of several years (van der Knaap et al. 2001, Romano et al. 2007), but in at least one instance there was a rapid evolution of characteristic features, prompting the suggestion that MRI analysis be periodically repeated for suspect cases that initially have equivocal findings (Huttner et al. 2007).

These MRI criteria have proved remarkably robust in the hands of neuroradiologists experienced with leukodystrophies (Rodriguez et al. 2001, Gorospe et al. 2002, Li et al. 2005). Subsequently, an MRI feature has been discovered in several later-onset patients that appears to be unique to Alexander disease – a scalloped garland-like signal enhancement on T2-weighting or FLAIR which lines the outer rim of the lateral ventricles (Fig. 7.1B) (van der Knaap et al. 2006). However, both the presence of the garland or the requirement for four of the five other features has been found to be too stringent a criterion for many of the later-onset cases. In these patients abnormalities in cerebral white matter may be in posterior rather than in prefrontal regions (Huttner et al. 2007, Farina et al. 2008), or white

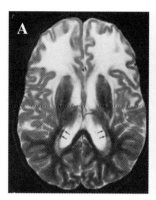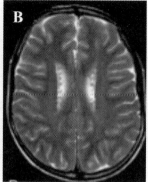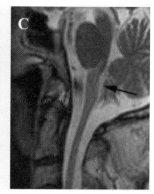

Fig. 7.1. MRIs of Alexander disease patients. **A**: Axial T2-weighted section demonstrating extensive signal abnormalities within the frontal white matter and a thin periventricular rim of low signal intensity (arrows). Both findings are commonly observed in patients with infantile- and juvenile-onset Alexander disease. **B**: Axial T2-weighted section displaying peculiar structures along the ventricular wall, resembling garlands. With the exception of signal abnormalities present in the medulla, hilus of dentate nucleus, and a thin periventricular rim (sections not shown), the remainder of the white matter appeared normal. **C**: Sagittal T2-weighted section characteristic of adult-onset Alexander disease showing atrophy and signal abnormalities in the medulla oblongata. Atrophy was also evident throughout the entire course of the spinal cord. Panel **A** is reproduced with permission from Figure 6A of van der Knaap et al. (2001); panel **B** from Figure 1D of van der Knaap et al. (2006), and panel **C** from Figure 1A of Pareyson et al. (2008).

matter deficits may be undetected. The MRI diagnostic for later-onset cases now appears to be simply brainstem and spinal cord atrophy (Fig. 7.1C) (van der Knaap et al. 2006, Ohnari et al. 2007, Balbi et al. 2008, Farina et al. 2008). Thus the MRI criteria of van der Knaap et al. (2001) have proved very powerful for the positive identification of Alexander disease among younger patients, but different criteria are required for later-onset cases. To date, brainstem and spinal cord atrophy has provided considerable predictive power (Farina et al. 2008), but its diagnostic efficacy for this evolving disease form needs additional verification.

Pathology
The defining feature of Alexander disease is the disseminated presence of Rosenthal fibers, named after the German neuropathologist who first described them in a syringomyelia in 1898 (Rosenthal 1898). The aggregates are eosinophilic and osmiophilic, rendering them readily visible by both light and electron microscopy (Wippold et al. 2006, Brenner et al. 2009). However, the "fiber" part of their designation is a misnomer, as Rosenthal fibers are not actually fibrous in appearance, but can be amorphous or ovoid, with widths ranging from 10 to 40 µm and lengths up to 100 µm. Rosenthal fibers are believed to form first as small clumps in the perinuclear region of the astrocyte, and then to increase in size as they migrate into the processes. These astrocytic inclusions are most often found in subpial, perivascular, and periventricular regions of the CNS, areas which normally show high GFAP levels. In early-onset cases the aggregates are particularly abundant in the more rostral

regions of the CNS; in later-onset cases they may be sparse in the cerebrum, but abundant in the brainstem, cerebellum and spinal cord. Although this suggests a general correlation between the presence of Rosenthal fibers and the affected brain regions, this match does not always hold (Crome 1953, Borrett and Becker 1985, Schwankhaus et al. 1995, Namekawa et al. 2002, Stumpf et al. 2003). Both immunohistochemistry and protein purification procedures have revealed GFAP to be the primary constituent of the aggregates, and the small stress proteins αB-crystallin and HSP27 also to be relatively abundant (Iwaki et al. 1993; Iwaki et al. 1989). More recently, additional proteins have been identified in the Rosenthal fibers, including plectin (Tian et al. 2006), the 20S proteasome subunit and phosphorylated c-Jun N-terminal kinase (Tang et al. 2006). Whether the sequestration of these, or yet to be discovered molecules, in the Rosenthal fibers is responsible for overt disease is an area of active research.

Alexander disease has been grouped within the leukodystrophies because, until recently, all cases displayed white matter lesions, particularly in the frontal lobes. In early-onset cases the deficits can be especially severe, and it is likely that the myelin never forms. In these cases the pathology can progress to a massive cystic lesion. However, later-onset cases have now been described in which no white matter pathology was discerned, and the only apparent pathology was atrophy of the brainstem, cerebellum, and/or spinal cord. This difference in pathology from the infantile form could depend on the relative timing of myelination and disease onset. The frontal lobes are one of the last regions to myelinate, with most myelination occurring during the first two years of age. Thus the frontal lobe myelination period corresponds to the onset period of the infantile form of Alexander disease.

The presence of Rosenthal fibers in astrocytes and the discovery that most cases of Alexander disease are caused by mutations in *GFAP* point to astrocytes as the primary target of the disease. There have been a few reports of decreased numbers of astrocytes in Alexander disease, but documentation of their loss is not generally reported. Similarly, both oligodendrocytes and neurons are clearly affected in this disease, but loss of these cells is also only occasionally mentioned. The astrocytes, particularly those harboring Rosenthal fibers, do appear highly reactive; and activation of microglia, perhaps mediated by the reactive astrocytes, has been observed in both a mouse model and human patients (Hagemann et al. 2005). However, immune infiltrates are not a general feature of the disorder, ruling out an inflammatory component such as is seen in multiple sclerosis.

Diagnosis

Because of its rarity, historically, the diagnosis of Alexander disease for a patient was pursued only after more common disorders with similar presentations had been excluded. The identification of MRI criteria for typical early-onset cases opened a more direct route to diagnosis for the majority of cases – those that present at a young age with typical clinical and MRI signs. The diagnosis can then be confirmed by *GFAP* gene sequencing, which has revealed a mutation in about 95% of cases analyzed (see below). For atypical and later-onset cases the diagnosis continues to be more serpentine. For these the clinical presentations are usually non-specific bulbar and pseudobulbar signs. However, even these have been absent from some adult-onset patients, who instead have presented with lower limb weakness (Pareyson et al. 2008). Multiple sclerosis or a tumor is sometimes the initial diagnosis. MRI findings are only sometimes helpful, as just one of the initially specified criteria may be met. Recently, authors have suggested that adult-onset Alexander disease should be considered for any patient displaying ataxia and palatal myoclonus (Delnooz et al. 2008, Howard et al. 2008) or simply atrophy of the brainstem, cerebellum, or spinal cord (Pareyson et al. 2008). Brainstem auditory evoked potentials were also found to be abnormal in all seven of a series of adult-onset cases examined (Pareyson et al. 2008), and observations in a mouse model of Alexander disease also suggested effects on the auditory brainstem response (Masuda et al. 2008). The auditory response was unaffected under normal conditions, but the mutant mice were more susceptible to noise-induced hearing loss due to cochlear damage, perhaps caused by Rosenthal fibers in the central portion of the cochlear nerve. The GFAP level has been found to be elevated in the cerebrospinal fluid (CSF) of three Alexander disease patients (Kyllerman et al. 2005), but is also increased in other instances of CNS disease or injury (Liem and Messing, 2009). The extent to which CSF levels of GFAP will prove useful for either diagnosis or monitoring the progression of treatment remains to be established. Thus, elimination of more common disorders continues to be the main route toward diagnosis of Alexander disease for these more challenging cases. Recent papers by Romano et al. (2007) and Farina et al. (2008) provide details for the differential diagnosis of adult-onset Alexander disease, and a review of all cases tested for *GFAP* mutations is presented in Pareyson et al. (2008).

Prior to development of reliable MRI criteria and the discovery of the association of *GFAP* mutations with Alexander disease, a biopsy or autopsy was necessary for a definitive diagnosis. This is still required for cases in which no *GFAP* mutation was found. However, biopsy results can be equivocal, because other disorders, such as pilocytic astrocytomas, can result in the focal appearance of Rosenthal fibers. Thus it is the widespread presence of the protein aggregates in at least some of the typical locations (subpial, perivascular, periventricular) that is diagnostic. A remaining complication is that disseminated Rosenthal fibers have also been found in persons who had autopsies for non-neurological conditions (Jacob et al. 2003). Whether this represents a subclinical stage of Alexander disease is not clear. It would be of considerable interest to determine if such persons carried *GFAP* mutations.

The presence of a de-novo *GFAP* mutation in a suspected Alexander disease patient is considered diagnostic proof of the disease. However, it is not always possible to test the parents of a patient to determine whether the mutation indeed newly occurred. Other criteria that can then be used to evaluate the disease association of the mutation are discussed in the following section. For the 5% of Alexander disease patients for whom *GFAP* mutations have not been found, definitive diagnosis presently can only be made at autopsy. A recent report for a single adult-onset patient raises the possibility that abnormal accumulation of F-18-ethyltyrosine in the medulla oblongata may assist diagnosis (Huttner et al. 2007).

When a *GFAP* mutation is discovered in an Alexander disease patient, the question arises as to whether other family members should be tested for its presence. As just noted, if the mutation has not previously been clearly linked to Alexander disease, testing of the parents can be important for determining causality. Testing of adult sibs of the patient may also be considered. Although most of the *GFAP* mutations arise de novo and are not detected in the parents, nearly all are likely to have originated in one of the parent's germ lines, particularly the father's (Li et al. 2006). This raises the possibility that additional children could carry the same mutation. The frequency of a second transmission of a mutation due to such germline mosaicism is as high as 30% for some genetic diseases (Zlotogora 1998), but has been extremely low for Alexander disease. Excluding identical twins, no instance has been reported of more than one affected child in over 50 instances in which the disease arose from a de-novo mutation (Table 7.3 of this chapter, and Table 24.3 in Brenner et al. 2009). Although the likelihood of having another affected child thus appears quite low, the severe consequences of Alexander disease may dissuade parents from having additional children. In such cases prenatal diagnosis is an option. The availability of fetal diagnosis may also prompt adult sibs of a patient to consider testing if they are of child- bearing age. Since there are no effective treatments for Alexander disease, non-symptomatic minor sibs of an affected child are not tested for ethical reasons (Duncan et al. 2008).

GFAP mutations

The chance observation that mice over-expressing GFAP produced abundant Rosenthal fibers led to investigation of *GFAP* as a candidate gene for Alexander disease. *GFAP* mutations were found in 12 of the 13 cases first studied (Brenner et al. 2001), all but one of which were early onset. These analyses were soon expanded to both additional infantile patients and those with the later-onset forms, with mutations being found in about 95% of the patients in each category (Rodriguez et al. 2001, Gorospe et al. 2002, Li et al. 2005). The positions of these mutations relative to the protein structure of GFAP are shown in Figure 7.2.

All of the mutations identified have been heterozygous, establishing a dominant mode of action. Most are simple mis-sense changes, in which one amino acid is substituted for another. A few small in-frame insertions or deletions have been also detected, as well as an intronic mutation resulting in an in-frame excision of exon 4. No mutation has been detected in the promoter of the gene, or that results in either a frame-shift or a termination codon, except at the extreme C-terminal region of the protein. This absence of truncated alleles (which would be expected to be recessive) argues that the mutations cause a dominant gain of function rather than loss of function. A gain of function is also supported by the findings that GFAP-null mice do not display signs of Alexander disease but instead are relatively healthy (Gomi et al. 1995, Pekny et al. 1995, McCall et al. 1996), and that the astrocytes of human patients have abundant quantities of normal-appearing GFAP filaments.

A number of the *GFAP* mutations are homologous to disease-causing mutations in other intermediate filaments. These include the hotspot mutations at R79 and R239 (Li et al. 2002). Curiously, *loss* of function has been inferred for these other intermediate filament mutations because the corresponding filament network is disrupted in the affected cells; some patients are homozygous for truncated alleles and null mice show similar disease characteristics (Fuchs 1996, Li et al. 2002). This apparent mechanistic contradiction between Alexander disease and other intermediate filament disorders has been explained by postulating that the mutations indeed affect a common polymerization step, but do so only

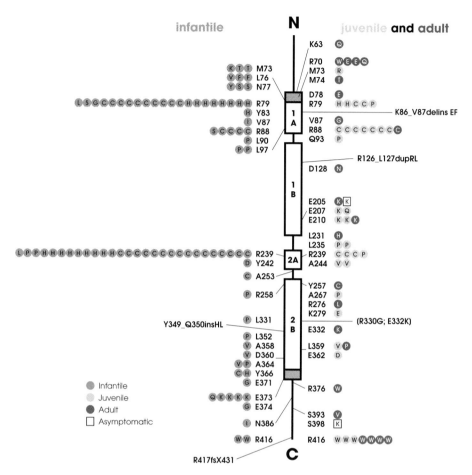

Fig. 7.2. Locations of *GFAP* mutations in Alexander disease in relation to the protein structure. The four open rectangular boxes represent the helical coiled–coil rod domains of GFAP; these structural motifs are highly conserved among most intermediate filament proteins. The solid lines joining these segments are non-helical linker regions, and the solid lines at either end are the non-conserved, random coil, N-terminal and C-terminal regions. The gray box just before segment 1A is a non-conserved prehelical sequence important for initiation of rod formation at the start of 1A; the gray box at the end of 2B represents the highly conserved 365TYRKLLEGEE374 sequence that includes the end of the coiled-coil 2B segment at E371. The wild-type amino acid is indicated next to the structure, and amino acid replacements within symbols on either side. Infantile cases are on the left, shown as blue circles; juvenile and adult cases are on the right, as orange and red circles, respectively, and asymptomatic cases as white squares. Each symbol represents a single patient, except that familial cases, including identical twins, are represented by a single symbol coded for the onset type of the proband. This figure is a modification and update of Figure 24.4 in Brenner et al. (2009) and a color version is available in the Plate section.

partially. The resultant biological effects of this kinetic bottle-neck then depend on the relative levels of the intermediate filament protein precursors as well as the biological roles of the assembled filaments (Li et al. 2002, Brenner et al. 2009).

Inspection of Figure 7.2 indicates some genotype–phenotype correlations among the mutations. For example, all R239H mutations identified have been associated with severe, rapid onset disease, whereas mutations in the 1B rod segment are associated with a later onset. On the other hand, other mutations such as R79C, R88C, and R416W are present in patients with both early and late onset Alexander disease, suggesting that additional genetic or environmental factors can significantly influence disease onset and progression. The possible structural basis for some of the genotype–phenotype correlations is discussed in Li et al. (2005) and Brenner et al. (2009).

Not all coding changes in the *GFAP* gene necessarily produce Alexander disease. Probable polymorphisms include P47L, D157N, E223Q, and D295N (E223Q is discussed below, for the others see Brenner et al. 2009.) Several criteria have been described to help determine whether a *GFAP* gene alteration is indeed disease-causing or is an innocuous variant (Brenner et al. 2009). The most powerful is finding that the mutation arose de novo; that is, it was not found in either of the parents. The probability that this would occur by chance for a gene the size of *GFAP* is less than 1 in 20 000 (Drake et al. 1998). Since nearly all known *GFAP* mutations are 100% penetrant (see below), parents are generally not tested if the mutation has previously been shown to arise de novo in another Alexander disease case. Even if a mutation has not been shown to arise de novo, there is still a high level of confidence that it is disease-causing: (a) if it affects an amino acid previously shown to be mutated de novo (but to a different amino acid); (b) if it is reported for two or more independent Alexander disease cases (especially if one or more displays typical clinical signs and MRIs); (c) if the mutant protein fails to form normal appearing filaments when expressed in cultured cells, or (d) if the mutation is present in sufficient numbers in an affected family.

Fulfilling one or more of these criteria should be a requirement for publishing a new *GFAP* mutation as disease-causing. The extent to which *GFAP* mutations associated with Alexander disease have met these criteria is documented in Table 23.4 of Brenner et al. (2009) for cases reported up to early 2007, and Table 7.3 of this chapter provides an update for subsequent reports through 2008.

Another criterion commonly cited in publications is the degree of conservation of the affected amino acid, but this appears of little value for ascertaining the role of a *GFAP* mutation in Alexander disease. On theoretical grounds, the underlying assumption is that a highly conserved residue has a critical function, so that its alteration would likely be deleterious. This logic is reasonable for loss-of-function mutations, but questionable for gain-of-function mutations such as occur in Alexander disease. On the practical side, there is 65% amino acid conservation among the six GFAP proteins listed in the ProSite database (human, mouse, rat, cow, orangutan, zebrafish; the identity is over 90% if zebrafish is excluded), so there is high probability that any amino acid selected at random will be conserved. Extending the homology to all species of the other type III intermediate filaments, viz. vimentin (12 species) and desmin (10 species), still leaves overall homology at 55%.

117

TABLE 7.3
Evidence for disease causality of new novel mutations

Mutation	Exon	De Novo?	Control Chromo	Func Test	Same Site?	Ref[6]
R70Q	1	Mo only[3]	210	ND	Yes	Caroli
R73K	1	Yes	210	ND	Yes	Caroli
M74T	1	ND	400	ND	No	Ohnari
R79P	1	Yes	210	ND	Yes	Caroli
Y83H[1]	1	Yes	100	ND	No	Wu
D128N*	1	ND	100	ND	No	Pareyson
E205K*	3	ND	100	ND	No	Pareyson
L231H*	4	ND	210	ND	No	Delnooz
Y257C	4	ND	ND	Yes	No	Howard
A267P	5	Yes	192	ND	No	Hinttala
R330G/E332K	6	ND	200	Yes	No	Balbi; Bachetti
E332K	6	ND	100	Yes	No	Pareyson; Bachetti
L359P	6	No[4]	210	ND	Yes	Romano; Caroli; Pareyson
A364V	6	Yes	250	ND	Yes	Hartmann
Y366C	6	Yes	250	ND	Yes	Hartmann
R376W*	7	ND	ND	ND	No	Hirayama
S393I*	8	ND	100	ND	No	Salmaggi
S398Y	8	ND	100	ND	Yes[5]	Pareyson
D417fs[2]	8	Yes	ND	ND	NA	Murakami

Data are presented for novel mutations reported since completion of Brenner et al. (2009) (see Table 24.3 of that reference for data for previously reported mutations). As discussed in the text, strong evidence that a mutation is disease-causing includes at least one of the following (column heading in parentheses): it arose de novo (De novo?); it was not present in at least 400 control chromosomes (Control chromo), the mutant protein assembles aberrantly in transfected cells (Func test) or a previously described Alexander disease mutation altered the same amino acid (Same site?). Newly described mutations that do not meet any of these criteria are indicated by an asterisk (*).

ND = not done.

1 Partial data previously reported in abstract form (Wu et al. 2006, Brenner et al. 2009)
2 Deletion of a G leading to a 14 amino acid frame-shift starting at position 417; shown to arise de novo in an independent case (D. Flint and M. Brenner, unpublished).
3 Only the mother was available for testing, and she was negative for the mutation.
4 An initial report in Caroli et al. (2007) that the mutation arose de novo was corrected in Pareyson et al. (2008).
5 Same mutation independently found in an unpublished patient (listed at http://www.waisman.wisc.edu/alexander/)
6 First author is listed; all dates are either 2007, 2008, or 2009.

It might be expected that the converse, lack of homology, might at least serve as an exclusionary criterion, but this also fails. Several of the de-novo mutations change amino acids that are not conserved among GFAP species (e.g., M74, A244, E332). It is even risky to assume that a mutation is innocuous because it changes an amino acid in human GFAP to one found in another species. An A53T change in α-synuclein produces Parkinson disease in humans (Polymeropoulos et al. 1997), but in mice, threonine is the normal amino acid at this position.

Absence of a mutation in ethnically matched controls is a criterion whose power increases with the number of chromosomes analyzed. As will be noted below, E223Q was given support as an Alexander disease mutation by its absence in 150 control chromosomes, but was subsequently detected when 400 additional controls were analyzed. The putative polymorphism D157N was not detected in 100 control chromosomes by Pareyson et al. (2008), but was found in 5 out of 100 control chromosomes by Li et al. (2005). On the other hand, Li et al. did not find the presumed polymorphism V115I in any of 100 control chromosomes. These limited examples suggest that in the order of 400 control chromosomes should be analyzed for a reasonable level of confidence that a mutation causes disease.

Criteria such as de-novo occurrence or grossly aberrant polymerization of the mutant protein provide strong assurance that a mutation is disease-causing. Their absence, however, is not compelling negative evidence. When a patient's gene-change is also found in a neuro-logically normal parent, it may be because it is just an innocuous variant, but it is also pos-sible that the mutation causes disease but is incompletely penetrant. For example, its effects could depend on other environmental or genetic factors, or the disease might appear as the individual ages. In several instances asymptomatic family members have been documented to carry the same mutation that is strongly implicated as being disease-causing for the affected proband (Brenner et al. 2009). Normal polymerization properties of an altered GFAP following cell transfection also does not rule out a disease-causing role, with the A244V mutation being an example (Li et al. 2005).

The E223Q coding change provides an illustrative example of the difficulty that can be encountered in trying to determine whether a GFAP alteration is disease-causing. This change was first reported as the sole coding difference present in an adult patient, suspected to have Alexander disease based on clinical signs and MRIs (Brockmann et al. 2003). Conservation of E223 among human, mouse, rat, and cow and its absence among 150 control chromosomes were cited to support a disease role for the change. However, it was present in the patient's mother, who did not display signs of Alexander disease, and aspects of the patient's medical history other than Alexander disease could have accounted for the clinical signs. The E223Q change was subsequently found in two independent patients, each of whom more clearly fit an Alexander disease diagnosis (Li et al. 2005, Dotti et al. 2009). However, in each case the E223Q was also present in an unaffected parent, and more importantly, each patient had an additional *GFAP* mutation which had arisen de novo. Thus it was not necessary to invoke a causative role for E223Q for either of these patients.

These findings prompted a further analysis of normal controls, with the discovery that one chromosome among the 400 additionally tested carried the E223Q change (Dotti et al. 2009), for a total frequency among controls of one in 550. The polymerization properties of the E223Q GFAP were also examined, with the ambiguous finding that normal filaments formed, but the bundles appeared somewhat thicker than those formed by the wild type. The presence of E223Q in a normal control strongly argues for the change being a rare but innocuous variant. But it is curious that E223Q appeared in three different patients with possible Alexander disease (a frequency of about 3 out of 280 chromosomes examined), but in only one out of 550 control chromosomes, a difference that is statistically significant. The possibility that E223Q has a role in disease under certain circumstances cannot therefore be completely excluded. A further discussion of mutations of uncertain consequence is provided in Brenner et al. (2009).

Cases without *GFAP* mutations

GFAP mutations have not been found in 7 of the 162 cases reported (Table 7.1 of this chapter and Table 24.1 of Brenner et al. 2009). The actual frequency could be greater, since a negative finding may be interpreted as eliminating Alexander disease as a diagnosis. In the absence of a *GFAP* mutation, only an autopsy can provide definitive evidence for Alexander disease. It is possible that these presumptive *GFAP*-negative cases actually do have mutations in the gene. Several different splice forms of GFAP have been described, including ones whose coding sequence includes regions within introns of the standard GFAP isoform, GFAPα (Quinlan et al. 2007). Perng et al. (2008) have recently shown that one of these, GFAPδ, is capable of co-assembly with GFAPα, and can affect the biological properties of the filaments formed. Interestingly, one of the patients lacking a standard *GFAP*-coding mutation is a compound heterozygote for nucleotide changes that would affect the sequence of GFAPδ, but not GFAPα (M. Brenner, unpublished observations). Whether either of these changes arose de novo, or affect the properties of GFAP filaments, is yet to be determined.

Another *GFAP* mutation that might be missed is one affecting splicing, either by causing exon skipping or introducing additional coding sequence through creation of new splice sites. Given that the *GFAP* mutations appear to act by a dominant gain of function, any such alteration would probably need to produce an in-frame coding change. Just such an event has been observed for a putative Alexander disease patient who carries a mutation that reduces the efficacy of the exon 4 splice acceptor site. The resultant occasional skipping of exon 4 produces an in-frame deleted protein which compromises assembly of normal GFAP (R. Li and M. Brenner, unpublished observations). Both GFAPδ and splicing mutations could escape detection because little if any of the intronic regions are generally sequenced during *GFAP* gene testing.

GFAP mutations could also be missed if the patient is mosaic. The finding that most of the de-novo mutations occur on the paternal chromosome has been interpreted to mean that most arise in the parental germline. However, some mutations could occur post-fertilization, during the development of the embryo. One such instance has been documented by the chance discovery that a *GFAP* mutation readily detected in buccal DNA was absent in blood DNA (D. Flint and M. Brenner, unpublished observations). Since astrocytes are of ectodermal origin, this suggests that buccal swabs (also ectoderm) are preferable to blood (mesodermal) as a DNA source for *GFAP* gene testing. Even with this precaution, more restricted mosaicism could still be missed.

A final class of *GFAP* mutations which could be overlooked is those that increase its expression at the transcriptional or translational level. Gene duplication has been implicated in several neurological disorders, including the gene for lamin B1 to produce adult-onset autosomal dominant leukodystrophy (Padiath et al. 2006), α-synuclein to produce Parkinson's disease (Chartier-Harlin et al. 2004), proteolipid protein to cause Pelizaeus–Merzbacher disease (Sistermans et al. 1998), and peripheral myelin protein 22 to cause Charcot–Marie–Tooth disease (Lupski et al. 1991). It is also possible that alterations as simple as point mutations could elevate GFAP levels by increasing mRNA translation, stability, processing, or synthesis. Finally, those cases of Alexander disease without *GFAP*-

coding mutations could be caused by mutations in other genes (Brenner et al. 2009), or have a non-genetic origin.

Recent cases

Characteristics of all Alexander disease patients through early 2007, who had undergone *GFAP* testing, were reported in Brenner et al. (2009). Table 7.1 provides the corresponding data for subsequently published cases through 2008. Several of these have unusual features.

Vazquez et al. (2008) reported the first instance in which suspicion of Alexander disease was raised by a fetal MRI, which was performed at 33 weeks of gestation following sonographic findings of ventricular enlargement. Two months after birth, DNA sequencing detected an M73T mutation to confirm the diagnosis.

Murakami et al. (2008) reported a 13-month-old boy whose only clinical presentation was psychomotor delay, but whose MRI was typical for infantile Alexander disease. This patient had a heterozygous single base deletion in exon 8 that predicts alteration of the 14 amino acids in positions 417 to 430, followed by a stop signal. Thus the predicted protein would have an altered C-terminal tail and would be 2 amino acids shorter than the wild type. No tests were performed to demonstrate that this frame-shift mutation is actually disease-causing, but we have encountered the identical mutation in another patient and found that it arose de novo (D. Flint and M. Brenner, unpublished observations).

Matej et al. (2008) reported an infantile patient with typical clinical signs and a previously known E373K mutation, but who had some unique pathological features. In addition to typical Rosenthal fibers, numerous large hyaline deposits were also present, with many deposits of both types being extracellular, presumably due to astrocyte deterioration. Rosenthal fibers were also found in the neurohypophyseal pituicytes, extending the reported range for these aggregates. A juvenile case with a novel A267P mutation was typical in most respects, but both MRI and the pathology showed the most severe effects were in the occipital rather than the frontal lobes (Hinttala et al. 2007).

MRI revealed the presence of tumor-like masses in two of the recent case reports. An infantile patient with typical clinical signs and the common R79C mutation appeared to have an optic chiasm tumor which later regressed (Mignot et al. 2009). An adult-onset patient with a novel R376W mutation had an intraventricular tumor with calcification around the foramen of Monro (Hirayama et al. 2008). The possibility that these tumors were coincidental events was raised in each account, but the authors also noted similar indications of tumors in other Alexander disease cases, which suggests that tumors may be an occasional feature of the disease. The patient with the R376W mutation also had an affected 4-year-old son. For both this mother-and-son pair and another with an S393I mutation reported by Salmaggi, et al. (2007), the mother did not display seizures but the son did. Neither the R376W nor the S393I mutation has been established as actually disease-causing (see Table 7.3).

Pareyson et al. (2008) described six new adult-onset Alexander disease cases along with five that had been previously reported. Interesting features of the six new cases include three having familial involvement, two being asymptomatic (one had an MRI for chronic headache and the other for a subarachnoid hemorrhage), and two not displaying the bulbar or pseudobulbar signs found in all previous adult-onset cases (Brenner et al. 2009), but instead presenting with lower limb weakness, presumably due to pyramidal involvement. One of these latter patients, with onset at age 62, is currently the oldest presenting Alexander disease patient with a genetic diagnosis.

Late-onset patients have also been reported by Howard et al. (2008) (58 years) and Balbi et al. (2008) (57 years for the proband of a familial case). This latter familial case has a number of additional unusual features. The *GFAP* alteration consists of a pair of closely linked coding changes, R330G and E332K. These appear to be in the same allele, as they were present in two sisters of the proband and his son. One of the sisters has clinical signs similar to her brother, whereas the other, presently aged 64, is asymptomatic (Table 7.1). The only symptom of the son is the novel presence of severe jabbing pain in the right retromandibular and auricular regions, which commenced at age 28 and later radiated to his shoulder and upper arm. Unique MRI findings included contrast enhancement in the inferior olives of the proband, and nodular T2-weighted hyperintensities in the brainstem of his son. Functional tests of the two coding changes in transfected cells suggested that the E332K alteration is primarily responsible for the disease phenotype (Bachetti et al. 2008), and the subsequent report by Pareyson et al. (2008) included a patient for whom E332K was the sole coding mutation.

Another unique adult-onset case was reported by Huttner et al. (2007). To our knowledge, this was the first patient to have presented with respiratory arrest. He was also the only one to experience severe heart arrhythmias and seizures (although mild cardiovascular abnormalities were noted for patient 11 of Pareyson et al. [2008] and one member of the family described by Stumpf et al. [2003] may have had seizures). This patient also had the shortest survival period for an adult case, dying from hyperthermia just 2 months after presentation. No *GFAP* mutation was found for this patient, but Alexander disease was diagnosed on the basis of several criteria. He displayed the common clinical signs of spasticity, bulbar/pseudobulbar signs and ataxia; his MRIs revealed brainstem and spinal cord lesions and bilateral signal hyperintensities in the basal ganglia, thalami, and periventricular regions; and most importantly, Rosenthal fibers and demyelination were present in multiple brain regions examined at autopsy. The unique clinical features of this patient and the absence of a *GFAP* mutation suggest the possibility of a variant form of Alexander disease.

Half of the 33 recently reported Alexander disease probands summarized in Table 7.1 are adult onset, far greater than the 5% they have historically represented. This increased percentage may in part be due to publication bias; such cases are more likely to be documented because they are still relatively novel, their highly variable nature makes discovery of unique (and thus publishable) clinical features more common than for infantile cases, and they display a greater frequency of novel mutations. But the increased percentage may also reflect evolving diagnostic sophistication. A gene testing service would not be expected to have a bias for onset form, yet between 2004 and 2008 over half (12 out of 21) of the proband Alexander disease cases found to have a *GFAP* mutation by such a laboratory in Genoa, Italy were of the adult-onset form (Pareyson et al. 2008). Given the increasing numbers of adult-onset cases being diagnosed – particularly familial cases in which some family members have mild or absent symptoms – it is possible that these later-onset forms will indeed prove far more common than previously appreciated.

GFAP mutations were found for all but two of the 33 newly reported probands, consistent with the 95% frequency rate previously observed. One of these had a number of unusual features, as discussed above (Hinttala et al. 2007). Novel *GFAP* mutations were detected in the majority of the newly reported cases: 4 out of 13 of the infantile, both of the juvenile and 12 out of the 15 mutations found in adult-onset cases. Again, these high percentages no doubt reflect publication bias, but they also indicate that multiple unique mutations are yet to be discovered. Point mutations have now been found at 66 different nucleotides, resulting in alterations of 46 of the 432 amino acids in the GFAP protein.

Disease mechanisms

It was noted above that Alexander disease is almost certainly not due to a loss of GFAP function, but instead the mutations endow GFAP with a gain of some toxic property. A dominant gain of function mechanism has also been found for several diseases due to mutations in the nuclear lamin intermediate filaments (Worman and Bonne 2007). However, GFAP appears to be unique among cytoplasmic intermediate filaments in this respect; other cytoplasmic intermediate filament disorders result in loss of function diseases (Fuchs 1996). A curious corollary of this difference is that although several of the Alexander disease *GFAP* mutations are highly homologous to ones that cause other cytoplasmic intermediate filament disorders in which normal-appearing intermediate filaments fail to form, in Alexander disease GFAP filaments are abundant (Wippold et al. 2006). Furthermore, these normal appearing filaments (as well as the Rosenthal fibers) have been shown to contain both wild type and mutant GFAP (Der Perng et al. 2006).

An explanation of these paradoxes is that the pathways to filament formation and aggregate formation are not mutually exclusive, but continually operate at relative rates that are dependent on the levels of GFAP monomer and other interacting proteins in the cell (Li et al. 2002, Tian et al. 2006, Mignot et al. 2007, Perng et al. 2008).

It has been suggested that the toxic species in Alexander disease is an intermediate in the GFAP polymerization process (Li et al. 2002), consistent with current thinking for other protein aggregate diseases such as Alzheimer disease (Santacruz et al. 2005), Parkinson disease (Nuber et al. 2008), and Huntington disease (Bodner et al. 2006). Supporting the possibility that a preaggregate form of mutant GFAP has biological effects is the observation of Yoshida et al. (2007) that only about 3% of U251 cells transfected with a mutant *GFAP* expression vector form aggregates, yet there is about a 50% increase in migration rate. Similarly, in a study of primary astrocytes derived from GFAP model mice, Cho and Messing (2008) found effects on cell division, viability, and hydrogen peroxide sensitivity that were disproportionate to the numbers of cells with aggregates. On the other hand, Mignot, et al. (2007) suggested that it is the aggregates that are toxic, because they observed that expression of mutant GFAP in primary astrocytes produced significant cell death only in cells with large, perinuclear aggregates. A caveat for the Mignot et al. and Yoshida et al. studies is that analyses were performed using green fluorescent protein (GFP)-tagged GFAP, which itself has been shown to have deleterious effects on GFAP assembly (Perng et al. 2008).

The nature of the toxic effect is an active area of investigation. The myelination defects are common in infantile cases, but mild or absent in the later-onset forms. This suggests that Alexander disease interferes with the myelination process, but not with its maintenance once formed. A possible target is the oligodendrocyte precursor. This cell type may be killed by elevated levels of iron, tumor necrosis factor-α, or glutamate, all of which may occur in Alexander disease (Brenner et al. 2009).

Prompted by their prior observations that Rosenthal fibers contain ubiquitin and the small stress proteins αB-crystallin and HSP27 (Iwaki et al. 1989, 1993), the Goldman laboratory investigated the possibility that the mutant GFAP induces a stress response and perturbs protein degradation. Both have been substantiated and also shown to be inter-connected (Liem and Messing 2009). Expression of Alexander disease mutant GFAP in cultured astrocytes activates the Jun N-terminal kinase (JNK) pathway, inhibits proteasome activity, and stimulates autophagy (Tang et al. 2006, 2008). Furthermore, potential positive feedback loops were discovered; both inhibition of proteasome activity and activation of JNK increased GFAP levels, with the JNK activation perhaps acting through its known inhibition of proteasome activity. Such positive-feedback loops could exacerbate disease progression. The extent to which these alterations contribute to the clinical features of Alexander disease is yet to be determined.

Several mouse models of Alexander disease have been developed to try to discern the disease mechanism (Brenner et al. 2009). The first of these was the human GFAP over-expressing mouse, whose Rosenthal fiber production led to the discovery of *GFAP* mutations in the disease. Additional models include a standard transgenic line expressing the mutant human R239H GFAP, and two mouse lines in which the mouse equivalent of the human R239H and R79H mutations have been inserted into the endogenous mouse gene. Each of these models displays abundant Rosenthal fibers, demonstrating that either overproduction of wild-type GFAP or the presence of mutant GFAP can generate these aggregates. However, none of the mice displays many of the other signs of Alexander disease. No myelin defects have been noted, there is no megalencephaly, and no seizures or movement disorders. The mice do display a strong oxidative stress response in their brains and excess accumulation of iron, especially in astrocytes. They are also much more prone to seizures following kainic acid treatment, which may be relevant to the seizure activity present in many Alexander disease patients.

The initiating lesion in Alexander disease occurs in astrocytes, but the clinical mani-festations reflect defective oligodendrocyte and neuronal functions. It is not known whether the connecting link is a loss of astrocytes, their aberrant function, or both. Loss of astrocytes has been documented only occasionally in patients' brains, but as noted above, decreased growth and viability have been observed in cell culture models (Mignot et al. 2007, Cho and Messing 2008). Possible aberrant functions that could be toxic to neurons and oligodendrocytes include decreased glutamate transport and increased release of cytokines. A significant reduction in the primary astrocyte glutamate transporter, Glt 1, has recently been observed in the mouse models (Hagemann et al. 2009). Given the multiple ways in which astrocytes are now considered to support oligodendrocyte and neuronal development, maintenance, and activity, it is possible that the clinical presentations of Alexander disease arise from many different failed functions of astrocytes.

Treatment

Presently there is neither a cure for Alexander disease nor a means to halt its relentless progression. Current treatment is targeted to palliative support and alleviating symptoms, such as drugs to control seizures or vomiting, and feeding tubes for nourishment. As the pathways that lead from the *GFAP* mutations to clinical signs become delineated, therapeutic targets may become evident. For example, should reduced glutamate transport prove to be a key factor, drugs to increase transport could be administered. Such drugs are already being developed for treatment of other neurological disorders, such as amyotrophic lateral sclerosis and neuropathic pain (Rothstein et al. 2005, Tawfik et al. 2008). Another potential therapeutic target is increased production of the small stress protein αB-crystallin, which has been found to have protective effects in mouse models of Alexander disease (Hagemann et al. 2009). On the other hand, as mentioned above, it is possible that multiple failed functions of astrocytes contribute to the disease. If this is the case, inhibiting *GFAP* expression may be the best therapy. This might be accomplished by limiting the reactive response of astrocytes, or by specifically targeting GFAP levels. The finding that GFAP-null mice show neither signs of Alexander disease nor display significant deficiencies suggests this approach may have benign side effects. A key assumption to this approach is that the toxic activities of the mutant GFAP, once in place, can be reversed. This seems likely, since reversal of protein aggregate disorders has been demonstrated in mouse models for liver disease (Mallory–Denk bodies) (Harada et al. 2008), spinocerebellar ataxia type 1 (Zu et al. 2004), and Huntington disease (Yamamoto et al. 2000). Furthermore, Mignot et al. (2007) observed that mutant GFAP aggregates sometimes spontaneously disappeared from transfected primary astrocytes. Dr Daniel Bonthius, at the University of Iowa, is investigating the use of virally delivered RNAi to knockdown synthesis of the mutant GFAP. Questions critical to this approach are what fraction of astrocytes must be rendered functionally normal to prevent clinical symptoms and can this level of conversion be achieved. Dr Albee Messing, at the University of Wisconsin, is screening an NINDS panel of drugs for their ability to reduce GFAP expression. Since these drugs are already approved for CNS use in humans, promising candidates could relatively quickly be used in the clinic.

Concluding remarks

Recognition of the multiple forms of Alexander disease continues to rapidly evolve. For example, the disorder can no longer be considered solely as a leukodystrophy or a disease of the young. Given the increasing numbers of later-onset cases reported and their frequent transmission, Alexander disease may also prove to be much more common than previously appreciated. Major questions remaining are the cause of the disease in patients who do not harbor a *GFAP* mutation, and how the known mutations result in the observed clinical deficits. Present knowledge of disease mechanisms, although currently limited, is already guiding translational research toward a cure.

Acknowledgments

We thank Dr Mark Beasley for statistical analyses and Dr Albee Messing for comments on the manuscript. This work was supported by an IDDRC grant P30HD038985 and NINDS grant P01NS42803.

REFERENCES

Alexander WS. (1949) Progressive fibrinoid degeneration of fibrillary astrocytes associated with mental retardation in a hydrocephalic infant. Brain 72(3): 373–81, 3 pl.

Bachetti T, Caroli F, Bocca P, et al. (2008) Mild functional effects of a novel GFAP mutant allele identified in a familial case of adult-onset Alexander disease. Eur J Hum Genet 16(4): 462–70.

Balbi P, Seri M, Ceccherini I, et al. (2008) Adult-onset Alexander disease: report on a family. J Neurol 255(1): 24–30.

Bodner RA, Outeiro TF, Altmann S, et al. (2006) Pharmacological promotion of inclusion formation: a therapeutic approach for Huntington's and Parkinson's diseases. Proc Natl Acad Sci USA 103(11): 4246–51.

Borrett D, Becker LE. (1985) Alexander's disease. A disease of astrocytes. Brain 108(Pt 2): 367–385.

Brenner M, Goldman JE, Quinlan RA, Messing A. (2009) Alexander disease: a genetic disorder of astrocytes. In: Parpura V, Haydon P, Eds. Astrocytes in (patho)Physiology of the Nervous System. New York: Springer, pp. 591–648.

Brenner M, Johnson AB, Boespflug-Tanguy O, Rodriguez D, Goldman JE, Messing A. (2001) Mutations in GFAP, encoding glial fibrillary acidic protein, are associated with Alexander disease. Nat Genet 27(1): 117–120.

Brockmann K, Meins M, Taubert A, Trappe R, Grond M, Hanefeld F. (2003) A novel GFAP mutation and disseminated white matter lesions: adult Alexander disease? Eur Neurol 50(2): 100–105.

Caroli F, Biancheri R, Seri M, et al. (2007) GFAP mutations and polymorphisms in 13 unrelated Italian patients affected by Alexander disease. Clin Genet 72(5): 427–433.

Chartier-Harlin MC, Kachergus J, Roumier C, et al. (2004) Alpha-synuclein locus duplication as a cause of familial Parkinson's disease. Lancet 364(9440): 1167–1169.

Cho W, Messing A. (2008) Properties of astrocytes cultured from GFAP over-expressing and GFAP mutant mice. Exp Cell Res 315: 1260–1272.

Crome L (1953) Megalencephaly associated with hyaline pan-neuropathy. Brain 76(2): 215–228.

Delnooz CC, Schelhaas JH, van de Warrenburg BP, de Graaf RJ, Salomons GS. (2008) Alexander disease causing hereditary late-onset ataxia with only minimal white matter changes: a report of two sibs. Mov Disord 23(11): 1613–1615.

Der Perng M, Su M, Wen SF, et al. (2006) The Alexander disease-causing glial fibrillary acidic protein mutant, R416W, accumulates into Rosenthal fibers by a pathway that involves filament aggregation and the association of alpha b-crystallin and HSP27. Am J Hum Genet 79(2): 197–213.

Dotti MT, Buccoliero R, Lee A, et al. (2009) An infantile case of Alexander disease unusual for its MRI features and a GFAP allele carrying both the p.Arg79His mutation and the p.Glu223Gln coding variant. J Neurol 256: 679–682.

Drake JW, Charlesworth B, Charlesworth D, Crow JF. (1998) Rates of spontaneous mutation. Genetics 148(4): 1667–1686.

Duncan RE, Gillam L, Savulescu J, Williamson R, Rogers JG, Delatycki MB. (2008) "You're one of us now": young people describe their experiences of predictive genetic testing for Huntington disease (HD) and familial adenomatous polyposis (FAP). Am J Med Genet C Semin Med Genet 148C(1): 47–55.

Farina L, Pareyson D, Minati L, et al. (2008) Can MR imaging diagnose adult-onset Alexander disease? AJNR Am J Neuroradiol 29(6): 1190–1196.

Fuchs E. 1996. The cytoskeleton and disease: genetic disorders of intermediate filaments. Annu Rev Genet 30: 197–231.

Gomi H, Yokoyama T, Fujimoto K, et al. (1995) Mice devoid of the glial fibrillary acidic protein develop normally and are susceptible to scrapie prions. Neuron 14(1): 29–41.

Gorospe JR, Maletkovic J. (2006) Alexander disease and megalencephalic leukoencephalopathy with subcortical cysts: leukodystrophies arising from astrocyte dysfunction. Ment Retard Dev Disabil Res Rev 12(2): 113–122.

Gorospe JR, Naidu S, Johnson AB, et al. (2002) Molecular findings in symptomatic and pre-symptomatic Alexander disease patients. Neurology 58(10): 1494–500.

Hagemann TL, Boelens WC, Wawrousek EF, Messing A. (2009) Suppression of GFAP toxicity by aB-crystallin in mouse models of Alexander disease. Hum Mol Genet 18(7):1190–1199.

Hagemann TL, Gaeta SA, Smith MA, Johnson DA, Johnson JA, Messing A. (2005) Gene expression analysis in mice with elevated glial fibrillary acidic protein and Rosenthal fibers reveals a stress response followed by glial activation and neuronal dysfunction. Hum Mol Genet 14(16): 2443–2458. E-pub 2005 Jul 13.

Harada M, Hanada S, Toivola DM, Ghori N, Omary MB. (20080 Autophagy activation by rapamycin eliminates mouse Mallory–Denk bodies and blocks their proteasome inhibitor-mediated formation. Hepatology 47(6): 2026–2035.

Hartmann H, Herchenbach J, Stephani U, et al. (2007) Novel mutations in exon 6 of the GFAP gene affect a highly conserved if motif in the rod domain 2B and are associated with early onset infantile Alexander disease. Neuropediatrics 38(3): 143–147.

Hinttala R, Karttunen V, Karttunen A, Herva R, Uusimaa J, Remes AM. (2007) Alexander disease with occipital predominance and a novel c.799G>C mutation in the GFAP gene. Acta Neuropathol 114(5): 543–545.

Hirayama T, Fukae J, Noda K, et al. (2008) Adult-onset Alexander disease with palatal myoclonus and intraventricular tumour. Eur J Neurol 15(2): e16–17.

Howard KL, Hall DA, Moon M, Agarwal P, Newman E, Brenner M. (2008) Adult-onset Alexander disease with progressive ataxia and palatal tremor. Mov Disord 23(1): 118–122.

Huttner HB, Richter G, Hildebrandt M, et al. (2007) Acute onset of fatal vegetative symptoms: unusual presentation of adult Alexander disease. Eur J Neurol 14(11): 1251–1255.

Iwaki T, Iwaki A, Tateishi J, Sakaki Y, Goldman JE. (1993) Alpha B-crystallin and 27-kd heat shock protein are regulated by stress conditions in the central nervous system and accumulate in Rosenthal fibers. Am J Pathol 143(2): 487–495.

Iwaki T, Kume-Iwaki A, Liem RK, Goldman JE. (1989) Alpha B-crystallin is expressed in non-lenticular tissues and accumulates in Alexander's disease brain. Cell 57(1): 71–78.

Jacob J, Robertson NJ, Hilton DA. (2003) The clinicopathological spectrum of Rosenthal fibre encephalopathy and Alexander's disease: a case report and review of the literature. J Neurol Neurosurg Psychiatry 74(6): 807–810.

Kyllerman M, Rosengren L, Wiklund LM, Holmberg E. (2005) Increased levels of GFAP in the cerebrospinal fluid in three subtypes of genetically confirmed Alexander disease. Neuropediatrics 36(5): 319–323.

Li R, Johnson AB, Salomons G, et al. (2005) Glial fibrillary acidic protein mutations in infantile, juvenile, and adult forms of Alexander disease. Ann Neurol 57(3): 310–326.

Li R, Johnson AB, Salomons GS, van der Knaap MS, et al. (2006) Propensity for paternal inheritance of de novo mutations in Alexander disease. Hum Genet 119(1–2): 137–144.

Li R, Messing A, Goldman J, Brenner M. (2002) GFAP mutations in Alexander disease. Int J Dev Neurosci 20(3–5): 259–268.

Liem RKH, Messing A. (2009) Dysfunctions of neuronal and glial intermediate filaments in disease. J Clin Invest 119(7): 1814–1824.

Lupski JR, de Oca-Luna RM, Slaugenhaupt S, et al. (1991) DNA duplication associated with Charcot–Marie–Tooth disease type 1A. Cell 66(2): 219–232.

Masuda M, Tanaka KF, Kanzaki S, et al. (2008) GFAP aggregates in the cochlear nerve increase the noise vulnerability of sensory cells in the organ of Corti in the murine model of Alexander disease. Neurosci Res 62(1): 15–24.

Matej R, Dvorakova L, Mrazova L, Houst'kova H, Elleder M. (2008) Early onset Alexander disease: a case report with evidence for manifestation of the disorder in neurohypophyseal pituicytes. Clin Neuropathol 27(2): 64–71.

McCall MA, Gregg RG, Behringer RR, et al. (1996) Targeted deletion in astrocyte intermediate filament (Gfap) alters neuronal physiology. Proc Natl Acad Sci USA 93(13): 6361–6366.

Messing A, Goldman JE. (2004) Alexander Disease. In: Lazzarini RA, Ed. Myelin and its Diseases. San Diego: Elsevier / Academic Press, pp. 851–866.

Mignot C, Delarasse C, Escaich S, et al. (2007) Dynamics of mutated GFAP aggregates revealed by real-time imaging of an astrocyte model of Alexander disease. Exp Cell Res 313(13): 2766–2779.

Mignot C, Desguerre I, Burglen L, Hertz-Pannier L, et al. (2009) Tumor-like enlargement of the optic chiasm in an infant with Alexander disease. Brain Dev 31(3): 244–247.

Murakami N, Tsuchiya T, Kanazawa N, Tsujino S, Nagai T. (2008) Novel deletion mutation in GFAP gene in an infantile form of Alexander disease. Pediatr Neurol 38(1): 50–52.

Namekawa M, Takiyama Y, Aoki Y, et al. (2002) Identification of GFAP gene mutation in hereditary adult-onset Alexander's disease. Ann Neurol 52(6): 779–785.

Nuber S, Petrasch-Parwez E, Winner B, et al. (2008) Neurodegeneration and motor dysfunction in a conditional model of Parkinson's disease. J Neurosci 28(10): 2471 2484.

Ohnari K, Yamano M, Uozumi T, Hashimoto T, Tsuji S, Nakagawa M. (2007) An adult form of Alexander disease: a novel mutation in glial fibrillary acidic protein. J Neurol 254(10): 1390–1394.

Okamoto Y, Mitsuyama H, Jonosono M, et al. (2002) Autosomal dominant palatal myoclonus and spinal cord atrophy. J Neurol Sci 195(1): 71–76.

Padiath QS, Saigoh K, Schiffmann R, et al. (2006) Lamin B1 duplications cause autosomal dominant leukodystrophy. Nat Genet 38(10): 1114–1123.

Pareyson D, Fancellu R, Mariotti C, et al. (2008) Adult-onset Alexander disease: a series of eleven unrelated cases with review of the literature. Brain 131(Pt 9): 2321–2331.

Pekny M, Leveen P, Pekna M, et al. (1995) Mice lacking glial fibrillary acidic protein display astrocytes devoid of intermediate filaments but develop and reproduce normally. Embo J 14(8): 1590–1598.

Perng MD, Wen SF, Gibbon T, et al. (2008) GFAP filaments can tolerate the incorporation of assembly-compromised GFAP-d, but with consequences for filament organization and aB-crystallin association. Mol Biol Cell 19: 4521–4533.

Polymeropoulos MH, Lavedan C, Leroy E, et al. (1997) Mutation in the alpha-synuclein gene identified in families with Parkinson's disease. Science 276(5321): 2045–2047.

Quinlan RA, Brenner M, Goldman JE, Messing A. (2007) GFAP and its role in Alexander disease. Exp Cell Res 313(10): 2077–2087.

Rodriguez D, Gauthier F, Bertini E, et al. (2001) Infantile Alexander disease: spectrum of GFAP mutations and genotype–phenotype correlation. Am J Hum Genet 69(5): 1134–1140.

Romano S, Salvetti M, Ceccherini I, De Simone T, Savoiardo M. (2007) Brainstem signs with progressing atrophy of medulla oblongata and upper cervical spinal cord. Lancet Neurol 6(6): 562–570.

Rosenthal W. (1898) Über eine eigenthümliche, mit syringomyelie complicirte geschwulst des rückenmarks. Bietr Pathol Anat 23: 111–143.

Rothstein JD, Patel S, Regan MR, Haenggeli et al. (2005) Beta-lactam antibiotics offer neuroprotection by increasing glutamate transporter expression. Nature 433(7021): 73–77.

Salmaggi A, Botturi A, Lamperti E, et al. (2007) A novel mutation in the GFAP gene in a familial adult onset Alexander disease. J Neurol 254(9): 1278–1280.

Santacruz K, Lewis J, Spires T, et al. (2005) Tau suppression in a neurodegenerative mouse model improves memory function. Science 309(5733): 476–481.

Schwankhaus JD, Parisi JE, Gulledge WR, Chin L, Currier RD. (1995) Hereditary adult-onset Alexander's disease with palatal myoclonus, spastic paraparesis, and cerebellar ataxia. Neurology 45(12): 2266–2271.

Shiihara T, Kato M, Honma T, Ohtaki S, Sawaishi Y, Hayasaka K. (2002) Fluctuation of computed tomographic findings in white matter in Alexander's disease. J Child Neurol 17(3): 227–230.

Sistermans EA, de Coo RF, De Wijs IJ, Van Oost BA. (1998) Duplication of the proteolipid protein gene is the major cause of Pelizaeus–Merzbacher disease. Neurology 50(6): 1749–1754.

Stumpf E, Masson H, Duquette A, et al. (2003) Adult Alexander disease with autosomal dominant transmission: a distinct entity caused by mutation in the glial fibrillary acid protein gene. Arch Neurol 60(9): 1307–1312.

Tang G, Xu Z, Goldman JE. (2006) Synergistic effects of the SAPK/JNK and the proteasome pathway on glial fibrillary acidic protein (GFAP) accumulation in Alexander disease. J Biol Chem 281(50) :38 634–38 643.

Tang G, Yue Z, Talloczy Z, Goldman JE. (2008) Adaptive autophagy in Alexander disease–affected astrocytes. Autophagy 4(5): 701–703.

Tawfik VL, Regan MR, Haenggeli C, et al. (2008) Propentofylline–induced astrocyte modulation leads to alterations in glial glutamate promoter activation following spinal nerve transection. Neuroscience 152(4): 1086–1092.

Tian R, Gregor M, Wiche G, Goldman JE. (2006) Plectin regulates the organization of glial fibrillary acidic protein in Alexander disease. Am J Pathol 168(3): 888–897.

van der Knaap MS, Naidu S, Breiter SN, et al. (2001) Alexander disease: diagnosis with MR imaging. Am J Neuroradiol 22(3): 541–552.

van der Knaap MS, Ramesh V, Schiffmann R, et al. (2006) Alexander disease: ventricular garlands and abnormalities of the medulla and spinal cord. Neurology 66(4): 494–498.

Vazquez E, Macaya A, Mayolas N, Arevalo S, Poca MA, Enriquez G. (2008) Neonatal Alexander disease: MR imaging prenatal diagnosis. AJNR Am J Neuroradiol 29(10): 1973–1975.

Wippold FJ, 2nd, Perry A, Lennerz J. (2006). Neuropathology for the neuroradiologist: Rosenthal fibers. AJNR Am J Neuroradiol 27(5): 958–961.

Worman HJ, Bonne G. (2007) "Laminopathies": a wide spectrum of human diseases. Exp Cell Res 313(10): 2121–2133.

Wu Y, Jiang YW, Wang JM, et al. (2006) GFAP mutations in 3 Chinese infantile Alexander disease patients. J Inherit Metab Dis 29(Suppl 1): 66.

Yamamoto A, Lucas JJ, Hen R. (2000) Reversal of neuropathology and motor dysfunction in a conditional model of Huntington's disease. Cell 101(1): 57–66.

Ye W, Qiang G, Jingmin W, Yanling Y, Xiru W, Yuwu J. (2008) Clinical and genetic study in Chinese patients with Alexander disease. J Child Neurol 23(2): 173–177.

Yoshida T, Tomozawa Y, Arisato T, Okamoto Y, Hirano H, Nakagawa M. 2007. The functional alteration of mutant GFAP depends on the location of the domain: morphological and functional studies using astrocytoma–derived cells. J Hum Genet 52(4): 362–369.

Zlotogora J. (1998) Germ line mosaicism. Hum Genet 102(4): 381–386.

Zu T, Duvick LA, Kaytor MD, et al. (2004) Recovery from polyglutamine–induced neurodegeneration in conditional SCA1 transgenic mice. J Neurosci 24(40): 8853–8861.

8
METACHROMATIC LEUKODYSTROPHY

Volkmar Gieselmann and Ingeborg Krägeloh-Mann

Classification and definition

Metachromatic leukodystrophy (MLD) is a lysosomal sphingolipid storage disorder. The disease is monogenic and is inherited in an autosomal recessive way. MLD is caused by the deficiency of the enzyme arylsulfatase A. The major substrate of arylsulfatase A is a membrane lipid, 3-*O*-sulfogalactosylceramide (sulfatide). The polar head of this sphingolipid consists of a galactose residue, which is sulfated in position 3. Arylsulfatase A removes this sulfate residue. If this step does not occur, owing to arylsulfatase A deficiency, the degradation of the lipid cannot proceed and it accumulates in oligodendrocytes, Schwann cells, and some neurons. The pathological hallmark of the disease is a progressive demyelination, which results in multiple neurological symptoms.

The degradation of sulfatide by arylsulfatase A depends on the presence of an activator protein, saposin B (Sandhoff et al. 2001). Therefore, deficiencies of saposin B also result in the inability to degrade sulfatide. Although very similar to MLD, this condition should not be considered identical to it, because saposin B is also involved in the degradation of lipids other than sulfatide which also accumulate in saposin B deficiency. Therefore the disease caused by saposin B deficiency should be considered as a variant form of MLD (Sandhoff et al. 2001).

Incidence and prevalence

The incidence of MLD was initially determined in Northern Sweden as 1 in 40 000 newborns (Gustavson and Hagberg 1971). More recent studies from Germany and the Netherlands determined the incidence as 0.6 per 100 000 (Heim et al. 1997) and 1.42 per 100 000 live births (Poorthuis et al. 1999), respectively. The discrepancy in the rates, although coming from two neighboring countries where a different gene pool is not very likely, indicates that different search strategies – through laboratories providing postnatal and prenatal diagnosis in the Netherlands, and through departments of pediatrics, neurology and neuropathology in Germany – may lead to different completeness or reliability of diagnosis. Results from a study performed in Portugal, searching through laboratories as in the Netherlands, suggest a birth prevalence of 1.85 in 100 000 (Pinto et al. 2004). Higher incidences were found in two ethnic groups. MLD is particularly frequent in Habbanite Jews, among whom the incidence is about 1 in 75 newborns, and Christian Arabs with an incidence of 1 in 10 000 (Zlotogora et al. 1994a).

It must be emphasized, however, that these epidemiological results were based on retrospective data. So far, no epidemiologically precise numbers for the incidence of MLD have been determined.

Genetics

The Arylsulfatase A Gene

The human arylsulfatase A gene is located on chromosome 22. The gene consists of 8 exons which encompass only about 3 kb of genomic sequence (Polten et al. 1991). It is a house-keeping gene, being expressed in all tissues. Three mRNAs of 2.1 kb, 3.7 kb, and 4.8 kb respectively, are transcribed from the gene. They are generated by the use of different polyadenylation signals located at different positions downstream of the termination codon. There is indirect evidence that these three mRNA species differ substantially in their translational efficacy (Gieselmann et al. 1989). Thus, although in total RNA the three species are almost equally abundant it seems that the smallest, 2.1 kb mRNA accounts for about 90% of enzyme synthesis. This may be due to differing extent of polyadenylation of the various mRNA species, since about 90% of the larger 3.7 kb and 4.8 kb mRNA species is lost during enrichment of polyadenylated mRNA, indicating a low degree of polyadeny-lation.

Arylsulfatase A Pseudodeficiency

Approximately 0.2 to 0.5% of the Caucasian population shows substantial arylsulfatase A deficiency with a residual enzyme activity of about 10% normal, but these individuals do not show any clinical symptoms related to this deficiency. Therefore this phenomenon has been termed arylsulfatase A pseudodeficiency. This nomenclature, however, is misleading since it suggests that the deficiency in these individuals is only apparent but not real. Pseudodeficiency is due to a frequent arylsulfatase A allele which bears two polymorphisms, one of which is causative for the low enzyme activity.

One of the polymorphisms of the pseudodeficiency allele results in the replacement of asparagine 350 by serine in the arylsulfatase A protein (Gieselmann et al. 1989). Since this asparagine bears an N-linked oligosaccharide side-chain, arylsulfatase A encoded by the pseudodeficiency allele has lost one of its three oligosaccharide side-chains and is therefore about 2 kDa smaller. The loss of an oligosaccharide side-chain, however, has only little impact on the enzyme. Individuals homozygous for an allele that bears just this polymor-phism still have about 60% of normal enzyme activity (Shen et al. 1993, Barth et al. 1994, Leistner et al. 1995). The reason for this has not been examined in detail but could be due to a slightly reduced stability. The second mutation in the arylsulfatase pseudodeficiency allele occurs in the first polyadenylation signal downstream of the termination codon. An A to G transition within this signal abolishes the polyadenylation consensus sequence causing the loss of this polyadenylation signal. Since this signal is necessary to synthesize the small, 2.1 kb mRNA species, this polymorphism leads to a complete deficiency of this mRNA species in pseudodeficient individuals. Because this mRNA accounts for 90% of arylsulfatase A synthesis, pseudodeficient individuals have a severe reduction of arylsul-fatase A synthesis. Thus, the loss of the N-glycosylation site reduces arylsulfatase A activity moderately, whereas the reduced synthesis of the enzyme due to the loss of the polyadeny-lation signal accounts for most of the loss of enzyme activity of pseudodeficient individuals (Barth et al. 1994, Leistner et al. 1995).

The frequency of the pseudodeficiency allele varies in different populations. Among Europeans its frequency has been estimated to be about 7.5% (Ott et al. 1997) to 13% (Barth et al. 1994), in India about 12.5% (Ott et al. 1997), whereas it is almost non-existent in Africans and Asians (Hwu et al. 1996, Ott et al. 1997). This allows the calculation that in Europe about 0.15% to 0.45% of the population is homozygous for the pseudodeficiency allele and such individuals are thus arylsulfatase A pseudodeficient. The polymorphism causing the loss of the N-glycosylation site can occur without the polymorphism in the polyadenylation signal (Ott et al. 1997). This allele is frequent in the African population (0.32 allele frequency) and less frequent among Europeans (0.06 allele frequency). An allele that bears only the polymorphism in the polyadenylation signal has so far not been described.

There is another allele which causes low enzyme activity but is not associated with MLD (Berger et al. 1999). Thus, it represents a second arylsulfatase A pseudodeficiency allele. This allele has been reported in a father and two healthy siblings of a MLD patient. Activity in these healthy individuals is substantially reduced but they show no clinical symptoms. The polymorphism found in the causative allele leads to substitution of alanine 464 by valine. In contrast to the pseudodeficiency allele described above, it is unknown why this substitution causes low enzyme actvity.

Various publications have associated arylsulfatase A pseudodeficiency with increased prevalence of neurological or psychiatric diseases (e.g., Mihaljevic-Peles et al. 2001, Alessandri et al. 2002). The issue has not been definitely resolved, however, and the link between pseudodeficiency and disease has so far not been generally accepted, largely because most studies did not provide convincing statistics that would unambiguously prove the claimed association.

MUTATIONS IN THE ARYLSULFATASE A GENE

More than 100 mutations in the arylsulfatase A gene causing MLD have been described (von Figura et al. 2001). Most of the defective arylsulfatase A alleles bear mis-sense mutations. Splice site mutations, deletions, or premature stop codons represent the minority of alleles. In addition, in some patients arylsulfatase A alleles were described that bear two deleterious mutations on the same allele (Kappler et al. 1994).

MLD is genetically very heterogeneous. The majority of mutations have only been found in a few, mostly single patients(e.g. Biffi et al. 2008). Among Caucasians only three MLD-causing alleles are frequent:

1. A splice donor site mutation of the exon 2/intron 2 border (IVS459+1A>G) has been found with a frequency of between 15% and 43%.
2. A mis-sense mutations causing a Pro426Leu amino acid substitution in between 16% and 25% of all MLD alleles, respectively (Polten et al. 1991, Barth et al. 1993, Berger et al. 1997).

The examination of various polymorphisms revealed that both alleles have a fixed haplotype and are in complete linkage disequilibrium (Zlotogora et al. 1994b, Coulter Mackie and Gagnier 1997, Gort et al. 2000). The most comprehensive determination of the frequency of the IVS459+1A>G and Pro426Leu allele was done by collection of data of 384 unrelated European patients (Lugowska et al. 2005b). In this group the IVS459+1G>A allele accounted for 25% of all alleles and the Pro426Leu for 18.6%, respectively.

3. A missense mutation causing an Ile179Ser substitution occurs with an allele frequency of about 12 to 13% in European patients (Berger et al. 1997, Lugowska et al. 2005a).

A few other alleles have been described in more than one patient (e.g., Biffi et al. 2008) but their exact frequencies have not been determined.

Defective arylsulfatatase A alleles in Japanese patients are different from those in European patients:

1. An allele causing a Gly99Asp substitution is the most frequent with 45% of all alleles detected.
2. Of the alleles coding for amino acid substitutions Gly245Arg and Thr409Ile, each accounts for about 10% of the defective alleles in Japanese patients (Kurosawa et al. 1998).

In five Chinese patients none of the most frequent European mutations was found but three rare mutations, which had previously been described in Caucasian patients, were also detected in Chinese patients (Wang et al. 2007). The amino acid substitution Ala212Val seems to be prominent among Canadian patients of Acadian or French ethnicity (Coulter-Mackie and Gagnier 2003), and a Thr274Met substitution has been found in several Lebanese patients in independent studies (Harvey et al. 1993, Hess et al. 1996a, Coulter-Mackie and Gagnier 2003).

GENOTYPE–PHENOTYPE CORRELATION

There is a genotype–phenotype correlation in MLD, which has been confirmed in various independent studies (Polten et al. 1991, Barth et al. 1993, Berger et al. 1997, Kurosawa et al. 1998). It is not so strict, however, that it would allow precise prediction of the clinical course of individual patients based on genetic analysis. This genotype–phenotype correlation can be summarized as follows:

- Patients homozygous for alleles that do not allow the expression of any enzyme activity (null alleles) always suffer from the most severe late-infantile form of disease.
- Heterozygosity for a null allele and an allele which allows for the expression of low amounts of enzyme activity is in many cases associated with the juvenile form of MLD but is occasionally found also in patients of adult onset.
- Homozygosity for the latter type of allele is most frequently associated with the most attenuated adult-onset form of MLD but may also be found in juveniles (Polten et al. 1991).

There are a few patients, however, who for unknown reasons do not fit in with this rule (Berger et al. 1997). Nevertheless, the genotype–phenotype correlation can be explained by the varying amount of residual enzyme activity associated with the genotype of the patient. In the case of homozygosity for a null allele, the patient expresses no enzyme activity and suffers from the most severe late-infantile form of MLD. One allele with some residual enzyme activity mitigates the course to the juvenile form and two alleles to the most attenuated, frequently the adult form of MLD. The correlation between phenotype and residual enzyme activity has not only been established from genetic studies, but has also been confirmed on the biochemical level (Conzelmann and Sandhoff 1991, Leinekugel et al. 1992).

Although it is difficult to measure residual enzyme activity in the low range precisely, a reasonable estimate is that late-onset adult patients have residual arylsulfatase A activities of about 2 to 4% of normal.

It is important to realize, however, that this genotype–phenotype correlation becomes obvious only when groups of patients are examined, but does not allow precise prediction of the clinical course for the individual patient. This is due to the fact that in the juvenile and adult forms of disease there is considerable heterogeneity among patients with the same arylsulfatase A genotype. Even among affected siblings bearing identical mutations the course of disease can be surprisingly different (Clarke et al. 1989, Arbour et al. 2000). Obviously there are other genetic or epigenetic factors, as yet unknown, which influence the course of disease substantially. These "factors" allow for only vague predictions of clinical course in late-onset patients based on genotype analysis. In contrast, the phenotype of late-infantile patients is rather uniform, with comparatively little variation of clinical course.

Genotype–phenotype correlation in MLD is not limited to age at onset. It is a well-known phenomenon that the adult forms of the disease may start either with primarily neurological or with psychiatric symptoms. These two groups of patients appear to have different genotypes. Homozygosity for the Pro426Leu allele – the most frequent allele among European adult patients – is found in those who primarily develop neurological symptoms (Rauschka et al. 2006). Patients heterozygous for a null allele and the Ile179Ser allele appear to develop initially psychiatric symptoms before neuromotor symptoms develop (Rauschka et al. 2006). It is also interesting to note that the latter genotype represents an exception to the genotype–phenotype correlation described above. The Ile179Ser allele is always found in late juvenile or adult patients but it occurs always in heterozygosity with a null allele (Fluharty et al. 1991, Gomez-Lira et al. 1998, Halsall et al. 1999). So far, no Ile179Ser homozygous patient has been identified. This is remarkable, given the frequency of this allele, and may suggest that the residual enzyme activity associated with this allele is sufficiently high, such that homozygosity does not cause disease. This theory is supported by the clinical course in the few patients who were described as being heterozygous for the Pro426Leu allele and the Ile179Ser allele. These patients developed their first symptoms at a comparatively old age (40–60 years) and showed a very mild progression (Duyff and Weinstein 1996, Perusi et al. 1999).

134

Individuals who are heterozygous for an arylsulfatase A pseudodeficiency allele and an MLD allele have even less residual arylsulfatase A activity than those who are homozygous for the pseudodeficiency allele. Therefore, it has been speculated whether individuals with such a genotype run the risk of developing clinical symptoms due to low arylsulfatase A activity (Hohenschutz et al. 1989). Frequencies of MLD alleles and the pseudodeficiency allele allow one to calculate that approximately 1 in 22 000 individuals will have such a genotype. Since it seems impossible to identify a sufficient number of such individuals by random screening, a systematic search was performed among relatives of MLD patients. This allowed the identification of 16 individuals who carried a mutation in one arylsulfatase A allele and the pseudodeficiency polymorphisms in the other (Penzien et al. 1993). Among these were two individuals with non-progressive neurological symptoms and two who showed magnetic resonance imaging (MRI) abnormalities without neurological symptoms. None of these patients excreted sulfatide in urine nor was their nerve conduction velocity decreased. This study therefore concluded that heterozygosity for arylsulfatase A pseudodeficiency allele and a MLD allele is not associated with any major health risk.

Biochemical background

BIOCHEMISTRY OF ARYLSULFATASE A

Arylsulfatase A is a lysosomal enzyme that catalyzes the first step in the degradation pathway of the sphingolipid 3-O-sulfogalactosylceramide, briefly called sulfatide. Sulfatide appears to be the major substrate of arylsulfatase A but the enzyme is also involved in the degradation of various other sulfolipids of less abundance (Sandhoff et al. 2002). Arylsulfatase A is synthesized at the rough endoplasmic reticulum as a precursor of 507 amino acids (Stein et al. 1989). It then receives three N-linked oligosaccharide side-chains at amino acid positions 158, 180, and 350, respectively, in a post-translational modification (Sommerlade et al. 1994). The fully glycosylated enzyme has a molecular weight of 62 kDa and forms non-covalently linked dimers. The enzymatic activity of arylsulfatase A depends critically on modification of a cysteine residue located in the active center (Dierks et al. 2003). This modification is not unique to arylsulfatase A but occurs in all sulfatases. This cysteine residue is converted to a formylglycine residue by a modifying enzyme called formyl glycine generating enzyme I (FGE I) which is located in the endoplasmic reticulum. The formylglycine contains an aldehyde which is essential for sulfatase activity and does not occur in any of the proteinogenic amino acids. Mutations in the gene coding for FGE I cause multiple sulfatase deficiency, a disease in which arylsulfatase A along with all other sulfatases are deficient. The clinical picture of this disease combines the symptoms of MLD with those of the diseases caused by deficiencies of other sulfatases – for example, glycosaminoglycan storage as a consequence of arylsulfatase B deficiency and ichthyosis as a consequence of steroidsulfatase deficiency.

From the endoplasmic reticulum, arylsulfatase A is transported to the Golgi apparatus. Here it is recognized as a lysosomal enzyme by a particular phosphotransferase, which initiates the synthesis of mannose-6-phosphate residues on the oligosaccharide side-chains.

These mannose-6-phosphate residues bind to mannose-6-phosphate receptors, which mediate the further vesicular transport of the enzyme to the lysosome. In the acidic environment of the lysosome the arylsulfatase A dimers associate reversibly to form octamers (von Bülow et al. 2002). The octamerization is important for the intralysosomal stability of the enzyme, since it makes a cathepsin L cleavage site located in the vicinity of the octamerization region inaccessible for the protease.

To degrade sulfatide, arylsulfatase A needs the assistance of a small activator protein called saposin B. This protein extracts sulfatide from the membranes and presents it to arylsulfatase A in a one-to-one complex. Saposin B is not specific for sulfatide, however, but is also involved in the degradation of other lipids by other enzymes. It can also extract globotriaosylceramide from membranes and present it to α-galactosidase A, the enzyme deficient in Fabry disease (Sandhoff et al. 2001). Deficiencies of saposin B are much rarer but also cause a disease that is clinically very similar to arylsulfatase necessary for the degradation of sulfatide but also of globotriaosylceramide, the latter lipid is also accumulated in saposin B deficiency, which distinguishes it from MLD.

BIOCHEMISTRY OF SULFATIDE

Sulfatide is synthesized from ceramide in a two-step process. In the first step a UDP-galactose-galactosyltransferase located in the endoplasmic reticulum transfers a galactose residue onto ceramide, generating galactosylceramide which is the most abundant glycolipid of myelin. In the second step a sulfotransferase located in the Golgi apparatus adds sulfate to the 3' hydroxyl group of the galactose moiety to generate sulfatide. This lipid is not ubiquitious but occurs only in particular tissues. Sulfatide is found, for example, in the epithelia of bile ducts, in renal tubules, and in particularly large amounts in myelin of the nervous system. In myelin, sulfatide accounts for about 3 to 4% of the total membrane lipids.

Although the exact function of sulfatide is yet to be revealed, mice which are not able to synthesize sulfatide and are thus completely devoid of this lipid allow for some insights into the function of this lipid. These mice appear normal at birth but develop hindlimb weakness at the age of 6 weeks. The structure of compact myelin is preserved in these mice but ultrastructural examination revealed disorganized lateral loops at the nodes of Ranvier (Honke et al. 2002). Within this region voltage-gated sodium and potassium channels, which normally cluster in the nodal and paranodal regions, respectively, were abnormally distributed in older mice (Ishibashi et al. 2002). Sodium channels were actually more dispersed along the axolemma than in wild-type mice and the potassium channels were abnormally localized in the paranodal region. Thus, sulfatide is important for the proper organization of the paranodal axoglial junctions and is essential for the correct localization of ion channels in this region. The incorrect localization of ion channels and the possible consequences for action potential propagation may explain the neurological symptoms that these mice develop.

Sulfatide is also involved in oligodendrocyte differentiation. When oligodendrocyte precursor cells of the sulfatide-deficient mice were examined in vivo and in vitro, the number of terminally differentiated oligodendrocytes at a given time-point was two to threefold higher than in normal mice. In addition, treatment of oligodendrocyte precursor cells in vitro with an anti sulfatide antibody results in reversible arrest of differentiation. When taken together, the data indicates that sulfatide seems to be an important negative regulator of oligodendrocyte differentiation (Hirahara et al. 2004).

In addition sulfatide has been shown to affect the biological activity of various proteins. It has been shown to be a cofactor of the Na^+/K^+-ATPase and be involved in the binding of serotonin, gamma-aminobutyric acic, and opiates to their respective receptors. Sulfatide can modulate the activity of a number of enzymes involved in different signal transduction cascades such as phospholipidase A2, PI3 kinase, certain phosphodiesterases. A considerable number of proteins are known which bind sulfatide such as laminin, proteolipid protein, MAL protein, tenascin R, and many others (for references see von Figura et al. 2001). Whether any of these protein–sulfatide interactions are of relevance in the pathophysiology of MLD has not been investigated.

Pathophysiology

Consequences of Mutations Underlying Null Alleles

It is obvious that frameshift-causing deletions and premature stop codons obviate the synthesis of any functional arylsulfatase A and cause null alleles. The most frequent allele found in late infantile patients is the IVS459+1A>G splice donor site mutation of exon 2. Since this mutation abolishes the use of this splice donor site completely, no detectable arylsulfatase A mRNA is generated from this allele. As a consequence no enzyme can be synthesized and this frequent allele qualifies as a null allele. Most of the mutations found in late-infantile patients are, however, mis-sense mutations. Some of them have been analyzed in detail for their biochemical consequences (e.g., Schestag et al. 2002, Poeppel et al. 2005). The results demonstrate that most mis-sense mutations causing null alleles lead to a misfolding of arylsulfatase A in the endoplasmic reticulum followed by proteasomal degradation. In these cases no functional enzyme can leave the endoplasmic reticulum and reach the lysosome. Therefore these mutations lead to null alleles

Consequences of Mutations Underlying Alleles With Residual Activity

In late-onset patients some residual enzyme activity must be expressed. This requires that some arylsulfatase A can reach the lysosome in a functionally active form. In MLD all alleles which fulfil these criteria bear mis-sense mutations. The most frequent of these alleles, which bears the Pro426Leu mis-sense mutation, has been extensively characterized at the biochemical level (von Bülow et al. 2002). The Pro426Leu substituted enzyme is not retained in the endoplasmic reticulum but is properly transported to the lysosome. In contrast to amino acid substitutions causing late-infantile MLD, there is no enhanced premature endoplasmic reticulum associated degradation. Wild-type arylsulfatase A is synthesized as a dimer. At the acidic lysosomal pH four of the dimers reversibly form an octamer. The Pro426Leu substitution interferes with the octamerization of arylsulfatase A upon arrival in the lysosome. The ability of the defective enzyme to form octamers is severely impaired. The area of the enzyme involved in octamerization includes a cleavage site for cathepsin L. Upon octamerization this cleavage site is covered and the wild-type enzyme is protected from proteolytic attack. Because the Pro426Leu-substituted enzyme does not octamerize its cathepsin L cleavage site remains exposed; cathepsin L can attack and the enzyme is rapidly degraded.

Although this reduces the half-life of the defective enzyme substantially, there are still low steady-state levels of enzymatically active arylsulfatase A present in the lysosome which are sufficient to continuously degrade small amounts of sulfatide. This retards lipid accumulation and provides an explanation for the attenuated phenotype of late-onset patients (Conzelmann and Sandhoff 1991).

The biochemical effects of other mis-sense mutations found in patients of late onset (e.g., Ile179Ser or Arg84Gln) have so far not been examined in detail, so that the molecular basis for the residual enzyme activity remains unclear.

CONSEQUENCES OF SULFATIDE ACCUMULATION

MLD is usually considered as a disease in which symptoms are solely caused by demyelination. Certainly the functional impairment of oligodendrocytes and Schwann cells most likely accounts for the majority of clinical symptoms. It must be kept in mind, however, that in the nervous system, sulfatide storage is not restricted to glial cells but also occurs in neurons (Peng and Suzuki 1987). This has been described in autoptic brain of humans and also in an arylsulfatase A -deficient mouse model (Wittke et al. 2004). This mouse model mimics human pathology with respect to the tissue pattern of sulfatide storage, but in contrast to humans arylsulfatase A-deficient mice do not demyelinate (Hess et al. 1996b). Nevertheless, these mice develop progressive neurological symptoms, which are easily recognizable in the second year of life but are not severe enough to limit life expectancy (D'Hooge et al. 2001, Stroobants et al. 2008). These include head tremor, ataxia, gait disturbance, and general impairment of motor function on functional measures such as the rotarod. These mice store sulfatide in various – although not all – neurons (Wittke et al. 2004). In old mice this results in degeneration of a number of axons, which can easily be detected in peripheral nerves. The development of neurological symptoms in the mice in the absence of demyelination can so far only be explained by the slowly increasing neuronal storage. This storage may affect neuronal function in at least two ways. First, storage may lead to alterations in the electrophysiological properties of neurons without apparent histopathological consequences. In the course of therapies these may still be fully reversible. Second, at later stages storage causes axonal degeneration which may be refractory to therapeutic interventions. Certainly, information from mouse models can only be extrapolated with caution to MLD patients. It seems possible that initial symptoms, in humans at least, may also be caused by neuronal storage rather than by demyelination. Later in the course of the disease, demyelination becomes prominent and its clinical consequences dominate the phenotype.

In addition, patients with MLD frequently suffer from epileptic seizures. In another arylsulfatase A-deficient mouse model in which neuronal sulfatide storage was increased by further genetic modification (Eckhardt et al. 2007) increased neuronal excitability was noted. In fact, these mice frequently died as a consequence of audiogenic seizures. Thus, it seems possible that neuronal storage contributes to the epilleptic seizures that occur in patients with MLD.

So far it remains unclear why storage in oligodendrocytes leads to demyelination. At the cellular level it is not understood how sulfatide interferes with oligodendrocyte and Schwann cell function. Nevertheless, mouse models allow for some insights into the pathophysiology. As mentioned above, the arylsulfatase A-deficient mouse model stores sulfatide but does not demyelinate (Hess et al. 1996b). Compared with normal animals, the level of sulfatide in brain of arylsulfatase A-deficient mice is only 1.5-fold increased (Ramakrishnan et al. 2007). Sulfatide levels have also been determined in brains of MLD patients. Here the increase in sulfatide level over normal varies from three- to eightfold, but in any case the extent of lipid accumulation is higher in humans than in mice. This suggests that the extent of sulfatide storage in mice does not suffice to trigger demyelination. Consequently, arylsulfatase A-deficient mice have been genetically modified so that sulfatide synthesis, and thus the sulfatide load in oligodendrocytes and Schwann cells, is increased (Ramakrishnan et al. 2007). These mice demyelinate in the second year of life and develop severe neurological symptoms. They thus represent a better animal model of MLD than the conventional arylsulfatase A-deficient mouse. Interestingly, sulfatide levels in the demyelinating mouse model are again just 1.5-fold higher than in the non-demyelinating model. This suggests that demyelination is triggered upon relatively slight increases in sulfatide levels. Although one should be critical when extending animal data to humans these data are in good agreement with the results of most recent studies of natural history of the disease. These have shown that the most prominent decline of neurological function in late infantile MLD patients occurs within a narrow time period of just 6 months (Kehrer et al. 2008a, b). This is consistent with the fact that an only a slight increase in sulfatide accumulation, which occurs during a time period of 6 months, triggers demyelination.

Slight increases of sulfatide occurring within 6 months result in dramatic alterations of clinical phenotype. With respect to possible future therapies this also means that only minor reductions of accumulation of sulfatide may result in considerable clinical improvement.

Typically in MLD patients there is not only an increase in the amount of sulfatide, but concomitantly the amount of galactosylceramide is substantially reduced. Galactosylceramide is the most abundant glycolipid of myelin and the immediate precursor of sulfatide. The reason for the diminution of galactosylceramide is unknown, but its decrease should also be considered in the pathophysiology.

In several glycosphingolipidoses not only sphingolipids accumulate, but also their respective lysosphingolipids, which have lost their amide-linked acyl side chain and are known to be biologically active compounds (Hannun and Bell 1987). For example, psychosine, the lysolipid form of galactosylceramide, is a potent inhibitor of proteinkinase C (Hannun and Bell 1987), interferes with IGF I mediated signal transduction pathways (Zaka et al. 2005), and is a non-physiological ligand of signal transduction receptors (Im et al. 2001). In brains of MLD patients increased levels of lysosulfatide have been detected. Although possible toxic effects of lysosulfatide have not been studied in particular, it is reasonable to presume that lysosulfatide shares some of the toxic properties of the well-examined psychosine, which is closely related structurally. Therefore lysosulfatide accumulation is likely to contribute to pathogenesis in MLD.

139

Clinical features

Clinically, MLD is heterogeneous with respect to the age at onset, the rate of progression, and the initial symptoms. In general three different clinical forms of MLD can be distinguished: a late-infantile form, a juvenile form, and an adult form. The literature is rather consistent that most children with a rapid early course develop symptoms in the second year life, and children with an onset beyond 3 years of age have a more protracted course (MacFaul et al. 1982, Lyon et al. 2006, Biffi et al. 2008). Thus, we would suggest the following age range:

- late-infantile form of disease presenting before the age of 3 years,
- juvenile form starting between 3 to 16 years, and
- adult forms developing first symptoms beyond the age of 16.

In a survey of 384 European patients, 48% of all patients suffered from the most severe late-infantile type of MLD, 31% from the juvenile type, and 21% from the adult type, respectively (Lugowska et al. 2005b). In the epidemiological studies mentioned above the proportion of late-infantile, juvenile, and adult types was 45%, 37%, and 18%, respectively, in Germany (Heim et al. 1997) and 41%, 40%, and 18%, respectively, in the Portuguese study (Poorthuis et al. 1999)

The distinction of the various forms of MLD is considered clinically helpful when it concerns the counseling of patients and their families and when treatment options are considered. The question arises, however, whether this classification is valid and describes different clinical entities or whether, in fact, the clinical presentation of MLD is a continuum ranging from severely affected infantile patients to individuals developing symptoms even beyond the age of 60 (Bosch and Hart 1978). The profile of first symptoms is, however, significantly different, especially between the late-infantile and juvenile forms: in late-infantile patients the most frequent first symptoms are abnormal movement patterns, gait disturbances, and developmental regression; whereas patients with juvenile onset more often have impaired fine motor skills, concentration and behavioral problems as the first symptoms (Kehrer et al. 2008a, b). In the adult forms, the initial symptoms often provoke the diagnosis of a psychiatric disease, especially schizophrenia, as psychotic symptoms and behavioral abnormalities often precede or accompany a decline of intellectual capacities (Kumperscak et al. 2007).

Most of the **late-infantile patients** become symptomatic at the age of 12 to 24 months. In a recent study of 16 late-infantile European patients, the average age at onset was 18.5 ± 4.5 months (Biffi et al. 2008). Such patients usually learn to walk, although a delay may be observed; they initially develop either muscular hypotonia or depressed deep tendon reflexes and weakness of the legs, leading to abnormal movement patterns and gait disturbances. The initially flaccid paresis converts later to a spastic quadriplegia with muscular atrophy. Occasionally, spastic paresis with muscular hypertonicity and hyperactive tendon reflexes and positive Babinski signs are the first neurological signs leading to abnormal posturing and equinus position of the feet (Case vignette 1 and Fig. 8.1). In the further course of disease patients regress with respect to language and then also cognitive

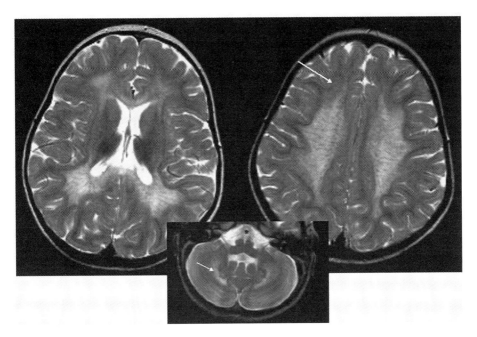

Fig. 8.1. MRI of a patient with late-infantile metachromatic leukodystrophy at a late stage of the disease (deterioration of motor functions without ability to sit, spastic tetraparesis, some communicative skills). T2-weighted axial images show widespread white matter hyperintensity involving the subcortical areas; U-fibers are partially affected (arrow on image to the right), the corpus callosum is clearly involved, the tigroid pattern is prominent. Cerebellar white matter is also affected (smaller arrow). There is still no atrophy.

development, speech becomes slow as movements do, fine motor skills deteriorate due to a mixture of peripheral neuropathy, spasticity, and also ataxia. In the later stage vision deteriorates due to optic atrophy, nystagmus develops; seizures are a late sign as is severe dementia. Patients finally die in a decerebrated state (von Figura et al. 2001, Lyon et al. 2006, Kehrer et al. 2008a, b).

CASE VIGNETTE 1: CLINICAL HISTORY OF A CHILD
WITH THE LATE-INFANTILE FORM OF MLD

Crawls at the age of 7 months, sits at 8 months, learns to walk with aid at 9 months but never learns to walk without aids; at the end of the first year, leg stiffness and equinus position of feet appears; at 25 months walking with aids is no longer possible, but crawling still is; this is lost at the age of 2.5 years and sitting without support 1 month later; 2 months after that, at the age of 2.75 years, head and trunk control is lost and hands have only holding function (pincer grip became clumsy due to spasticity at around 2.25 years). First language acquisition is normal (short sentences before 2 years), but at around 2 years there is stagnation of vocabulary spurt; at 2.5 years speech consists of single, dyslalic words, which is lost 4 months later. At the age of 3 years there is spastic tetraparesis, tendon reflexes are abolished; the child turns the head, looks at and follows close objects, laughs when kindly talked to. (See also Fig. 8.1.)

In the **juvenile patients** the onset of disease may not be dominated by neurological symptoms but, rather, starts insidiously with poor school performance, inadequate behaviour, or psychiatric symptoms (Hyde et al. 1992, Fukutani et al. 1999, Halsall et al. 1999, Colsch et al. 2008, Kehrer et al. 2008b). There are some examples in which these patients were misdiagnosed as being schizophrenic, depressive, or affected with Alzheimer disease (e.g., Sadovnick et al. 1993, Suzuki et al. 2008). In most patients, gross motor function becomes mildly impaired with some "coordination problems," and neurological signs may include reduced deep tendon reflexes indicating peripheral nerve involvement and also a positive Babinski sign but without much spastic posturing. This situation may remain rather stable for several months or even a few years. Once clear neurological signs such as spastic posturing and muscle hypertonicity develop, however, a rapid decline of gross motor function occurs, which may be as rapid as that in the late-infantile form (Case vignette 2 and Fig. 8.2). In some patients, this decline may not occur before reaching early or even later adulthood (I. Krägeloh-Mann, personal observation).

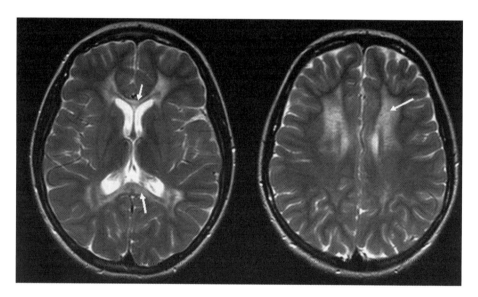

Fig. 8.2. MRI of a patient with juvenile metachromatic leukodystrophy at an early stage of the disease (some cognitive problems, no neurological signs). T2-weighted axial images show periventricular hyperintensity in the parieto-occipital and frontal areas; corpus callosum is already affected (genu and splenium, arrows); the tigroid pattern is just starting to show up (arrow on image to the right).

CASE VIGNETTE 2: CLINICAL HISTORY OF A
CHILD WITH THE JUVENILE FORM OF MLD

First signs are noticed at the beginning of the fifth year in the form of behavioral changes (regressing to infantile behaviour) and concentration problems leading to the diagnosis of a "hyperkinetic syndrome." At school entry examination (age 6 years) gait appears broad based and there is some uncertainty when climbing stairs, walking on heels becomes difficult and then impossible. Loss of language skills starts at around 6.75 years, at 7.5 years only single words are used. At that time the child walks only some steps and fine motor coordination is described as clumsy (inability for sequential finger opposition). At 8 years the child does not even walk with aid and at 8.25 years locomotion such as crawling or rolling is lost as well as active speech. At 8.5 years grasping is no longer possible and at 9.5 years sitting without support is lost and at 12.33 years head control. (See also Fig. 8.2.)

In the **adult patients** the disease is characterized by a slow decline in intellectual capabilities, emotional instability, abnormal behaviour, and memory deficits. Polyneuropathy is rarely an initial clinical symptom (Hageman et al. 1995). In general the course of disease is much slower than in the late-infantile form, and adults may survive even for decades after the diagnosis has been made. In addition, various patients have been described who developed first symptoms at a quite advanced age (Bosch and Hart 1978, Duyff and Weinstein 1996, Perusi et al. 1999). Mean survival time of adult MLD patients after the timepoint of diagnosis is about 12 years (Hageman et al. 1995).

SPECIFIC CLINICAL SIGNS

In most patients demyelination affects the central as well as the peripheral nervous systems but a number of patients have been described who presented with demyelination at the timepoint of diagnosis, which was prominent either in the central nervous system or peripheral nervous system (Haberlandt et al. 2008). In some patients the MRI even appeared normal although the peripheral nervous system was clearly affected (Felice et al. 2000, Comabella et al. 2001, Coulter Mackie et al. 2002). Given the rarity of these phenotypes and the genetic heterogeneity of MLD, it is difficult to correlate such particular clinical courses with the presence of certain alleles. It is, however, remarkable that two independent patients of Asian/Indian descent clinically presented with peripheral neuropathy alone and had the same mutation causing a Thr286Pro amino acid substitution (Felice et al. 2000, Coulter Mackie et al. 2002). At the other end of the phenotypic spectrum there are patients in whom demyelination of the central nervous system predominates in the absence of peripheral involvement (Cengiz et al. 2002, Gallo et al. 2004, Marcao et al. 2005).

Nevertheless the peripheral nervous system is involved in most patients as shown by the pathological features of various electrophysiological parameters. Thus, peripheral neuropathy results in a reduction of nerve conduction velocity, in prolonged peak latency, temporal dispersion, and diminished amplitude of the compound action potential (Cameron et al. 2004). The sensory fibers are frequently more severely affected than the motor fibers (Bindu et al. 2005). Conduction is also impaired in the central nervous system, as shown by the delay in interpeak latencies of brainstem auditory-evoked potentials. In late-infantile patients this delay may already be present in early stages of the disease (Brown et al. 1981) but it may be absent in late-onset patients (Clark et al. 1979, Wulff and Trojaborg 1985).

MLD is dominated by neurological symptoms, but some patients suffer from cholecystitis and gall bladder polyps (e.g., Ries and Deeg 1993). These symptoms are most likely due to the affection of autonomous nervous system in the course of disease. Although parts of the kidney tubular system also store significant amounts of sulfatide, patients do not develop any renal symptoms.

MRI AND MAGNETIC RESONANCE SPECTROSCOPY

Alterations in the white matter of late-infantile MLD patients are already detectable early in the course of the disease, but after initial symptoms are presented (Zafeiro et al. 1999). In MRI symmetrical, confluent high-signal density regions on T2-weighted images develop first in periventricular regions (see Fig. 8.2). With disease progression, high-signal density regions spread into the hemispheres and the cerebellar white matter (Kim et al. 1997, Faerber et al. 1999). Cortical atrophy with significant enlargement of the ventricles can also occur (Zafeiro et al. 1999). Although the arcuate fibers are typically spared in MLD they may be involved in later stages of the disease (Kim et al. 1997, Zafeirio et al. 1999).

Within the abnormal white matter low-density tigroid stripes can frequently be seen which extend radially. These stripes are typical for MLD but not specific, as they can also be seen in other leukodystrophies. Based on microscopic examination this pattern has been explained by myelin breakdown products which are stored in perivascular macrophages and by sparing of myelin sheaths (van der Voorn et al. 2005). The corpus callosum is involved early in the disease whereas subcortical white matter is spared until late stages. Demyelination can also be seen in the posterior limbs of the internal capsule, descending pyramidal tracts, and the cerebellar white matter. There is no contrast enhancement of the abnormal white matter (Kim et al. 1997)

Proton magnetic resonance spectroscopy of MLD patients shows an elevation of choline. This has been interpreted as a sign of enhanced membrane turnover associated with demyelination. Reduction of *N*-acetyl aspartate in gray and white matter is due to neuronal and axonal loss and the increase of myo-inositol is ascribed to the accompanying gliosis (Kruse et al. 1993, Sener 2003).

Laboratory and genetic diagnosis

On clinical suspicion of MLD, arylsulfatase A enzymatic activity is usually measured in blood leukocytes using artificial water-soluble substrates. Determination of the enzyme in other body fluids, in particular urine, does not yield reliable results and cannot be used to diagnose MLD.

Recently, a procedure has been described that allows determination of arylsulfatase A in dried blood spots (Tan et al 2008) and may be applicable to newborn screening. In addition to the determination arylsulfatase A activity, the quantification of sulfatide excretion in urine is also a very valuable parameter in the diagnosis of MLD.

PROBLEMS IN THE DIAGNOSIS OF MLD

It is important to realize that the determination of arylsulfatase A activity in leukocytes will in no case give a definite answer as to whether or not the patient is affected with MLD (Francis et al. 1993, Rafi et al. 2003). Although finding very little arylsulfatase A activity is highly suggestive of MLD, in particular the late-infantile form, neither a normal arylsulfatase A activity nor a reduced arylsulfatase A activity will exclude or prove a classical or variant form of MLD. For the non-specialist this statement is important to remember. The situation is due to the following circumstances.

DIFFERENTIAL DIAGNOSIS OF MLD AND SAPOSIN B DEFICIENCY

One has to keep in mind that in order to cleave its natural substrate sulfatide, arylsulfatase A depends on the assistance of the activator protein saposin B (Sandhoff et al. 2001). If saposin B is deficient, sulfatide cannot be degraded, resulting in a variant form of MLD (e.g., Deconinck et al. 2008). Since the routine determination of arylsulfatase A activity is assayed with a water-soluble artificial substrate where the monitored hydrolysis does not depend on saposin B, the enzyme activity remains normal when saposin B is deficient. Therefore, if arylsulfatase A activity is normal but the clinical picture strongly suggests MLD (Deconinck et al. 2008) a saposin B deficiency must be excluded. There is no simple biochemical assay for demonstration of saposin B deficiency. When suspecting MLD due to saposin B deficiency, the most meaningful test to perform is determination of sulfatide in urine. High sulfatide excretion in urine without arylsulfatase A deficiency is particularly suggestive of saposin B deficiency.

Direct demonstration of saposin B deficiency can preferably be done by Western Blot Analysis in leukocytes or cultured fibroblasts and/or identification of mutations in the part of the prosaposin gene coding for saposin B. Alternatively, the in-vivo sulfatide degradation capacity of cultured patient fibroblasts can be determined. This so-called sulfatide loading assay, however, depends on a skin biopsy and radioactively labelled sulfatide. Therefore, this assay is unsuitable for routine diagnostic purposes and its application is rather restricted.

DIFFERENTIAL DIAGNOSIS OF MLD AND ARYLSULFATASE A PSEUDODEFICIENCY

The second essential aspect in the diagnosis of MLD is the fact that the demonstration of reduced arylsulfatase A activity alone does not prove MLD. As discussed earlier in this chapter about 0.2% to 0.5% of the normal population is arylsulfatase A pseudodeficient. Thus, enzyme deficiency due to arylsulfatase A pseudodeficiency is about 200-fold more frequent than a deficiency associated with MLD. Therefore, pseudodeficieny must always be excluded in a case where MLD is suspected (Francis et al. 1993, Rafi et al. 2003). Therefore, any time an individual has been found to be arylsulfatase A deficient, the possibility that he/she is homozygous for the pseudodeficiency allele (which displays either one or two polymorphic variations of the arylsulfatase A gene – see section on Genetics) must be excluded. This can be done by polymerase chain reaction / restriction enzyme digestion methods, which allow detection of the polymorphism in the polyadenylation signal. Since one of the two polymorphic variations, the substitution of asparagine 350 by serine, affects the enzyme activity only to a negligible extent, it is not necessary to include this polymorphism in the genetic diagnosis of arylsulfatase A pseudodeficiency. Another possibility to support the assumption of arylsulfatase A pseudodeficiency is to show the absence of massive sulfatide excretion in a 24-hour urine sample (see below). As arylsulfatase A pseudodeficiency may be accompanied by slightly increased sulfatide excretion, molecular genetic testing is mandatory in these cases.

MLD-causing Mutations and the Arylsulfatase A Pseudodeficiency Allele

Unfortunately, the demonstration of the presence of the pseudodeficiency allele in an individual does not definitely exclude MLD. Because the pseudodeficiency allele is so frequent, it is not surprising that mutations causing MLD have also occurred on the backgound of the pseudodeficiency allele (e.g., Gieselmann et al. 1991, Regis et al. 1998). Thus, the presence of one or two of the polymorphic variations defining a pseudodeficiency allele does not exclude the presence of mutations in this allele. This also has to be kept in mind when diagnosing MLD.

Given these problems, the biochemical diagnosis of MLD is not straightforward. Most of the problems described can be circumvented by a simple test which, in these times of molecular genetic diagnosis, may seem to be archaic: the determination of sulfatide in urine. Independent of whether the disease is due to arylsulfatase A or saposin B deficiency, and independent of the presence of pseudodeficiency polymorphisms in an allele causing MLD, the demonstration of the excretion of high amounts of sulfatide in urine is a proof of MLD, including its variants. Therefore the demonstration of increased sulfatide concentration in a 24-hour urine sample is a "must" in the diagnosis of MLD. Diagnosis of MLD by biochemical means is preferable to genetic diagnosis. Owing to the large variety of mutations it is usually necessary to sequence the entire gene, and this diagnostic test is therefore of limited value in the routine diagnosis of MLD.

Genetic Counseling for MLD

Identification of MLD carriers among relatives of patients by determination of arylsulfatase A activity in blood leukocytes is possible, but given the wide range of arylsulfatase A activities in the normal population (e.g., Barth et al. 1994) the reliability of this procedure is restricted. Reliability can be increased, however, if enzyme activities are measured not only in leukocytes of the relative in question, but also in parents and control individuals.

Also, in genetic counseling the arylsulfatase A pseudodeficiency allele must be considered; this is important. Since about 10% of all MLD carriers are also carriers of the arylsulfatase A pseudodeficiency allele, reduced enzyme activity in a putative carrier among siblings of a patient must not be interpreted as proof of carrier status when the presence of an arylsulfatase A pseudodeficiency allele was not excluded in the parents. Therefore, also in genetic counseling it is a "must" to determine arylsulfatase A activity in the patient's parents. A determined value that is clearly below approximately 50% of normal suggests

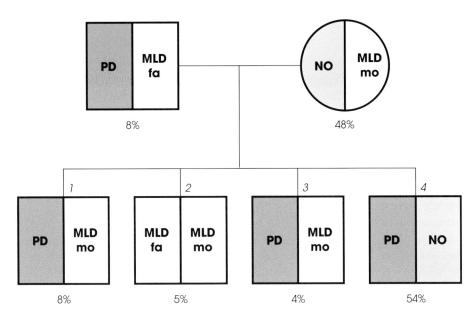

Fig. 8.3. Genealogical tree of a family in which pseudodeficiency and metachromatic leukodystrophy alleles are inherited. PD, pseudodeficiency allele; MLD, metachromatic leukodystrophy allele; NO, normal arylsulfatase A allele; fa, father; mo, mother. Values below the symbols of the individuals give the percentage of residual arylsulfatase A activity. Thus, the father has low arylsulfatase A activity because he is heterozygous for a pseudodeficiency and a MLD allele. In spite of the low activity the father is healthy. The mother is a classical heterozygote with 48% of enzyme activity. Three of the children (*1, 2, 3*) have a substantial arylsulfatase A deficiency. Children *1* and *3* inherited the pseudo-deficiency allele from the father and the MLD allele from the mother and have the same genotype as their father. The arylsulfatase A activity associated with this genotype suffices to ensure a normal life. These children are not affected. Only child *2* has inherited the MLD allele from the father and the mother and is thus affected with MLD. The different genotypes cannot be reliably differentiated by enzyme activity determination. Child *4* inherited the pseudodeficiency allele from the father and the normal allele from the mother. Although this child has arylsulfatase A activity in the range typical for a carrier (compare to the mother) he will not be a carrier for MLD since he has not inherited an MLD allele. Reduced activity is due to the pseudodeficiency allele.

compound heterozygosity for an MLD and a pseudodeficiency allele in the parents. In this case a reduced arylsulfatase A activity in the person seeking genetic counseling can also be due to heterozygosity for the pseudodeficiency allele rather than a MLD allele (Fig. 8.3). Therefore, whenever possible, identification of carriers should be based on DNA sequencing rather than arylsulfatase A activity determination.

PRENATAL DIAGNOSIS
Prenatal diagnosis of MLD is possible and depends on the determination of arylsulfatase A activity in cultured amniotic fluid cells, chorionic villi biopsies, or cells cultured from chorionic villi (von Figura et al. 2001). Before a prenatal diagnosis is initiated it is of utmost importance to clarify whether one of the parents is a carrier of a pseudodeficiency allele

(Fig. 8.3). If this is the case, low arylsulfatase A activity in the amniotic or chorionic samples does not prove MLD. The fetus in question may be a compound heterozygote for a MLD allele inherited from one parent and the pseudodeficiency allele inherited from the other parent. Such an individual is not at risk for any severe neurological disorder related to the low arylsulfatase A activity. In this case it is necessary to prove or exclude the presence of a pseudodeficiency allele in the fetus before the definite diagnosis is made.

Therapy

HEMATOPOETIC STEM CELL TRANSPLANTATION

Stem cell transplantation is considered an option for at least partial endogenous and continuous enzyme replacement. The interpretation of the outcome of patients who had hematopoetic stem cell transplantation in the past has been a matter of debate for many years, but the experience accumulated allows some generally accepted conclusions. Thus, transplantation of patients suffering from the late-infantile form of disease has no beneficial effect, even when conducted before the onset of symptoms (Malm et al. 1996, Bredius et al. 2007) because the progression of disease is too rapid. It is unclear, however, whether neonatal or very early infantile transplantation is of a beneficial effect similar to that shown for Krabbe disease (Escolar et al. 2005). Late-onset patients who have already developed substantial neurological deficits should also not undergo transplantation.

The only group in which hematopoetic stem cell transplantation is considered potentially beneficial comprises late juvenile or adult patients in the early stages of disease, well before major cognitive or motoric deficits occur (Krivit et al. 1999a, b, Krivit 2004). Thus, due to the progressive nature of the disease, there is a limited window of opportunity for hematopoetic stem cells transplantation in MLD, and within this time a suitable donor must be identified.

Two reports have documented a clinical stabilization of transplanted patients with juvenile MLD. All disease parameters investigated 8 and 13 years after bone marrow transplantation, respectively, did not show progression of disease (Kidd et al. 1998, Görg et al. 2007). Long-term stabilization in these patients appears likely to be due to bone marrow transplantation.

In some cases the course of disease in patients who underwent transplantation appeared clearly different to that in their non–transplant-treated siblings (Kapaun et al. 1999, Görg et al. 2007). One has to keep in mind, however, that phenotypic variability of MLD can even occur within the same family. Improvements seen in the treated sibling may therefore not be due to bone marrow transplantation but merely reflect intrafamilial variability.

A co-transplantation of traditional human stem cell transplantation and multipotent mesenchymal stroma cells could give better results, as the aim is to optimize the efficiency of enzyme release in the various tissues of the recipient (Müller et al. 2006). Proof-of-principle is, however, not yet available.

Currently, various therapeutic approaches are in clinical and preclinical development, which may offer therapeutic options for MLD patients. Of these, enzyme replacement trials are already in clinical phase I/II studies. Hematopoetic stem cell based gene therapies and direct injection of adeno-associated virus based vectors into the brain of patients are in a late stage of preclinical development, whereas therapies based on the direct transplantation of cells derived from embryonic stem cells or oligodendrocyte precurors are still in the experimental phase. Here we will only discuss work in early clinical and late preclinical development. For a complete discussion of experimental therapies in MLD, see the review by Sevin et al. (2007b).

Enzyme replacement therapy

Enzyme replacement therapy has been established for various lysosomal storage diseases, most successfully in Gaucher disease. In diseases with severe involvement of the central nervous system such as MLD, the efficacy of enzyme replacement therapies seems questionable because it is likely that the intravenously administered enzyme cannot pass the blood–brain barrier. As far as clinical development is concerned, however, enzyme replacement therapy is most advanced. This therapy is based on preclinical work performed in the non-demyelinating arylsulfatase A-deficient mouse model (Matzner et al. 2005). Treatment of these mice with four repetitive weekly injections of recombinant human arylsulfatase A (20 mg/kg body weight) resulted in a reduction of sulfatide storage in kidney, peripheral nervous system and, surprisingly, also in the central nervous system. When considering the latter it must be kept in mind, however, that the doses applied to the mice are high. The therapy was also accompanied by functional improvement in neuromotor abilities and electrophysiological parameters. These experiments have laid the basis for phase I clinical trials, which are currently ongoing and for which no data have been published so far.

Gene therapy

The other still-experimental approaches are based on gene therapy. Two strategies are being pursued and are past the stage of proof-of-principle in mouse models. One approach involves autologous hematopoetic stem cell transplantation after ex-vivo retroviral or lentiviral vector based modification to over-express arylsulfatase A, respectively (Matzner et al. 2002, Biffi et al. 2006). This approach is based on the rationale that part of the central nervous system microglia is thought to differentiate from blood-derived monocytes. Thus, it is assumed that arylsulfatase A over-expressing and secreting monocytes after bone marrow transplantation invade the brain, differentiate into microglia, and supply enzyme to deficient resident glia and possibly neurons. The feasibility of this approach was examined in the non-demyelinating arylsulfatase A-deficient mouse model with very different results. Whereas one group did not see any improvement of sulfatide storage in brain (Matzner et al. 2002), the other group demonstrated substantial improvements (Biffi et al. 2006). Based on the latter results a gene therapy trial in humans will be launched soon.

An alternative approach is to inject viral vectors conferring arylsulfatase A expression directly into the brain to achieve long-term genetic correction of resident central nervous system cells. Using adeno-associated virus based vectors the feasibility has been examined in mice and resulted in substantial reduction of sulfatide storage in the central nervous system (Sevin et al. 2006, 2007a, b, Kurai et al. 2007). This was accompanied by substantial improvements in behavioral performance of the treated mice. As soon as ongoing toxicological studies have been completed an adeno-associated virus based clinical trial will be initiated in near future.

In conclusion, various therapeutic approaches are currently under development for MLD. The years to come will show which of these has the potential to positively influence the disease outcome in the patients.

REFERENCES

Alessandri MG, De Vito G, Fornai F. (2002) Increased prevalence of pervasive developmental disorders in children with slight arylsulfatase A deficiency. Brain Dev 24: 688–692.

Arbour LT, Silver K, Hechtman P, Treacy EP, Coulter-Mackie MB. (2000) Variable onset of metachromatic leukodystrophy in a Vietnamese family. Pediatr Neurol 23: 173–176.

Barth ML, Fensom A, Harris A. (1993) Prevalence of common mutations in the arylsulphatase A gene in metachromatic leukodystrophy patients diagnosed in Britain. Hum Genet 91: 73–77.

Barth ML, Ward C, Harris A, Saad A, Fensom A. (1994) Frequency of arylsulphatase A pseudodeficiency associated mutations in a healthy population. J Med Genet 31: 667–671.

Berger J, Loschl B, Bernheimer H, et al. (1997) Occurrence, distribution, and phenotype of arylsulfatase A mutations in patients with metachromatic leukodystrophy. Am J Med Genet 69: 335–340.

Berger J, Gmach M, Mayr U, Molzer B, Bernheimer H. (1999) Coincidence of two novel arylsulfatase A alleles and mutation 459+1G>A within a family with metachromatic leukodystrophy: molecular basis of phenotypic heterogeneity. Hum Mutat 13: 61–68.

Biffi A, Capotondo A, Fasano S, et al. (2006) Gene therapy of metachromatic leukodystrophy reverses neurological damage and deficits in mice. J Clin Invest 116: 3070–3082.

Biffi A, Cesani M, Fumagalli F, et al. (2008) Metachromatic leukodystrophy – mutation analysis provides further evidence of genotype–phenotype correlation. Clin Genet 74: 349–357.

Bindu PS, Mahadevan A, Taly AB, Christopher R, Gayathri N, Shankar SK. (2005) Peripheral neuropathy in metachromatic leucodystrophy. A study of 40 cases from south India. J Neurol Neurosurg Psychiatry 76: 1698–1701.

Bosch EP, Hart MN. (1978) Late adult-onset metachromatic leukodystrophy. Dementia and polyneuropathy in a 63-year-old man. Arch Neurol 35: 475–477.

Bredius RG, Laan LA, Lankester AC, et al. (2007) Early marrow transplantation in a pre-symptomatic neonate with late infantile metachromatic leukodystrophy does not halt disease progression. Bone Marrow Transplant 39: 309–310.

Brown FR, 3rd, Shimizu H, McDonald JM, et al. (1981) Auditory evoked brainstem response and high-performance liquid chromatography sulfatide assay as early indices of metachromatic leukodystrophy. Neurology. 31: 980–985.

Cameron CL, Kang PB, Burns TM, Darras BT, Jones HR, Jr. (2004) Multifocal slowing of nerve conduction in metachromatic leukodystrophy. Muscle Nerve 29: 531–536.

Cengiz N, Ozbenli T, Onar M, Yildiz L, Ertas B. (2002) Adult metachromatic leukodystrophy: three cases with normal nerve conduction velocities in a family. Acta Neurol Scand 105: 454–457.

Clark JR, Miller RG, Vidgoff JM. (1979) Juvenile-onset metachromatic leukodystrophy: biochemical and electrophysiologic studies. Neurology 29: 346–353.

Clarke JT, Skomorowski MA, Chang PL. (1989) Marked clinical difference between two sibs affected with juvenile metachromatic leukodystrophy. Am J Med Genet 33: 10–13.

Colsch B, Afonso C, Turpin JC, Portoukalian J, Tabet JC, Baumann N. (2008) Sulfogalactosylceramides in motor and psycho-cognitive adult metachromatic leukodystrophy: relations between clinical, biochemical analysis and molecular aspects. Biochim Biophys Acta 1780: 434–440.

Comabella M, Waye JS, Raguer N, et al. (2001) Late-onset metachromatic leukodystrophy clinically presenting as isolated peripheral neuropathy: compound heterozygosity for the IVS2+1G—>A mutation and a newly identified missense mutation (Thr408Ile) in a Spanish family. Ann Neurol 50: 108–112.

Conzelmann E, Sandhoff K. (1991) Biochemical basis of late-onset neurolipidoses. Dev Neurosci 13: 197–204.

Coulter-Mackie M, Gagnier L. (1997) Two new polymorphisms in the arylsulfatase A gene and their haplotype associations with normal, metachromatic leukodystrophy and pseudodeficiency alleles. Am J Med Genet 73: 32–35.

Coulter-Mackie MB, Applegarth DA, Toone JR, Gagnier L, Anzarut AR, Hendson G. (2002) Isolated peripheral neuropathy in atypical metachromatic leukodystrophy: a recurrent mutation. Can J Neurol Sci 29: 159–163.

Coulter-Mackie MB, Gagnier L. (2003) Spectrum of mutations in the arylsulfatase A gene in a Canadian DNA collection including two novel frameshift mutations, a new missense mutation (C488R) and an MLD mutation (R84Q) in cis with a pseudodeficiency allele. Mol Genet Metab 79: 91–98.

Deconinck N, Messaaoui A, Ziereisen F, et al. (2008) Metachromatic leukodystrophy without arylsulfatase A deficiency: a new case of saposin-B deficiency. Eur J Paediatr Neurol 12: 46–50.

D'Hooge R, Van Dam D, Franck F, Gieselmann V, De Deyn PP. (2001) Hyperactivity, neuromotor defects, and impaired learning and memory in a mouse model for metachromatic leukodystrophy. Brain Res 907: 35–43.

Dierks T, Schmidt B, Borissenko LV, et al. (2003) Multiple sulfatase deficiency is caused by mutations in the gene encoding the human C (alpha)-formylglycine generating enzyme. Cell 113: 435–444.

Duyff RF, Weinstein HC. (1996) Late-presenting metachromatic leukodystrophy. Lancet. 348: 1382–1383.

Eckhardt M, Hedayati KK, Pitsch J, et al. (2007) Sulfatide storage in neurons causes hyperexcitability and axonal degeneration in a mouse model of metachromatic leukodystrophy. J Neurosci 27: 9009–9021.

Escolar ML, Poe MD, Provenzale JM, et al. (2005) Transplantation of umbilical-cord blood in babies with infantile Krabbe's disease. N Engl J Med 352: 2069–2081.

Faerber EN, Melvin JJ, Smergel EM. (1999) MRI appearances of metachromatic leukodystrophies. Pediatr Radiol 29: 669–672.

Felice KJ, Gomez Lira M, Natowicz M, et al. (2000) Adult-onset MLD: a gene mutation with isolated polyneuropathy. Neurology 55: 1036–1039.

Fluharty AL, Fluharty CB, Bohne W, von Figura K, Gieselmann V. (1991) Two new arylsulfatase A (ARSA) mutations in a juvenile metachromatic leukodystrophy (MLD) patient. Am J Hum Genet 49: 1340–1350.

Francis GS, Bonni A, Shen N, et al. (1993) Metachromatic leukodystrophy: multiple nonfunctional and pseudodeficiency alleles in a pedigree: problems with diagnosis and counseling. Ann Neurol 34: 212–218.

Fujii T, Kobayashi T, Honke K, et al. (1992) Proteolytic processing of human lysosomal arylsulfatase A. Biochim Biophys Acta 1122: 93–98.

Fukutani Y, Noriki Y, Sasaki K, et al. (1999) Adult-type metachromatic leukodystrophy with a compound heterozygote mutation showing character change and dementia. Psychiatry Clin Neurosci 53: 425–428.

Gallo S, Randi D, Bertelli M, Salviati A, Pandolfo M. (2004) Late onset MLD with normal nerve conduction associated with two novel missense mutations in the arylsulfatase A gene. J Neurol Neurosurg Psychiatry 75: 655–657.

Gieselmann V, Fluharty AL, Tonnesen T, von Figura K. (1991) Mutations in the arylsulfatase A pseudo-deficiency allele causing metachromatic leukodystrophy. Am J Hum Genet 49: 407–413.

Gieselmann V, Polten A, Kreysing J, von Figura K. (1989) Arylsulfatase A pseudodeficiency: loss of a polyadenylylation signal and N-glycosylation site. Proc Natl Acad Sci USA 86: 9436–9440.

Görg M, Wilck W, Granitzny B, et al. (2007) Stabilization of juvenile metachromatic leukodystrophy after bone marrow transplantation: a 13-year follow-up. J Child Neurol 22: 1139–1142.

Gomez-Lira M, Perusi C, Mottes M, et al. (1998) Molecular genetic characterization of two metachromatic leukodystrophy patients who carry the T799G mutation and show different phenotypes; description of a novel null-type mutation. Hum Genet 102: 459–376.

Gort L, Coll MJ, Chabas A. (2000) Metachromatic leukodystrophy: a novel mutation (c237delC) and extension of the haplotype associated with the P426L mutation. Hum Mutat 16: 375–.

Gustavson KH, Hagberg B. (1971) The incidence and genetics of metachromatic leucodystrophy in northern Sweden. Acta Paediatr Scand 60: 585–590.

Haberlandt E., Scholl-Bürgi S, Neuberger J, et al. (2008) Peripheral neuropathy as the sole initial finding in three children with infantile metachromatic leukodystrophy. Eur J Paediatr Neurol 13: 257–260.

Hageman AT, Gabreels FJ, de Jong JG, et al. (1995) Clinical symptoms of adult metachromatic leukodystrophy and arylsulfatase A pseudodeficiency. Arch Neurol 52: 408–413.

Halsall DJ, Halligan EP, Elsey TS, Cox TM. (1999) Metachromatic leucodystrophy: a newly identified mutation in arylsulphatase A, D281Y, found as a compound heterozygote with I179L in an adult onset case. Hum Mutat 14: 447.

Hannun YA, Bell RM. (1989) Functions of sphingolipids and sphingolipid breakdown products in cellular regulation. Science 243: 500–507.

Harvey JS, Nelson PV, Carey WF, Robertson EF, Morris CP. (1993) An arylsulfatase A (ARSA) missense mutation (T274M) causing late-infantile metachromatic leukodystrophy. Hum Mutat 2: 261–267.

Heim P, Claussen M, Hoffmann B, et al. (1997) Leukodystrophy incidence in Germany. Am J Med Genet. 71: 475–478.

Hess B, Kafert S, Heinisch U, Wenger DA, Zlotogora J, Gieselmann V. (1996a) Characterization of two arylsulfatase A missense mutations D335V and T274M causing late infantile metachromatic leukodystrophy. Hum Mutat 7: 311–317.

Hess B, Saftig P, Hartmann D, et al. (1996b) Phenotype of arylsulfatase A-deficient mice: relationship to human metachromatic leukodystrophy. Proc Natl Acad Sci USA. 93: 14 821–14 826.

Hirahara Y, Bansal R, Honke K, Ikenaka K, Wada Y. (2004) Sulfatide is a negative regulator of oligodendrocyte differentiation: development in sulfatide-null mice. Glia 45: 269–.

Hohenschutz C, Eich P, Friedl W, Waheed A, Conzelmann E, Propping P. (1989) Pseudodeficiency of arylsulfatase A: a common genetic polymorphism with possible disease implications. Hum Genet 82: 45–48.

Honke K, Hirahara Y, Dupree J, et al. (2002) Paranodal junction formation and spermatogenesis require sulfoglycolipids. Proc Natl Acad Sci USA 99: 4227–4232.

Hwu WL, Tsai LP, Wang WC, Chuang SC, Wang PJ, Wang TR. (1996) Arylsulfatase A pseudodeficiency in Chinese. Hum Genet 97: 148–149.

Hyde TM, Zeigler JC, Weinberger DR. (1992) Psychiatric disturbances in metachromatic leukodystrophy, insights into the neurobiology if psychosis. Arch Neurol 49: 401–406.

Im DS, Heise CE, Nguyen T, O'Dowd BF, Lynch KR. (2001) Identification of a molecular target of psychosine and its role in globoid cell formation. J Cell Biol 153: 429–434.

Ishibashi T, Dupree JL, Ikenaka K, et al. (2002) A myelin galactolipid, sulfatide, is essential for maintenance of ion channels on myelinated axon but not essential for initial cluster formation. J Neurosci 22: 6507–6514.

Kapaun P, Dittmann RW, Granitzny B, et al. (1999) Slow progression of juvenile metachromatic leukodystrophy 6 years after bone marrow transplantation. J Child Neurol. 14: 222–228.

Kappler J, Sommerlade HJ, von Figura K, Gieselmann V. (1994) Complex arylsulfatase A alleles causing metachromatic leukodystrophy. Hum Mutat 4: 119–127.

Kehrer C, Kustermann-Kuhn B, Krägeloh-Mann I. (2008a) Clinical course of metachromatic leucodystrophy (MLD) in children – an analysis using standardized functional motor scores. Neuropediatrics 39; DOI: 10.1055/s-2008-1079467.

Kehrer C, Kustermann-Kuhn B, Raabe C, Krägeloh-Mann I. (2008b) Natural history of metachromatic leucodystrophy (MLD) – clinical course. Eur J Pediatr 167: 361–376.

Kidd D, Nelson J, Jones F, et al. (1998) Long-term stabilization after bone marrow transplantation in juvenile metachromatic leukodystrophy. Arch Neurol 55: 98–99.

Kim TS, Kim IO, Kim WS, et al. (1997) MR of childhood metachromatic leukodystrophy. AJNR Am J Neuroradiol 18: 733–738.

Krivit W, Aubourg P, Shapiro E, Peters C. (1999a) Bone marrow transplantation for globoid cell leukodystrophy, adrenoleukodystrophy, metachromatic leukodystrophy, and Hurler syndrome. Curr Opin Hematol 6: 377–382.

Krivit W, Peters C, Shapiro EG. (1999b) Bone marrow transplantation as effective treatment of central nervous system disease in globoid cell leukodystrophy, metachromatic leukodystrophy, adrenoleukodystrophy, mannosidosis, fucosidosis, aspartylglucosaminuria, Hurler, Maroteaux-Lamy, and Sly syndromes, and Gaucher disease type III. Curr Opin Neurol 12: 167–176.

Krivit W. (2004) Allogeneic stem cell transplantation for the treatment of lysosomal and peroxisomal metabolic diseases. Springer Semin Immunopathol 26: 119–132.

Kruse B, Hanefeld F, Christen HJ, et al. (1993) Alterations of brain metabolites in metachromatic leukodystrophy as detected by localized proton magnetic resonance spectroscopy in vivo. J Neurol 241: 68–74.

Kumperscak HG, Plesnicar BK, Zalar B, Gradisnik P, Seruga T, Paschke E. (2007) Adult metachromatic leukodystrophy: a new mutation in the schizophrenia-like phenotype with early neurological signs. Psychiatr Genet 17: 85–91.

152

Kurai T, Hisayasu S, Kitagawa R, et al. (2007) AAV1 mediated co-expression of formylglycine-generating enzyme and arylsulfatase a efficiently corrects sulfatide storage in a mouse model of metachromatic leukodystrophy. Mol Ther 15: 38–43.

Kurosawa K, Ida H, Eto Y. (1998) Prevalence of arylsulphatase A mutations in 11 Japanese patients with metachromatic leukodystrophy: identification of two novel mutations. J Inherit Metab Dis 21: 781–782.

Leinekugel P, Michel S, Conzelmann E, Sandhoff K. (1992) Quantitative correlation between the residual activity of beta-hexosaminidase A and arylsulfatase A and the severity of the resulting lysosomal storage disease. Hum Genet 88: 513–523.

Leistner S, Young, E, Winchester B. (1995) Pseudodeficiency of arylsulfatase A: strategy for clarification of genotype in families of subjects with low arylsulfatase A activity and neurologic symptoms. J Inherit Metab Dis 18: 710–716.

Lugowska A, Berger J, Tylki-Szymańska A, et al. (2005a) Molecular and phenotypic characteristics of metachromatic leukodystrophy patients from Poland. Clin Genet 68: 48–54.

Lugowska A, Amaral O, Berger J, et al. (2005b) Mutations c.459+1G>A and p.P426L in the ARSA gene: prevalence in metachromatic leukodystrophy patients from European countries. Mol Genet Metab 86: 353–359.

Lyon G, Kolodny EH, Pastores GM. (2006) Neurology of Hereditary Metabolic Diseases of Children, 3rd edn. New York: McGraw Hill.

MacFaul R, Cavanagh N, Lake BD, Stephens R, Whitfield AE. (1982) Metachromatic leucodystrophy: review of 38 cases. Arch Dis Child 57: 168–175.

Malm G, Ringden O, Winiarski J, et al. (1996) Clinical outcome in four children with metachromatic leukodystrophy treated by bone marrow transplantation. Bone Marrow Transplant 17: 1003–1008.

Marcao AM, Wiest R, Schindler K, et al. (2005) Adult onset metachromatic leukodystrophy without electroclinical peripheral nervous system involvement: a new mutation in the ARSA gene. Arch Neurol 62: 309–313.

Matzner U, Hartmann D, Lullmann-Rauch R, et al. (2002) Bone marrow stem cell-based gene transfer in a mouse model for metachromatic leukodystrophy: effects on visceral and nervous system disease manifestations. Gene Ther 9: 53–63.

Matzner U, Herbst E, Hedayati KK, et al. (2005) Enzyme replacement improves nervous system pathology and function in a mouse model for metachromatic leukodystrophy. Hum Mol Genet 14: 1139–1152.

Mihaljevic-Peles A, Jakovljevic M, Milicevic Z, Kracun I. (2001) Low arylsulphatase A activity in the development of psychiatric disorders. Neuropsychobiology 43: 75–78.

Müller I, Kustermann-Kuhn B, Holzwarth C, et al. (2006) In vitro analysis of multipotent mesenchymal stroma cells as potential cellular therapeutics in neurometabolic diseases in pediatric patients. Exp Hematol. 34: 1413–1419.

Ott R, Waye JS, Chang PL. (1997) Evolutionary origins of two tightly linked mutations in arylsulfatase-A pseudodeficiency. Hum Genet 101: 135–140.

Peng L, Suzuki, K. (1987) Ultrastructural study of neurons in metachromatic leukodystrophy. Clin Neuropathol 6: 224–230.

Penzien JM, Kappler J, Herschkowitz N, et al. (1993) Compound heterozygosity for metachromatic leukodystrophy and arylsulfatase A pseudodeficiency alleles is not associated with progressive neurological disease. Am J Hum Genet 52: 557–564.

Perusi C, Lira MG, Duyff RF, et al. (1999) Mutations associated with very late-onset metachromatic leukodystrophy. Clin Genet 55: 130.

Pinto R, Caseiro C, Lemos M, et al. (2004) Prevalence of lysosomal storage diseases in Portugal. Eur J Hum Genet 12: 87–92.

Poeppel P, Habetha M, Marcao A, Bussow H, Berna L, Gieselmann V. (2005) Missense mutations as a cause of metachromatic leukodystrophy. Degradation of arylsulfatase A in the endoplasmic reticulum. FEBS J 272: 1179–1188.

Polten A, Fluharty AL, Fluharty CB, Kappler J, von Figura K, Gieselmann V. (1991) Molecular basis of different forms of metachromatic leukodystrophy. N Engl J Med. 324: 18–22.

Poorthuis BJ, Wevers RA, Kleijer WJ, et al. (1999) The frequency of lysosomal storage diseases in The Netherlands. Hum Genet 105: 151–156.

Rafi MA, Coppola S, Liu SL, Rao HZ, Wenger DA. (2003) Disease-causing mutations in cis with the common arylsulfatase A pseudodeficiency allele compound the difficulties in accurately identifying patients and carriers of metachromatic leukodystrophy. Mol Genet Metab 79: 83–90.

153

Ramakrishnan H, Hedayati KK, Lüllmann-Rauch R, Wessig C, Fewou SN, Maier H, Goebel HH, Gieselmann V, Eckhardt M. (2007) Increasing sulfatide synthesis in myelin-forming cells of arylsulfatase A-deficient mice causes demyelination and neurological symptoms reminiscent of human metachromatic leukodystrophy. J Neurosci. 27: 9482–9490.

Rauschka H, Colsch B, Baumann N, et al. (2006) Late-onset metachromatic leukodystrophy: genotype strongly influences phenotype. Neurology 67: 859–863.

Regis S, Filocamo M, Stroppiano M, Corsolini F, Caroli F, Gatti R. (1998) A 9-bp deletion (2320del9) on the background of the arylsulfatase A pseudodeficiency allele in a metachromatic leukodystrophy patient and in a patient with nonprogressive neurological symptoms. Hum Genet 102: 50–53.

Ries M, Deeg KH. (1993) Polyposis of the gallbladder associated with metachromatic leukodystrophy. Eur J Pediatr 152: 450–451.

Sadovnick AD, Tuokko H, Applegarth DA, Toone JR, Hadjistavropoulos T, Beattie BL. (1993) The differential diagnosis of adult onset metachromatic leukodystrophy and early onset familial Alzheimer disease in an Alzheimer clinic population. Can J Neurol Sci 20: 312–318.

Sandhoff R, Hepbildikler ST, Jennemann R, et al. (2002) Kidney sulfatides in mouse models of inherited glycosphingolipid disorders: determination by nano-electrospray ionization tandem mass spectrometry. J Biol Chem 277: 20 386–20 398

Sandhoff K, Kolter T, Harzer K. (2001) Sphingolipid Activator Protein. In: Scriver CR, Beaudet AL, Sly, WS, Valle D, Eds. The Metabolic and Molecular Bases of Inherited Disease. New York: McGraw Hill, pp. 3371–3388.

Schestag F, Yaghootfam A, Habetha M, et al. (2002) The functional consequences of mis-sense mutations affecting an intra-molecular salt bridge in arylsulphatase A. Biochemistry 367: 499–504.

Sener RN. (2003) Metachromatic leukodystrophy: diffusion MR imaging findings. AJNR Am J Neuroradiol. 23: 1424–1426.

Sevin C, Benraiss A, Van Dam D, et al. (2006) Intracerebral adeno-associated virus-mediated gene transfer in rapidly progressive forms of metachromatic leukodystrophy. Hum Mol Genet 15: 53–64.

Sevin C, Verot L, Benraiss A, et al. (2007a) Partial cure of established disease in an animal model of metachromatic leukodystrophy after intracerebral adeno-associated virus-mediated gene transfer. Gene Ther 14: 405–414.

Sevin C, Aubourg P, Cartier N. (2007b) Enzyme, cell and gene-based therapies for metachromatic leukodystrophy. J Inherit Metab Dis 30:175–183

Shen N, Li ZG, Waye JS, Francis G, Chang PL. (1993) Complications in the genotypic molecular diagnosis of pseudo arylsulfatase A deficiency. Am J Med Genet 45: 631–637.

Sommerlade HJ, Selmer T, Ingendoh A, et al. (1994) Glycosylation and phosphorylation of arylsulfatase A. J Biol Chem 269: 20 977–20 981.

Stein C, Gieselmann V, Kreysing J, et al. (1989) Cloning and expression of human arylsulfatase A. J Biol Chem 264: 1252–.

Stroobants S, Leroy T, Eckhardt M, Aerts JM, Berckmans D, D'Hooge R. (2008) Early signs of neurolipidosis-related behavioural alterations in a murine model of metachromatic leukodystrophy. Behav Brain Res 189: 306–316.

Suzuki C, Watanabe M, Tomiyama M, et al. (2008) A novel mutation in the arylsulfatase A gene associated with adult-onset metachromatic leukodystrophy without clinical evidence of neuropathy. Eur Neurol. 60: 310–311.

Tan MA, Dean CJ, Hopwood JJ, Meikle PJ. (2008) Diagnosis of metachromatic leukodystrophy by immune quantification of arylsulphatase A protein and activity in dried blood spots. Clin Chem 54: 1925–1927.

von Bülow R, Schmidt B, Dierks T, et al. (2002) Defective oligomerization of arylsulfatase A as a cause of its instability in lysosomes and metachromatic leukodystrophy. J Biol Chem 277: 9455–9461.

van der Voorn JP, Pouwels PJ, Kamphorts W, et al. (2005) Histopathological correlates of radial stripes on MR images in lysosomal storags disorders. Am J Neuroradiol 26: 442–446.

von Figura K, Gieselmann V, Jaeken J. (2001) Metachromatic leukodystrophy. In: Scriver CR, Beaudet AL, Sly WS, Valle D, Eds. The Metabolic and Molecular Bases of Inherited Disease. New York: McGraw Hill, pp. 3695–3724.

Wang J, Zhang W, Pan H, et al. (2007) ARSA gene mutations in five Chinese metachromatic leukodystrophy patients. Pediatr Neurol 36: 397–401.

Wittke D, Hartmann D, Gieselmann V, Lullmann-Rauch R. (2004) Lysosomal sulfatide storage in the brain of arylsulfatase A-deficient mice: cellular alterations and topographic distribution. Acta Neuropathol (Berl) 108: 261–271.

Wulff CH, Trojaborg W. (1985) Adult metachromatic leukodystrophy: neurophysiologic findings. Neurology 35: 1776–1778.

Zafeiriou DI, Kontopoulos EE, Michelakakis HM, Anastasiou AL, Gombakis NP. (1999) Neurophysiology and MRI in late-infantile metachromatic leukodystrophy. Pediatr Neurol 21: 843–846.

Zaka M, Rafi MA, Rao HZ, Luzi P, Wenger DA. (2005) Insulin-like growth factor-1 provides protection against psychosine-induced apoptosis in cultured mouse oligodendrocyte progenitor cells using primarily the PI3K/Akt pathway. Mol Cell Neurosci 30: 398–407.

Zlotogora J, Gieselmann V, von Figura K, Zeigler M, Bach G. (1994a) Late infantile metachromatic leukodystrophy in Israel. Biomed Pharmacother 48: 347–350.

Zlotogora J, Furman-Shaharabani Y, Harris A, Barth ML, von Figura K, Gieselmann V. (1994b) A single origin for the most frequent mutation causing late infantile metachromatic leucodystrophy. J Med Genet 31: 672–674.

9
CANAVAN DISEASE

Kimberlee Michals and Reuben Matalon

Introduction

In 1931, M. M. Canavan described spongy degeneration of the white matter of the brain in a patient who was thought to have Schilder disease (Canavan 1931). An earlier report had described a similar brain pathology, which was also thought to be a case of Schilder disease (Globus and Strauss 1928). The recognition that the cases described by these authors represented a distinct disease entity came in 1949, when van Bogaert and Bertrand prepared a detailed report of three Jewish children with spongy degeneration of the brain (van Bogaert and Bertrand 1949). They suggested an autosomal recessive mode of inheritance for a disease that was more common among Jewish individuals (Fig. 9.1). The term "Canavan disease" prevailed for the spongy degeneration of the brain described by van Bogaert and

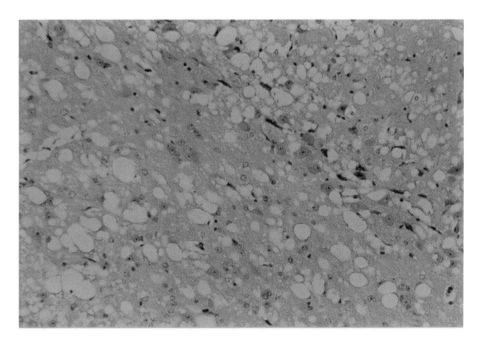

Fig. 9.1. Brain biopsy of a patient with Canavan disease, showing spongy degeneration of the brain. This procedure is no longer necessary, since diagnosis can be made by urine analysis for excessive amount of *N*-acetylaspartic acid. (A color version of this figure is available in the Plate section.)

Bertrand. Since then, numerous cases have been reported, with an increased prevalence among Jewish individuals (Banker and Victor 1979).

The identification of aspartoacylase as the enzyme defective in Canavan disease, with high concentrations of *N*-acetylaspartic acid in urine and brain, was discovered in 1988 by Matalon and colleagues (Matalon et al. 1988, 1989). Subsequent reports confirmed that elevated *N*-acetylaspartic acid is diagnostic for Canavan disease (Echenne et al. 1989, Elpeleg et al. 1989). The deficiency of aspartoacylase leads to the accumulation of *N*-acetylaspartic acid in the brain and increased concentration of *N*-acetylaspartic acid in cerebrospinal fluid (CSF), plasma, and urine.

The diagnosis of Canavan disease can be readily ascertained from elevated levels of urinary *N*-acetylaspartic acid, without the need for brain biopsy. Since 1988, Canavan disease has been diagnosed frequently and with certainty in many ethnicities, not only in Jewish patients. The gene for Canavan disease was cloned in 1993 and localized to the short arm of chromosome 17 (Kaul et al. 1994a). Mutations that lead to Canavan disease can be determined in patients, family members, and at-risk populations (Kaul et al. 1993, Matalon et al. 1995). Aspartoacylase has been shown to be dimeric with zinc at the active site, similar to the carboxypeptidase A family (Hershfield et al. 2007).

Molecular basis

The human aspartoacylase gene consists of 20 kb of genomic DNA, localized to the short arm of chromosome 17 (17p13-ter) (Kaul et al. 1994a). The cDNA for the open reading frame of aspartoacylase is 639 bp long, predicting 313 amino acids with a molecular mass of 36 kDa. The gene is comprised of six exons and is conserved among species. There is a great deal of homology of the coding sequences of the bovine, mouse, and human aspartoacylase gene (Kaul et al. 1994a).

There are two common mutations among Ashkenazi Jewish individuals. A mis-sense mutation on codon 285 (exon 6) with substitution of glutamic acid to alanine (E285A) accounting for 84% of mutations identified in a large number of Jewish patients, and a nonsense mutation, tyrosine to termination, on codon 231 (exon 5) (Y231X) accounts for 13.4% of Jewish patients (Kaul et al. 1994b, Matalon 1997). Together these two mutations account for over 97% of the alleles in Jewish patients with Canavan disease (Kaul et al. 1994b).

Canavan disease is less frequent among non-Jewish individuals. The most common causative mutation, found in about 30% of non-Jewish patients, is in codon 305 (exon 6), a mis-sense mutation substituting alanine to glutamic acid (A305E) (Kaul et al. 1994b, c, Shaag et al. 1995, Kaul et al. 1996, Matalon and Michals-Matalon 1998, 1999, Sistermans et al. 2000). There are more than 50 other mutations described, including deletions of the aspartoacylase gene, all in non-Jewish individuals (Elpeleg and Shaag 1999, Rady et al. 1999, 2000, Sistermans et al. 2000).

Clinical features

The triad of hypotonia, head lag, and macrocephaly suggests Canavan disease. Newborns with Canavan disease do not have distinctive clinical features. In the first few months of life

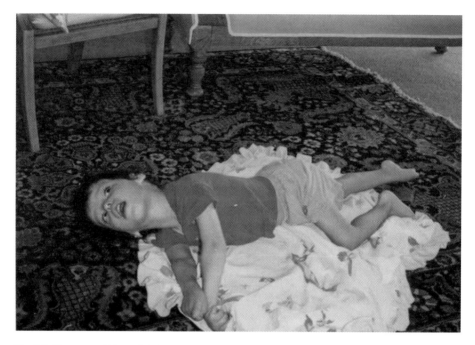

Fig. 9.2. Five-year-old boy with Canavan disease with macrocephaly. In infancy he was very hypotonic; now he has spasticity and similar characteristics to patients with cerebral palsy.

delayed development may be minimal. In early infancy the head circumference may be normal, or in some cases remains at the upper limit of normal. However, in the majority of cases head circumference increases after the age of 6 months, and by the first year it is above the 90th percentile. As the infant grows older it becomes obvious that developmental milestones are delayed. Head control remains poor, and inability to support the head is a constant feature of Canavan disease. Seizures and optic atrophy usually develop in the second year of life. Patients with Canavan disease often become irritable and exhibit sleep disturbance. As the disease progresses, problems with gastroesophageal reflux become prominent, leading to feeding difficulties and poor weight gain. Swallowing deteriorates, and some of the children require nasogastric feeding or permanent feeding gastrostomies. Most patients with Canavan disease die in the first decade of life. However, with improved medical and nursing care a larger number of children survive beyond the first decade. As children with Canavan disease get older, joint stiffness increases, so that these children look more like patients with cerebral palsy (Fig. 9.2) (Matalon and Michals-Matalon 2000, 2003). Patients with Canavan disease remain totally dependent on others for their daily living activities.

Variant forms of the disease
Prior to the biochemical identification of Canavan disease, Adachi and colleagues described three forms of Canavan disease: congenital, infantile, and juvenile (Adachi et al. 1973).

These forms were not clearly distinguished but the congenital form was a more readily recognizable disease, and probably was the same as the infantile form. Most cases of the congenital form were later confirmed by increased urinary *N*-acetylaspartic acid and deficiency of aspartoacylase (Matalon et al. 1993).

The juvenile form of Canavan disease suggested by Adachi in 1973 was difficult to confirm, since *N*-acetylaspartic aciduria and aspartoacylase deficiency had not yet been discovered. Toft et al. (1973) described two children with the juvenile form of Canavan disease based on magnetic resonance imaging and spectroscopy (MRI/MRS) findings of increased *N*-acetyaspartic acid. Other patients with mild manifestations of Canavan disease have been reported, and confirmed by biochemical and genetic analysis. The first case had slightly elevated urine *N*-acetylaspartic acid and was a compound heterozygote with mild mutation in one allele of the aspartoacylase gene, Y288C, and a severe mutation, A305E, on the other allele. This patient had a large head, retinitis pigmentosa, and mild developmental delay, but did not have mental retardation, and was able to go to a normal school. The MRI of the patient showed no sponginess of the brain but did show increased signal intensity in the basal ganglia, similar to mitochondrial disease (Surendran et al. 2003a). Other patients with mutation Y288C presenting similar MRI findings have since been reported (Yalcinkaya et al. 2005).

Two siblings were identified to have mild elevation of urine *N*-acetylaspartic acid. They had one mild mutation, R71H on one allele, with another mutation, A305E, on the other allele (Fig. 9.3). These patients were mildly affected, the slight increase of *N*-acetylaspartic

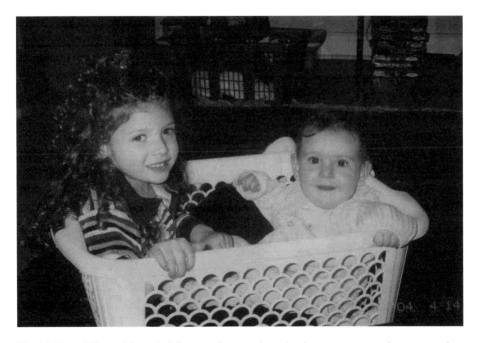

Fig. 9.3. Two siblings with atypical Canavan disease, whose development was very close to normal.

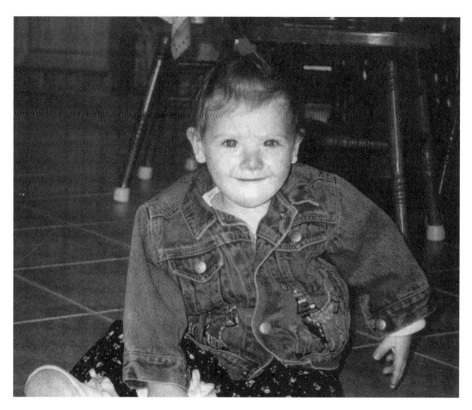

Fig. 9.4. Girl with atypical Canavan disease. Development appears normal and there is no macrocephaly.

acid was discovered accidentally on routine urine testing. Their developmental milestones were normal or minimally delayed, they had no macrocephaly (Fig 9.4), and the MRI did not show spongy degeneration of the brain. However, they had changes in the basal ganglia and no increase in cerebral *N*-acetylaspartic acid by MRS. In these two siblings mitochondrial disease was suggested (Janson et al. 2006, Matalon 2006).

Diagnostic workup
The triad of megalencephaly, head lag, and hypotonia in early life should initiate the workup. The computed tomography (CT) scan and MRI of the brain reveal diffuse white matter degeneration in Canavan disease (Rushton et al. 1981, Brismar et al. 1990, McAdams et al. 1990, Matalon and Michals-Matalon 2000). The white matter involved is primarily in the cerebral hemispheres, with similar changes in the cerebellum and brainstem (Fig. 9.5). However, because the MRI or CT may be interpreted as normal early in life, follow-up evaluations are indicated (Matalon and Michals-Matalon 2000). An early MRI of a 2-year-old child with Canavan disease revealed severe white matter degeneration; the child was initially thought to have periventricular leukomalacia caused by an ischemic episode at birth. Diagnosis was established by urine examination which showed a very high level of

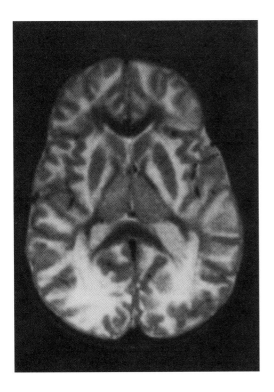

Fig. 9.5. The MRI shows universal white matter involvement in Canavan disease, including the internal and external capsules and the U-fibers.

N-acetylaspartic acid. In Canavan disease there is an increase of *N*-acetylaspartic acid when compared with the level in normal brain, as shown by MRS (Grodd et al. 1990, Wittsack et al. 1996). This technology can be helpful but is not always definitive, especially in mild cases of Canavan disease (Matalon 2006).

The specific tests that lead to the diagnosis of Canavan disease are biochemical. Levels of urine *N*-acetylaspartic acid are elevated greatly: 1440.5 ± 873.1 mmol/mmol creatinine compared with controls of 23.5 ± 16.1 mmol/mmol creatinine. A new method using liquid chromatography–tandem mass spectrometry (LC-MS/MS) is being developed to test urine without special extraction (Al-Dirbashi et al. 2007). Aspartoacylase activity is not present in the blood. Cultured skin fibroblasts manifest the enzyme deficiency with very low level of activity of aspartoacylase, viz. 0.005 ± 0.009 mU/mg protein, while normal fibroblasts have a higher activity, around 0.240 ± 0.095 mU/mg protein. Enzyme determination may be difficult, because the level of aspartoacylase activity fluctuates depending on culture conditions. However, enzyme determination is not needed for the diagnosis of Canavan disease: *N*-Acetylaspartic acid is also elevated in blood and in CSF but the strikingly high concentration of this analyte in urine is the only test required for diagnosis. Brain biopsy is not required to confirm the diagnosis.

Once the diagnosis of Canavan disease is reached, DNA mutation analysis should be performed on the proband as well as on family members, for counseling and preventive measures. Blood specimens on filter paper can be used for DNA analysis. New mutations leading to aspartoacylase deficiency are being discovered among non-Jewish patients (Elpeleg and Shaag 1999, Rady et al. 1999, 2000, Sistermans et al. 2000). Determining the genotype is important for counseling and prenatal detection.

Differential diagnosis

Macrocephaly, which is characteristic of Canavan disease, can also be found in Alexander disease, Krabbe disease, vacuolating leukodystrophy, Tay–Sachs disease, and other neurodegenerative disorders (Goutieres et al. 1996, van der Knaap et al. 1996). Other diseases that can lead to spongy degeneration of the brain include L-2-hydroxyglutaric acidemia, homocystinuria, viral infections, and mitochondrial disease (Chou and Waisman 1965, Rushton 1968, Lisson et al. 1981, Walter 1982, Egger et al. 1992, Topcu et al. 1996). Autosomal-dominant megalencephaly may also be confused with Canavan disease. Increased levels of *N*-acetylaspartic acid in the urine establish the diagnosis of Canavan disease and this increase is not found in any of the other conditions (Matalon and Michals-Matalon 2003).

Pathogenesis and pathophysiology

Canavan disease is an autosomal recessive disorder caused by aspartoacylase deficiency. The enzyme deficiency leads to inability to hydrolyze *N*-acetylaspartic acid, resulting in increased concentrations of this compound, which is the hallmark for diagnosis of the disease. *N*-Acetylaspartic acid is abundant in mammalian brain, only slightly less than glutamic acid (Tallan et al. 1956, McIntosh and Cooper 1965). *N*-Acetylaspartic acid is synthesized primarily in the mitochondria of neuronal cells, but aspartoacylase is found distally, in the oligodendroglia that synthesize myelin. This biochemical compartmentation seems to suggest that the substrate for the enzyme is important for the maintenance and synthesis of white matter (Ory-Lavollee et al. 1987, Kaul et al. 1991, Chakraborty et al. 2001). The role of *N*-acetylaspartic acid is still unclear; that it has has a dual role as an osmolyte and a source of acetate for the white matter is a possibility. In the aspartoacylase-deficient brain, there is increase in water content, sponginess, and decreased concentrations of acetate (Madhavarao et al. 2005).

As Canavan disease progresses the brain becomes atrophic, and the gray matter becomes involved as well. Microscopy shows spongy degeneration throughout the white matter in the subcortical regions. The astrocytes are swollen, and electron microscopy shows distorted and elongated mitochondria (Adachi et al. 1972, Adornato et al. 1972, Luo and Huang 1984, DeCoo et al. 1991). The spinal cord also becomes involved with sponginess of the spinal tracts (Surendran et al. 2005).

Prognosis

There is no specific treatment for Canavan disease. Management is symptomatic and palliative. Physical therapy may help prevent contractures. Seizures need to be controlled. Special care is needed when patients are fed in order to avoid aspiration. Nasogastric feeding or gastrostomy feeding will be needed in many of these children. The prognosis for typical Canavan disease is poor. These children remain retarded, unable to hold up their head or sit without support. Sleep disorders, feeding difficulties, and seizure disorders usually complicate the disease. Most children die in the first decade, and only a few have survived beyond 20 years of age.

Epidemiology

Canavan disease is panethnic, although it is most prevalent among Ashkenazi Jews of Eastern European extraction, most of whom have two specific mutations (Kaul et al. 1994b). In non-Jewish patients the mutations are different and more diverse.

Studies of blood specimens from over 5000 healthy Ashkenazi Jews indicated that 1 out of 37.7 were carriers for these two mutations. The incidence of Canavan disease in this population, including other mutations, was estimated to be 1 in 5600 births (Matalon 1997). A study of the carrier frequency in New York metropolitan Ashkenazi Jewish population was found to be 1 in 40 (Kronn et al. 1995). Studies from Canada showed the rate of carrier for Canavan disease to be 1 in 57 (Feigenbaum et al. 2004). A more recent study of carrier frequency of a group of diseases found in the Jewish population in Israel was 1 in 82 (Fares et al. 2008).

These predictions of carrier frequencies depend on the Jewish population tested and their countries of origin. Ashkenazi Jewish people from Ukraine or Lithuania are probably the main founders of the Jewish mutations. While "Ashkenazi Jews" from other countries in Europe have less frequency of Canavan disease, so the term "Ashkenazi" does not indicate that the population is homogenous.

Canavan disease is being diagnosed at increased frequency among non-Jewish individuals. Cases of non-Jewish Canavan disease have been reported from Turkey, France, Saudi Arabia, Japan, and other countries (Ozand et al. 1990, Yalaz et al. 1990, Shaag et al. 1995, Kaul et al. 1996, Rady et al. 1999, Rady et al. 2000, Sistermans et al. 2000, Tahmaz et al. 2001, Zeng et al. 2002). Some non-Jewish patients with milder clinical features of Canavan disease have also been reported (Goutierea et al. 1996, Sistermans et al. 2000, Tacke et al. 2005, Janson et al. 2006).

Gene therapy

The knock-out mouse for Canavan disease was created to try gene therapy (Matalon et al. 2000). However, even prior to the mouse trials, gene therapy was tried in Canavan disease patients. Two children with Canavan disease were the first to have such a trial (Leone et al. 2000). The results or this trial were not encouraging (Fink 2000, Leone et al. 2000).

There is a clinical protocol describing gene therapy of Canavan disease using AAV-2 as a vector for aspartoacylase (Janson et al. 2002).

Adeno-associated virus-2 (AAV-2) with aspartoacylase has been injected into the brain of 10 patients with Canavan diseases. The data from this trial suggest that there were no neutralizing antibodies in 7 out of 10 patients, whereas 3 had antibodies to AAV-2. This is a phase 1 study and further studies will be needed regarding the safety and efficacy of this method (McPhee et al. 2006). At this point it seems clear that gene therapy for Canavan disease, the way it has been practiced, is not a viable treatment option.

A knock-out mouse for Canavan disease was created to help explore therapeutic modalities for Canavan disease (Fig. 9.6) (Matalon et al. 2000). The knock-out mouse has a phenotype and spongy degeneration that are similar to the human disease (Fig. 9.7) (Matalon et al. 2000, Surendran et al. 2003 b, c). Studies on the knock-out mouse showed an impact on reproduction (Surendran et al. 2005).

A vector, AAV2, carrying the aspartoacylase gene was injected into the corpus striatum and mice were clinically observed, and sacrificed at different time intervals. Enzyme activity was present several weeks after the injection and the reporter gene seemed to spread to a short distance beyond the site of injection. Although the results were encouraging a better vector that spreads throughout the brain is needed (Matalon et al. 2003).

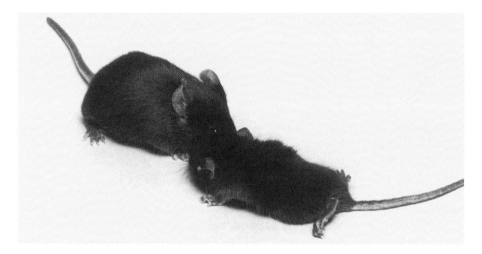

Fig. 9.6. A normal mouse (left) and a knock-out mouse (right) can be clearly distinguished.

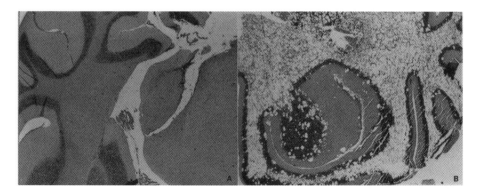

Fig. 9.7. Cerebellum of the knock-out mouse with spongy degeneration of the white matter is seen onthe right while on the left is a normal cerebellum. (A color version of this figure is available in the Plate section.)

Stem cell therapy was tried with the knock-out mouse and some of the stem cells converted to oligodendrocytes, but not enough to cure the disease. The fact that oligodendrocytes are involved in myelin synthesis is encouraging, but more such cells will be needed to correct the defect in Canavan disease. (Surendran et al. 2004).

Acetate supplementation using glycerol triacetate is being tried in mice with Canavan disease. Early results suggest improved MRI imaging and decreased sponginess in the mouse brain (R. Matalon, unpublished data). Studies are being planned in order to find out whether such a trial is applicable to human patients (Mathew et al. 2005).

A new, promising method of therapy is currently under experiment on the knock-out mouse for Canavan disease. Recombinant aspartoacylase is injected into the mouse intraperitoneally with or without hyaluronidase. Each mouse received three treatments on successive days. One hour after the last treatment mice were perfused and brains were assayed for aspartoacylase activity. The activity of enzyme increased, 25% above baseline in animals treated with aspartoacylase alone and 50% above baseline in those treated with both aspartoacylase and hyaluronidase. These experiments are being extended and they hold promise for an effective enzyme replacement therapy for Canavan disease (Matalon et al. 2008).

A complex of polyethyleneglycol with aspartoacylase (PEG-ASPA) was injected into the peritoneum of the mouse, and it seems to cross the blood–brain barrier without hyaluronidase. The enzyme activity in the brain increased two- to threefold (R. Viola and R. Matalon unpublished data). These experiments are also encouraging for the possible use of enzyme replacement therapy for the treatment of Canavan disease.

A report of a naturally occurring tremor rat may be a model for Canavan disease (Kitada et al. 2000). Baslow and colleagues used lithium chloride for 5 days and showed 13% reduction of N-acetylaspartic acid in the brain of tremor rats (Baslow et al. 2002).

Prevention

The risk in an affected newborn is 1 to 4 if both parents are carriers of the disease. Carrier determination and preventive counseling can now be attained with the help of DNA analysis (Matalon et al. 1995, Matalon and Michals-Matalon 1999, Matalon and Michals 2002). The high carrier rate observed in Ashkenazi Jews warrants screening of this population similar to screening programs for Tay–Sachs disease. The Committee on Genetics of the American College of Obstetrician Gynecologists has recommended screening of Canavan disease in Jewish couples (ACOG 1999). Carrier testing for Canavan disease, however, requires DNA analysis because the enzyme, aspartoacylase, is not detectable in blood. In a couple where both are carriers with informative DNA findings, prenatal diagnosis can be offered using DNA analysis. Other methods of prenatal diagnosis may include determination of N-acetylaspartic acid in amniotic fluid, which may be increased in an affected pregnancy (Jacobs et al. 1991, 1992, Bennett et al. 1993, Kelley 1993, Rolland et al. 1993, Elpeleg et al. 1994). Levels of N-acetylaspartic acid in amniotic fluid may also be problematic (Besley et al. 1999).

Preimplantation genetics as a method of preimplantation diagnosis using a single cell for diagnosis of Canavan disease has been practiced, determining the specific risk mutations. The mutation-free egg was fertilized and successfully implanted (Yaron et al. 2005).

REFERENCES

ACOG committee opinion. (1999) Screening for canavan disease. Committee on Genetics. Number 212; November, 1998. American College of Obstetrician Gynecologists. Int J Gynaecol Obstet 1: 91–92.

Adachi M, Schneck L, Cazara J, Volk BW. (1973) Spongy degeneration of the central nervous system (van Bogaert and Bertrand type; Canavan's disease). Hum Pathol 4: 331–346.

Adachi M, Torii J, Schneck L, Volk BW. (1972) Electron microscopic and enzyme histochemical studies of the cerebellum in spongy degeneration (van Bogaert and Bertrand type). Acta Neuropathol 20: 22–31.

Adornato BT, O'Brien JS, Lampert PW, Roe TF, Neustein HB. (1972) Cerebral spongy degeneration of infancy: a biochemical and ultrastructural study of affected twins. Neurology 1972;22: 202–210.

Al-Dirbashi OY, Rashed MS, Al-Qahtani K, Al-Mokhadab MA, Kurdi W, Al-Sayed MA. (2007) Quantification of N-acetylaspartic acid in urine by LC-MS/MS for the diagnosis of Canavan disease. J Inherit Metab Dis 30(4): 612.

Banker BQ, Victor H. (1979) Spongy degeneration of infancy. In: Goodman RM, Motulsky AG, Eds. Genetic Diseases Among Ashkenazi Jews. New York: Raven, pp. 201–217.

Baslow MH, Kitada K, Suckow RF, Hungund BL, Serikawa T. (2002) The effects of lithium chloride and other substances on levels of brain N-acetyl-L-aspartic acid in Canavan disease-like rats. Neurochem Res 27: 403–406.

Bennett MJ, Gibson KM, Sherwood WG, et al. (1993) Reliable prenatal diagnosis of Canavan disease (aspartoacylase deficiency): comparison of enzymatic and metabolite analysis. J Inherit Metab Dis 16: 831–836.

Besley GT, Elpeleg ON, Shaag A, Manning NJ, Jakobs C, Walter JH. (1999) Prenatal diagnosis of Canavan disease – problems and dilemmas. J Inherit Metab Dis 22: 263–266.

Brismar J, Brismar G, Gascon G, Ozand P. (1990) Canavan disease: CT and MR imaging of the brain. AJNR Am J Neuroradiol 11: 805–810.

Canavan MM. (1931) Schilder's encephalitis periaxialis diffusa. Arch Neurol Psychiatr 25: 299–308.

Chakraborty G, Mekala P, Yahya D, Wu G, Ledeen RW. (2001) Intraneural N-acetylaspartate supplies groups for myelin lipid synthesis: evidence for myelin-associated aspartoacylase. J Neurochem 78: 736–745.

Chou SM, Waisman H. (1965) Spongy degeneration of the central nervous system, case of homocystinuria. Arch Pathol 79: 357–363.

De Coo IF, Gabreels FJ, Renier WO, et al. (1991) Canavan disease: neuromorphological and biochemical analysis of a brain biopsy specimen. Clin Neuropathol 10: 73–78.

Echenne B, Divry P, Vianey-Liaud C. (1989) Spongy degeneration of the neuraxis (Canavan–van Bogaert disease) and N-acetylaspartic aciduria. Neuropediatrics 20: 79–81.

Egger J, Wayne-Williams CJ, Erdohazi M. (1992) Mitochondrial cytopathy or Leigh's syndrome? Mitochondrial abnormalities in spongiform encephalopathies. Neuropediatrics 13: 219–224.

Elpeleg ON, Amir N, Barash V, et al. (1989) Canavan disease and N-acetylaspartic aciduria. Neuropediatrics 20: 238.

Elpeleg ON, Shaag A. (1999) The spectrum of mutations of the aspartoacylase gene in Canavan disease in non-Jewish patients. J. Inherit Metab Dis 22: 531–534.

Elpeleg ON, Shaag A, Anikster Y, Jakobs C. (1994) Prenatal detection of Canavan disease (aspartoacylase deficiency) by DNA analysis. J Inherit Metab Dis 17: 664–666.

Fares F, Baderneh K, Abosaleh M, Harari-Shaham A, Diukman R, David M. (2008) Carrier frequency of autosomal-recessive disorders in the Ashkenazi Jewish population: should the rationale for mutation choice for screening be reevaluated? Prenat Diagn 28(3): 236–241.

Feigenbaum A, Moore R, Clarke J, et al. (2004). Canavan disease: carrier-frequency determination in the Ashkenazi Jewish population and development of a novel molecular diagnostic assay. Am J Med Genet A 124A(2): 142–147.

Fink DJ. (2000) Gene therapy for Canavan disease? Ann Neurol 48: 9–10.

Globus JH, Strauss I. (1928) Progressive degenerative subcortical encephalopathy (Schilder's disease). Arch Neurol Psychiatr 20: 1190–1228.

Goutieres F, Boulloche J, Bourgeois M, Aicardi J. (1996) Leukoencephalopathy, megalencephaly, and mild clinical course. A recently individualized familial leukodystrophy. Report on five new cases. J Child Neurol 11: 439–444.

Grodd W, Krageloh-Mann I, Peterson D, Trefz FK, Harzer K. (1990) In vivo assessment of N-acetylaspartate in brain in spongy degeneration (Canavan disease) by proton spectroscopy. Lancet 336: 437–438.

Hershfield JR, Pattabiraman N, Madhavarao CN, Namboodiri MA. (2007) Mutational analysis of aspartoacylase: Implications for Canavan disease. Brain Res 1148: 1–14.

Jacobs C, ten Brink HJ, Divry P, Rolland Mo. (1992) Prenatal diagnosis of Canavan disease. Eur J Pediatr 151: 620.

Jacobs C, ten Brink HJ, Langelaar SA, et al. (1991) Stable isotope dilution analysis of N-acetylaspartic acid in CSF, blood, urine and amniotic fluid: accurate postnatal diagnosis and the potential for prenatal diagnosis of Canavan disease. J Inherit Metab Dis 14: 653–660.

Janson CG, Kolodny EH, Zeng BJ, et al. (2006) Mild-onset presentation of Canavan's disease associated with novel G212A point mutation in aspartoacylase gene. Ann Neurol 59: 428–431.

Janson C, McPhee S, Bilaniuk L, et al. (2002) Clinical protocol. Gene therapy of Canavan disease: AAV-2 vector for neurosurgical delivery of aspartoacylase gene (ASPA) to the human brain. Hum Gene Ther 13: 1391–1412.

Kaul R, Balamurugan K, Gao GP, Matalon R. (1994a) Canavan disease: genomic organization and localization of human ASPA to 17p13-ter and conservation of the ASPA gene during evolution. Genomics 21: 364–370.

Kaul R, Casanova J, Johnson A, Tang P, Matalon R. (1991) Purification, characterization and localization of aspartoacylase from bovine brain. J Neurochem 56L: 129–135.

Kaul R, Gao GP, Aloya M, et al. (1994b) Canavan disease: mutations among Jewish and non-Jewish patients. Am J Hum Genet 55: 34–41.

Kaul R, Gao GP, Balamurugan K, Matalon R. (1993) Human aspartoacylase cDNA and mis-sense mutation in Canavan disease. Nat Genet 5: 118–123.

Kaul R, Gao GP, Balamurugan K, Matalon R. (1994c) Canavan disease: molecular basis of aspartoacylase deficiency. J Inherit Metab Dis 17: 295–297.

Kaul R, Gao GP, Matalon R, et al. (1996) Identification and expression of eight novel mutations among non-Jewish patients with Canavan disease. Am J Hum Genet 59: 95–102.

Kelley RI. (1993) Prenatal diagnosis of Canavan disease by measurement of N-acetyl-L-aspartate in amniotic fluid. J Inherit Metab Dis 16: 918–919.

Kitada K, Akimitsu T, Shigematsu Y, et al. (2000) Accumulation of N-acetyl-L-aspartate in the brain of the tremor rat, a mutant exhibiting absence-like seizure and spongiform degeneration in the central nervous system. J Neurochem 74: 2512–2519.

Kronn D, Oddoux C, Phillips J, Ostrer H. (1995) Prevalence of Canavan disease heterozygotes in the New York metropolitan Ashkenazi Jewish population. Am J Hum Genet 57: 1250–1252.

Leone P, Janson CG, Bilaniuk L, et al. (2000) Aspartoacylase gene transfer to the mammalian central nervous system with therapeutic implications for Canavan disease. Ann Neurol 48: 27–38.

Lisson G, Leupold D, Bechinger D, Wallesch C. (1981) CT findings in a case of deficiency of 3-hydroxy-3-methylglutaryl CoA lyase. Neuroradiology 22: 99–101.

Luo Y, Huang K. (1984) Spongy degeneration of the CNS in infancy. Arch Neurol 41: 164–170.

Madhavarao CN, Arun P, Moffett JR, et al. (2005) Defective N-acetylaspartate catabolism reduces brain acetate levels and myelin lipid synthesis in Canavan's disease. Proc Natl Acad Sci USA 102: 5221–5226.

Matalon R. (1997) Canavan disease: diagnosis and molecular analysis. Genet Test 1: 21–25.

Matalon R. (2006) Canavan disease. In: Medlink Neurology, Sid Gilman, Editor in Chief. July 2006, database online. Available at http://www.medlink.com

Matalon R, Bhatia G, Suzucs S, Michals-Matalon K, Tyring S, Grady J. (2008) Aspartoacylase entry to the brain of Canavan mouse with hyaluronidase. J Inherit Metab Dis 31(Suppl 1): 28

Matalon R, Kaul R, Casanova J, et al. (1989) SSIEM Award. Aspartoacylase deficiency: The enzyme defect in Canavan disease. J. Inherit Metab Dis 12(2): 329–331.

Matalon R, Kaul R, Gao GP, et al. (1995) Prenatal diagnosis for Canavan disease: the use of DNA markers. J Inherit Metab Dis 18: 215–217.

Matalon R, Kaul R, Michals K. (1993) Canavan disease: biochemical and molecular studies. J Inherit Metab Dis 16: 744–752.

Matalon R, Michals KM. (2002) Canavan disease prenatal diagnosis and genetic counseling. Obstet Gynecol Clin Am 29: 297–304.

Matalon R, Michals K, Kaul R. (1995) Canavan Disease: from spongy degeneration to molecular analysis. J. Pediatr 127: 511–517.

Matalon R, Michals-Matalon K. (1999) Prenatal diagnosis in Canavan disease. Prenat Diagn 19: 669–670.

Matalon R, Michals K, Sebasta D, Deanching M, Gashkoff P, Casanova J. (1988) Aspartoacylase deficiency and N-acetylaspartic aciduria in patients with Canavan disease. Am J Med Genet 29: 463–471.

Matalon R, Michals-Matalon K, Surendran S, Tyring SK. (2006) Canavan disease: studies on the knockout mouse. Adv Exp Med Biol 576: 77–93; 361–363.

Matalon R, Michals-Matalon K. (1998) Molecular basis of Canavan disease. Eur J Paediatr Neurol 2: 69–76.

Matalon R, Michals-Matalon K. (1999) Recent advances in Canavan disease. Adv Pediatr 6: 493–506.

Matalon R, Michals-Matalon K. (2000) Spongy degeneration of the brain, Canavan disease: biochemical and molecular findings. Front Biosci 5: D307–D311.

Matalon R, Michals-Matalon K. (2003) Canavan disease. In: Rosenberg RN, Prusiner SB, DiMauro S, Barchi R, Nestler EJ, Eds. The Molecular Genetic Basis of Neurological and Psychiatric Disease, 3rd edn. Philadelphia: Butterworth-Heinemann, pp. 383–387.

Matalon R, Rady PL, Platt KA, et al. (2000) Knock-out mouse for Canavan disease: a model for gene transfer to the central nervous system. J Gene Med 2: 165–175.

Matalon R, Surendran S, Rady P, et al. (2003) Adeno-associate virus-mediated aspartoacylase gene transfer to the brain of knockout mouse for Canavan disease. Mol Ther 5: 580–587.

Mathew R, Arun P, Madhavarao CN, Moffett JR, Namboodiri MA. (2005) Progress toward acetate supplementation therapy for Canavan disease: glyceryl triacetate administration increases acetate, but not N-acetylaspartate, levels in brain. J Pharmacol Exp Ther 315: 297–303.

McAdams HP, Geyer CA, Doe SL, Deigh D, Mitchell M. Ghaed VN. (1990) CT and MR imaging of Canavan disease. Am J Neuroradiol 11: 397–399.

McIntosh JM, Cooper JR. (1965) Studies on the function of N-acetylaspartic acid in the brain. J Neurochem 12: 825–835.

McPhee S, Janson C, Li C, et al. (2006) Immune responses to AAV in a phase I study for Canavan disease. J Gene Med 8: 577–588.

Ory-Lavollee L, Blakely RD, Coyle JT. (1987) Neurochemical and immunocytochemical studies on the distribution of N-acetylaspartylglutamate and N-acetyl-aspartate in rat spinal cord and some peripheral nervous tissues. J Neurochem 48: 895–899.

Ozand PT, Gascon CG, Dhalla M. (1990) Aspartoacylase deficiency and Canavan disease in Saudi Arabia. Am J Med Genet 35: 266–268.

Rady PL, Penzien JM, Vargas T, Tyring SK, Matalon R. (2000) Novel splice site mutation of aspartoacylase gene in a Turkish patient with Canavan disease. Europ J Paediatr Neurol 4: 27–30.

Rady PL, Vargas T, Tyring SK, Matalon R, Langenbeck U. (1999) Novel missense mutation (Y231C) in a Turkish patient with Canavan disease. Am J Med Genet 87L: 273–275.

Rolland MO, Divry P, Mandon G, Thoulon JM, Fiumara A, Mathieu M. (1993) First trimester prenatal diagnosis of Canavan disease. J Inherit Metab Dis 16: 581–583.

Rushton AR, Shaywitz BA, Duncan CC, Geehr RB, Manuelidis EE. (1981) Computerized tomography in the diagnosis of Canavan's disease. Ann Neurol 10: 57–60.

Rushton DI. (1968) Spongy degeneration of the white matter of the central nervous system associated with hyperglycinuria. J Clin Pathol 21: 456–462.

Shaag A, Anikster Y, Christensen E, et al. (1995) The molecular basis of Canavan (aspartoacylase deficiency) disease in European non-Jewish patients. Am J Hum Genet 57: 572–580.

Sistermans EA, de Coo RF, van Beerendonk HM, Poll-The BT, Kleijer WJ, van Oost BA. (2000) Mutation detection in the aspartoacylase gene in 17 patients with Canavan disease: four new mutations in the non-Jewish population. Eur J Hum Genet 8: 557–560.

Surendran S, Bamforth FJ, Chan A, Tyring SK, Goodman SI, Matalon R. (2003a) Mild elevation of N-acetylaspartic acid and macrocephaly: diagnostic problem. J Child Neurol 18: 809–812.

Surendran S, Campbell GA, Tyring SK, Matalon R. (2005) Aspartoacylase gene knockout results in severe vacuolation in white matter and gray matter of the spinal cord in the mouse. Neurobiol Dis 18: 385–389.

Surendran S, Matalon KM, Szucs S, Trying S, Matalon R. (2003b) Metabolic changes in the knockout mouse for Canavan's disease: implications for patients with Canavan's disease. J Child Neurol 18: 611–615.

Surendran S, Matalon KM, Trying S, Matalon R. (2003c) Molecular basis of Canavan's disease: from human to mouse. J Child Neurol 18: 604–610.

Surendran S, Michals-Matalon K, Quast M, et al. (2003d) Canavan disease: a monogenic trait with complex genomic interaction. Mol Genet Metab 80: 74–80.

Surendran S, Rady P, Michals-Matalon K, et al. (2003e) Expression of glutamate transporter, GABRA6, serine proteinase inhibitor 2 and low levels of glutamate and GABA in the brain of knock-out mouse for Canavan disease. Brain Res Bull 61: 427–435.

168

Surendran S, Shihabuddin LS, Clarke J, et al. (2004) Mouse neural progenitor cells differentiate into oligoden-drocytes in the brain of a knockout mouse model of Canavan disease. Dev Brain Res 153: 19–27.

Surendran S Szucs S Tyring SK Matalon R. (2005) Aspartoacylase gene knockout mouse: impact on reproduction. Reprod Toxicol 20: 281–283.

Tacke U, Olbrich H, Sass JO, et al. (2005) Possible genotype-phenotype correlations in children with mild clinical course of Cavavan disease. Neuropediatrics 36: 252–255.

Tahmaz FE, Sam S, Hoganson GE, Quan F. (2001) A partial deletion of the aspartoacylase gene is the cause of Canavan disease in a family from Mexico. J Med Genet 38: E9.

Tallan HH, Moore S, Stein WH. (1956) N-Acetyl-L-aspartic acid in brain. J Biol Chem 219: 257–264.

Toft PB, Geib-Holtorff R, Rolland MO, et al. (1993) Magnetic resonance imaging in juvenile Canavan disease. Eur J Pediatr 152: 750–753.

Topcu M, Erdem G, Saatci I, et al. (1996) Clinical and magnetic resonance imaging features of L-2-hydroxyglutaric acidemia: report of three cases in comparison with Canavan disease. J Child Neurol 11: 373–377.

Van Bogaert L, Bertrand I. (1949) Sur une idiotie familiale avec degerescence songlieuse de neuraxe (note preliminaire). Acta Neurol Belg 49: 572–587.

Van der Knaap MS, Barth PG, Vrensen GF, Valk J. (1996) Histopathology of an infantile-onset spongiform leukoencephalopathy with a discrepantly mild clinical course. Acta Neuropathol 92: 206–212.

Walter GF. (1982) Molecular pathological aspects in spongy encephalopathies. Wien Klin Wochenschr 94: 375–376.

Wittsack HJ, Kugel H, Roth B, Heindel W. (1996) Quantitative measurements with localized 1H MR spectroscopy in children with Canavan's disease. J Magn Reson Imaging 6: 889–893.

Yalaz K, Topcu M, Topalglu H, et al. (1990) N-Acetylaspartic aciduria in Canavan disease: another proof in two infants. Neuropediatrics 21: 140–142.

Yalcinkaya C, Benbir G, Salomons GS, et al. (2005) Atypical MRI findings in Canavan disease: a patient with a mild course. 36: 336–339.

Yaron Y, Schwartz T, Mey-Raz N, Amit A, Lessing JB, Malcov M. (2005) Preimplantation genetic diagnosis of Canavan disease. Fetal Diagn Ther 20: 465–468.

Zeng BJ, Wang ZH, Ribeiro LA, et al. (2002) Identification of novel mutations of the aspartoacylase gene in non-Jewish patients with Canavan disease. J Inherit Metab Dis 25: 557–570.

169

10
PELIZAEUS–MERZBACHER DISEASE: GENETIC MODELS AND MECHANISMS

Klaus-Armin Nave and Ajit Singh Dhaunchak

In 1895, F. Pelizaeus reported a neurological disorder in a family in which male children were affected by nystagmus, ataxia, spasticity, and developmental delay (Pelizaeus 1885). L. Merzbacher investigated the same family 25 years later and described a diffuse hypomyelination of the central nervous system (CNS) of these patients (Merzbacher 1910). More than 100 years later, the Pelizaeus–Merzbacher disease (PMD) is genetically well-defined, but there is no treatment for patients, except for medications counteracting seizures and spasticity. With the discovery of naturally occurring animal models (*jimpy*) of the disease (Phillips 1954), the identification of the *jimpy* disease gene as *Plp1* (Dautigny et al. 1986, Nave et al. 1986), and following the development of new *Plp1* mutant mouse models, the underlying molecular and cellular mechanisms of human PMD are becoming evident. It is now established that duplications of the human gene, *PLP1*, are the most frequent cause of PMD. Both PMD and its milder allelic disorder, spastic paraplegia type-2 (SPG-2), are X-linked recessive disorders of CNS myelination and cover a broad spectrum of disease severity. Our current understanding of the molecular and cellular pathomechanisms of PMD/SPG2 is discussed in this chapter.

Involvement of myelin proteolipid protein

PMD is caused by abnormal expression of proteolipid protein (PLP), an abundant membrane protein of CNS myelin. Since myelin membranes can be efficiently purified by sucrose gradient centrifugation, this protein was first analyzed and entirely sequenced at the amino acid level (Lees et al. 1983, Stoffel et al. 1984), that is, well before the association with PMD was clear. Also, post-translational modifications were established, including the removal of the N-terminal methionine, formation of two disulfide bonds between two pairs of extracellular cysteine residues (Fig. 10.1), and the acylation of six cysteine residues in the intracellular loop regions of PLP (Popot et al. 1991, Weimbs and Stoffel 1992, 1994). The covalent linkage of fatty acids adds to the hydrophobic nature of the molecule and might play a role in myelin targeting of PLP (Schneider et al. 2005). By mapping tryptic peptides under reducing and non-reducing conditions (Weimbs and Stoffel 1992), the location of both disulfide bridges could be determined to be within the extracellular loop EC2 (C183–C227 and C200–C219). Thus, PLP is a highly hydrophobic protein with four transmembrane (TM) domains and two extracellular loop regions (EC1, EC2) that interact with the opposing membrane in compact myelin (Stoffel et al. 1989, Popot et al. 1991). Both N- and C-terminus of PLP protrude into the cytosol (Fig. 10.1).

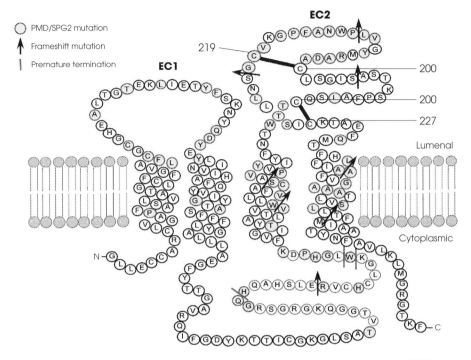

Fig. 10.1. Topological model of PLP/DM20 and position of amino acid changes in PMD/SPG2. Two-dimensional model of proteolipid protein (PLP) (276 residues as black beads) and its splice isoform DM20, lacking 35 residues (marked in gray) from an intracellular loop. The orientation of four transmembrane domains positions both N- and C-terminus into the glial cytoplasm. Within the second extracellular domain (EC2), the position of two disulfide-bridges is indicated. Positions of amino acids in EC2 which are substituted in patients with Pelizaeus–Merzbacher disease (PMD) are marked in yellow. The single-letter code of the wild-type sequence is shown. Disulfide bonds in extracellular loop 2 (EC2) are critical for PLP folding (Dhaunchak and Nave 2007) and indicated by black lines. Many substitutions within EC2 lead to abnormal PLP crosslinks that result in protein retention in the endoplasmic reticulum and activation of the unfolded-protein response. (A color version of this figure is available in the Plate section.)

After synthesis in the endoplasmic reticulum (ER), PLP traffics through the Golgi apparatus, where it associates with cholesterol and galactocerebrosides. Here, PLP also partitions into membrane lipid rafts and is delivered to the cell surface for targeting and incorporation into the growing myelin membrane (Gow et al.1997, Wahle and Stoffel 1998, Simons et al. 2000). Thus membrane raft formation and association of PLP with cholesterol are initial and critical steps of myelin assembly in the CNS. Indeed, cholesterol availability is a rate-limiting factor in myelin synthesis (Saher et al. 2005). A single oligodendrocyte can myelinate several axons in vivo and the synthesis of an entire myelin sheath occurs within a few days. At this developmental stage, the metabolic activity of oligodendrocytes must be extremely high, as approximately 10^5 myelin-specific proteins are synthesized per minute per cell, in addition to myelin lipids that outweigh myelin proteins by three- to fourfold (reviewed in Pfeiffer et al. 1993).

Like most membrane proteins, PLP becomes co-translationally inserted into the bilayer. In the oxidative environment of the ER, numerous chaperones catalyze the proper folding of the growing polypeptide (Mothes et al. 1997). Before exiting the ER, new proteins are screened by a quality control system that retains unfolded or misfolded proteins and marks them for degradation (Ellgaard et al. 1999, Ellgaard and Helenius 2003). Some membrane proteins, including ion channels and connexins, further form homo- and hetero-oligomers in the ER and can exit only when properly assembled (Hurtley and Helenius 1989). Monomeric or incompletely assembled subunits are retained by stable interactions with ER-resident chaperones (Kleizen and Braakman 2004). Mutant proteins that are retained in the ER can induce the unfolded protein response (UPR), which includes ER growth and transcriptional activation of genes encoding chaperones (Patil and Walter 2001, Rutkowski and Kaufman 2004). In mammalian cells, the UPR can also trigger apoptosis (Harding et al. 2002, Federovitch et al. 2005). ER stress has been suggested to be involved in many neurological disorders, including PMD, Parkinson disease, and Alzheimer disease. The exact mechanism and underlying cause for such neurological disorders remains poorly understood owing to lack of appropriate animal models except for PMD. For this disease, the cause of ER stress, downstream mechanism, and pathophysiology are becoming clear, mainly due to the availability of excellent in-vitro and in-vivo models (described in later section).

The *PLP1* gene

Proteolipid protein remained exceptionally well-conserved during vertebrate evolution, with the *PLP1* gene in human and *Plp1* in rodents encoding the same protein sequence. *PLP1* is an X-chromosome-linked gene (at locus Xq22.2) that spans about 17 kb and is composed of seven exons and a 5′ promoter region (Diehl et al. 1986, Macklin et al. 1987a, Ikenaka et al. 1988). An additional 5′ exon with a leader sequence and an alternate amino terminus generates soma-restricted PLP. The mRNA for soma-restricted PLP was reported in mouse brain (Bongarzone et al. 1999, 2001) but is not found in the human transcriptome, leaving its function unclear. Alternative splicing within PLP exon 3 generates a shorter mRNA for DM20 which lacks exon 3B (Nave et al. 1987). Identical in topology, DM20 is 35 residues shorter in the cytosolic loop (see Fig. 10.1), which might explain subtle differences of conformation and in subcellular sorting (Gow and Lazzarini 1996, Gow et al. 1997). Under reducing conditions both proteolipids show an increased electrophoretic mobility and migrate as 25 kDa (PLP) and 20 kDa proteins (DM20). Together they constitute reportedly 50% of total myelin protein by mass (Lees and Brostoff 1984), but recent estimates based on mass spectroscopy are considerably lower (H. B. Werner and K-A. Nave, unpublished data).

Expression of PLP and DM20 is spatially and temporally tightly regulated (Campagnoni and Skoff 2001). PLP is predominantly expressed in oligodendrocytes and is the major isoform expressed during myelination and adulthood. In contrast, DM20 is (relatively) more abundant than PLP in oligodendrocyte precursor cells prior to myelination as well as in some non-myelinating cells, including the heart, spleen, thymus, and lymph nodes (Campagnoni et al. 1992, Pribyl et al. 1996a, b, Campagnoni and Skoff 2001). The spatial and temporal regulation of the *PLP* gene is controlled in addition to its promoter by a regulatory region within the large first intron (Wight et al. 1993, Spassky et al. 1998, Fuss et al. 2000).

Genetics of PMD/SPG-2

PMD exhibits a variable clinical course, ranging from patients with disease symptoms apparent at birth to milder forms with a late onset. In the more frequent type I ("classical") form, affected boys reach a few motor development milestones up to about 10 years of age, but after a plateau show slow deterioration (at ages 15–20 years) and death occurs often in the fourth decade (Nave and Boespflug-Tanguy 1996). In the most severe type II ("connatal") form of PMD, neonates show virtually no psychomotor development and death occurs in the first decade. Motor performance varies between families (i.e., specific mutations) but also between affected males of the same pedigree. This suggests the existence of yet unidentified disease modifier genes, which have also been noted for *Plp1* mutations in different lines of inbred mice.

Clinically distinct from either type of PMD is X-linked spastic paraplegia type 2 (SPG-2) which is a milder, allelic form at the *PLP1* locus (Johnston and Mc 1962, Saugier-Veber et al. 1994). Patients with SPG-2 have progressive gait abnormalities after almost normal motor development during infancy. This makes SPG-2 a late-onset disease that, nevertheless, shares clinical features with PMD (nystagmus, cerebellar ataxia, pyramidal syndrome). Myelination may not be severely affected and progressive axonal involvement may be largely responsible for the clinical picture of SPG-2, similar to findings in specific mouse mutants of the *Plp1* gene.

Genetic defects in PMD/SPG-2 can be grouped into four categories: (1) *PLP1* gene duplications, (2) *PLP1* coding region mutations, (3) *PLP1* null mutations, and (4) undetectable changes in *PLP1*. The following is a brief overview of genetic findings.

The most common cause of PMD is a duplication of the *PLP1* gene, which accounts for about 70% of all patients (Raskind et al. 1991, Inoue et al. 1996a, Sistermans et al. 1998). The majority are tandem duplications, involving a large genomic segment that also includes neighboring genes (Inoue et al. 1996a, Inoue et al. 1999a, Woodward et al. 1999). The duplicated segments vary in size from hundreds of kilobases to a few megabases with several neighboring genes inevitably being over-expressed. Irrespective of the breakpoint, *PLP1* duplications result in a uniform phenotype in PMD patients, pointing to the fact that at locus Xq22.2 only *PLP1* is sensitive to gene dosage. The more severe phenotype of patients with three copies of *PLP1* also shows the dosage effects of *PLP1* on the clinical onset of PMD (Woodward et al. 1998). Occasionally, the duplicated gene is found translocated to a different locus on the X chromosome (Hodes et al. 2000). Earlier animal studies had shown that over-expression of *Plp1* is sufficient to cause CNS hypomyelination in transgenic mice (Mastronardi et al. 1993, Kagawa et al. 1994, Readhead et al. 1994, Gow et al. 1998). Clinical phenotypes associated with increased gene dosage are variable, suggest a direct correlation between the level of Plp1 expression and disease severity (Inoue et al. 1996b, Anderson et al. 1998, Edgar et al. 2010), and includes neuroinflammation (Ip et al. 2006). T-cell infiltration into the CNS of mice is not a general feature of myelin gene mutations and its significance for PMD remains to be determined.

The second major genetic defect in PMD involves coding region mutations in *PLP1* gene, arising from nonsense, mis-sense and splice-site mutation causing frameshifts. More than 60 different *PLP1* mutations have been identified that alter PLP and DM20; most are mis-sense point mutations that result in amino acid substitutions, but also nonsense and frameshift mutations that produce abnormal PLP/DM20 proteins have been defined (Hodes et al. 1993, Garbern 2007). Mutations are found over the entire length of PLP with an over-representation in the second extracellular loop and codon 202 representing a mutational "hot spot." The codon D202 was subjected to five different mis-sense mutations and this aspartate residue was changed to a histidine, glycine, valine, asparagine, or glutamate residue in different patients. Susceptibility of this region hints at structural and conformational cues that might be important for protein interactions in *cis* or in *trans*, that is, with the opposing membrane in compact myelin (Stoffel et al. 1989, Popot et al. 1991).

PLP1-null mutations have been identified in several patients, ranging from complete deletion of the gene to an in-frame stop codon (Raskind et al. 1991, Sistermans et al. 1996, Garbern et al. 1997, Garbern et al. 2002). Incidence of such mutations is rare when compared to *PLP1* duplications (Raskind et al. 1991, Inoue and Lupski 2002). Only a few deletion cases have been reported and the missing genomic segments have been relatively small, containing up to two genes (Inoue and Lupski 2002). Most likely, larger deletions cause an early lethality.

The remaining patients with clinical features of PMD have no detectable sequence abnormality, suggesting mutations in regulatory parts of the gene (Kawanishi et al. 1996) or other disease genes involved. Regulatory defects may also arise from mutations in genes encoding transcriptional factors that control myelin gene expression, including Sox10 and Nkx2.2. One Sox10 mutation combines features of PMD, Charcot–Marie–Tooth disease type 1, and Waardenburg–Hirschsprung syndrome (Inoue et al. 1999b, Inoue et al. 2002).

Genetic models

Spontaneous point mutations of the *Plp1* gene were identified in several species and can be considered animal models of PMD. They cover a wide spectrum of disease phenotypes, similar to human PMD/SPG-2. In addition, *Plp1*-transgenic and *Plp1*-null mutants have been generated as models for the corresponding forms of the human disease

THE *JIMPY* MOUSE AND ITS ALLELES

The *jimpy* mutation, discovered as a lethal X-linked trait (Phillips 1954, Sidman et al. 1964), provided the first animal model for human PMD. With clinical symptoms apparent during the second postnatal week, and coinciding with the onset of myelination in the CNS, *jimpy* presents the most severe (connatal) form of PMD. Affected males are smaller in size than wild-type males and develop a generalized body tremor, ataxia, and seizures, followed by premature death at 3 to 4 weeks of age (Sidman et al. 1964).

The molecular defect in *jimpy* mice is an A to G point mutation in *Plp1* that destroys the splice acceptor site of intron 4, thereby causing an abnormal loss of exon 5 from mature

PLP and DM20 mRNA. This in turn leads to a frameshift of translation and truncated PLP/DM20 proteins that lack the last transmembrane domain (Dautigny et al. 1986, Morello et al. 1986, Nave et al. 1986, Macklin et al. 1987b). The histological phenotype is a complete lack of myelin in the CNS, associated with lack of mature oligodendrocytes (Hirano et al. 1969, Kraus-Ruppert et al. 1973, Meier and Bischoff 1974, Meier and Bischoff 1975). Increased rate of oligodendrocyte cell death resembles apoptosis (Skoff 1982, Skoff and Ghandour 1995) in some but not all aspects (Knapp et al. 1999). A small percentage of *jimpy* oligodendrocytes survive and generate patches of myelin for 1 to 2% of axons. Ultrastructurally, the intraperiod line, normally a double-line with irregular appearance, appears fused in *jimpy* to a single electron-dense structure that is indistinguishable from the major dense line.

Jimpy has become the prototype of allelic mutants in mouse and rat that share a similar phenotype. In the *myelin synthesis deficient* mutant (*Plp*[jp-msd]) (Eicher and Hoppe 1973), slightly more spinal cord axons become ensheathed (Billings-Gagliardi et al. 1980). The mutation causes a substitution (A242V) in the fourth transmembrane domain (Gencic and Hudson 1990). The same mutation has been identified in a human family with connatal PMD (Komaki et al. 1999), and a related one (A242E) has been described (Seeman et al. 2002). The mutation *jimpy-4J* (*Plp*[jp-4J]) has the most severe histological phenotype (Billings-Gagliardi et al. 1995) and results from the substitution A38S (Pearsall et al. 1997).

A myelin-deficient rat model (termed *md rat*) (Csiza and de Lahunta 1979, Dentinger et al. 1982) has also become a widely studied model for the connatal form of PMD. The primary defect here is a point mutation in exon 3 of *Plp1* causing a non-conservative substitution (T74P) and predicting a break in the second transmembrane domain of PLP (Koeppen et al. 1987). The complete lack of PLP from compact myelin results in a characteristic decrease of myelin periodicity (Duncan et al. 1987). Clinically, *md rat*s are similar to *Plp1* mutant mice with tremors, tonic seizures, and premature death. A longer-lived mutant substrain has been isolated, with affected males surviving for about 80 days (Nadon and Duncan 1995), suggesting the role of an unknown disease modifier gene.

THE *RUMPSHAKER* MOUSE

The *rumpshaker* (*Plp*[jp-rsh]) mutation is single residue substitution (I186T) in extracellular domain 2 of PLP/DM20 and is associated with a much milder phenotype on its original mixed genetic background (Schneider et al. 1992). On the 101/C3H mixed background, *rumpshaker* animals are long lived and reproduce well, showing only ataxia and mild tremor with a little seizure activity. The spinal cord axons in *rumpshaker* mice are thinly myelinated, and there are both unmyelinated and normally myelinated axons in the optic nerve (Fanarraga et al. 1992). The mutant proteolipids are also incorporated into the myelin, with the DM20 isoform predominating (Fanarraga et al. 1992, Karthigasan et al. 1996). It is known that the expression of misfolded PLP in mutant mice activates the transcription of *chaperone* genes and the transcription factor *chop* (Southwood et al. 2002). Unexpectedly, 'chop' deficiency in *rumpshaker* mice further worsened the phenotype, implicating 'chop' in the pathogenesis of dysmyelination. Moreover, the clinical severity of *rumpshaker* mice is markedly influenced by the genetic background: on the C57BL background the *rumpshaker* mutation is lethal within a few weeks, similar to *jimpy*. The responsible modifier gene(s) is still unknown (Al-Saktawi et al. 2003). McLaughlin et al. (2006) demonstrated that PLP processing and incorporation into myelin is similar in both C3H and C57BL6 backgrounds. Although 'chop' levels were significantly increased in C57BL6 (thus correlating with disease severity), there was no difference in the expression of two other markers of the "unfolded protein response," namely BIP and xbp1-splicing (McLaughlin et al. 2007). Except for the unexplained sensitivity to genetic background, *rumpshaker* animals are a genuine model for SPG-2 in humans; in fact the same *PLP1* mutation was identified later in the index family of this human disease (Kobayashi et al. 1994, Naidu et al. 1997).

TRANSGENIC *PLP1* OVER-EXPRESSION

Another *PLP1* mutation, and in fact the most common mechanism underlying PMD, involves the duplication of the entire gene, corresponding to a predicted twofold over-expression of PLP and its splice isoform DM20. Mouse models of this type of PMD had been generated incidentally, even before *PLP1* duplication became known, during an attempt to rescue the gene defect of *jimpy* mice with a wild-type *Plp1* transgene (Kagawa et al. 1994, Readhead et al. 1994). An unexpected observation was the severely dysmyelinated phenotype of all those transgenic mice that over-expressed wild-type *Plp1* by at least twofold (quantified at the level of *Plp1* transcripts; Readhead et al. 1994). These transgenic rodents are a valid model of PMD as a *PLP1* gene dosage disease (Inoue et al. 1999a). Mice homozygous for a genomic *Plp1* transgene (and over-expressing more than 200%) develop a novel phenotype in mice, less severe than *jimpy* with a survival time of about 6 months (Readhead et al. 1994). The shorter lived and more severely affected *Plp1* transgenic mice generated by Kagawa et al. (1994) over-express at even higher levels and exhibit a pronounced oligodendrocyte death.

Mice with only one autosomal *Plp1* (transgenic) allele over-express PLP/DM20 less than twofold and develop quite normally. However, these mice have a delayed onset of disease with progressive ataxia and behavioral abnormalities evident at 12 to 16 months of age. A striking feature is the vacuolization of the subcortical white matter (Anderson et al. 1998), the cause of which is not well understood. Moreover, there is a secondary immune response that includes the recruitment of activated CD8+ T cells into the brain (Ip et al. 2006, Leder et al. 2007). We have speculated that the underlying pro-inflammatory milieu in this and other leukodystrophy models is caused by abnormal lipid metabolism in the white matter (Kassmann et al. 2007, Kassmann and Nave 2008). In PLP over-expressing mice, this may be a direct consequence of mis-targeting PLP-containing membrane microdomains and myelin membranes.

PLP normally interacts with cholesterol (Simons et al. 2000) and other lipids to form myelin rafts. These are subsequently transported to the plasma membrane, most likely for endosomal sorting into the growing myelin sheath. In cultured oligodendrocytes, over-expression of PLP results in accumulation of this protein and associated lipids in the late endosome/lysosome, causing aberrant raft membrane trafficking (Simons et al. 2002). Indeed the incorporation of PLP/DM20 into myelin is reduced despite an elevated level of *Plp1* gene expression (Karim et al. 2007). Also a *PLP*-transgenic rat model exhibited intracellular accumulation of PLP (together with other membrane proteins, such as myelin associated glycoprotein [MAG] and myelin oligodendrocyte glycoprotein [MOG], but not with myelin basic protein), suggesting a more generalized perturbation of myelin and non-myelin protein transport (Bauer et al. 2002).

PLP/DM20-DEFICIENT MICE

Various laboratories have used gene targeting technologies and homologous recombination of mouse embryonic stem cells to ablate the expression of PLP and/or DM20 (Boison and Stoffel 1994, Klugmann et al. 1997, Stecca et al. 2000, Sporkel et al. 2002). These studies provided yet another novel model of PMD, as human *PLP1*-null mutations show a relative mild clinical course of disease (Raskind et al. 1991, Sistermans et al. 1996). Surprisingly, from a cell-biological point of view, PLP/DM20 is not required for myelin formation.

Stoffel and co-workers reported the first targeting of the *Plp1* gene and obtained mice with a severe perturbation of *Plp1* gene expression (close to null mutation), resulting from the combination of a splice defect and an anti-sense silencing defect (Boison and Stoffel 1994). This mutation did not interfere with myelination but caused highly disordered myelin. Myelin lamellae were loosely wrapped and lacked the intraperiod line. This led to a profound reduction of conduction velocity in the CNS, impaired neuromotor coordination, and behavioral changes (Boison and Stoffel 1994, Gutierrez et al. 1995). Large-diameter axons were loosely myelinated, and small diameter axons were even unmyelinated. The suggestion that adhesive properties of PLP caused the tight apposition of membrane in compact myelin (Boison et al. 1995) was only partly confirmed by the analysis of a true *Plp1*-null mutation (Klugmann et al. 1997). Indeed, the compaction defects along the intraperiod line were highly variable with findings of absent, condensed, and normal intraperiod lines and an overall propensity of mutant myelin for fixation artifacts (Klugmann et al. 1997, Yool et al. 2002, Rosenbluth et al. 2006).

Later, we observed that *Plp1*-null mice develop widespread axonal swellings (Griffiths et al. 1998) that are caused by perturbed fast axonal transport (Edgar et al. 2004) and that lead to progressive neurodegeneration, predominantly of small caliber axons. This feature of length-dependent axon loss was also found in human PMD patients with a *PLP1*-null mutation (Garbern et al. 2002). Consistent with these observations, Stecca et al. (2000) demonstrated that genetic ablation of PLP isoforms, expressing only DM20 at normal levels, resulted in a phenocopy of the combined PLP/DM20-null phenotype (Griffiths et al. 1998, Stecca et al. 2000). This suggests that PLP or PLP plus DM20, but not DM20 alone, is required for oligodendrocytes to maintain axonal integrity. In contrast, when Sporkel et al. (2002) also created a PLP-isoform-specific mouse mutant, they found minimal phenotypic abnormalities, suggesting that DM20 is sufficient. Currently, these discrepancies, which may rest on expression-level differences, cannot be explained. However, Griffiths et al. (1998) noted that both PLP and DM20 cDNA based transgenes, when expressed in PLP/DM20-null mice, reduce the extent of axonal pathology, which agrees better with the findings of Sporkel et al. (2002).

All mammals are in principle sensitive to mutation of the X-linked *Plp1* gene, as illustrated by a mutation in dogs with a generalized body tremor, and the pup's ability to suckle, walk, and maintain sternal recumbency (Greene et al. 1977). Head, neck, and limbs oscillated rhythmically when it attempted to perform any motor function. This canine mutation (later named *shaking pup*; *shp*) is a mutation in exon 2 of *Plp1*, with a substitution (H36P) in the first transmembrane domain (Nadon et al. 1990). The same position is substituted in the *paralytic tremor* (*pt*) mutation of rabbit (H36N), causing a coarse body tremor and limb paresis as a result of CNS dysmyelination (Tosic et al. 1993). It is hoped that larger animals will be useful for specific therapeutic approaches that might give misleading results within small rodent brains, such as the efficacy of glial cell transplants.

Subcellular mechanisms of disease development

PLP1 GENE MUTATIONS AND OLIGODENDROCYTE APOPTOSIS

The classical neurological mouse mutant *jimpy* lacks CNS myelin almost completely. Underlying this condition is a paucity of mature oligodendrocytes and signs of increased oligodendrocyte death, such as pyknotic cells and TUNEL-positive oligodendroglial nuclei (Skoff 1982, Knapp et al. 1986). Transplantation experiments of oligodendrocytes from *jimpy* brains into wild-type (or *shiverer*) host brains have confirmed that cell death is cell-autonomous at an early stage of development (Lachapelle et al. 1994). It coincides with increasing expression of the mutant *Plp1* gene and it is important to note that the misfolded protein never accumulates to significant levels (Vermeesch et al. 1990). Collectively, these studies have provided evidence that mutant oligodendrocytes differentiate to the stage of myelin protein synthesis, but undergo apoptosis later, presumably following a threshold expression of mutant PLP. However, Beesley et al. (2001) noticed that *Plp1* mutant oligodendrocytes (from *md* rats) fail to express MOG. Even when oligodendrocyte apoptosis was suppressed by a caspase 3 inhibitor, the expression of MOG could not be detected suggesting a direct effect of mutant PLP also on oligodendrocyte differentiation (Beesley et al. 2001). Oligodendrocyte death as a result of "toxic gain of function effect" from aberrant *Plp1* expression is evidenced by oligodendrocyte survival in *Plp*-null mutant mice.

Analyzing the outcome of transient PLP cDNA expression in heterologous non-glial cells, Gow et al. (1994) established a genotype–phenotype correlation between endoplasmic reticulum (ER) retention of mutant PLP and disease severity of a particular mutation. PLP and DM20 from mutant mice are indeed physically misfolded, as demonstrated by a monoclonal antibody (O10) that defines a conformational sensitive epitope of PLP/DM20 that is lost from virtually all PMD-mutant isoforms (Jung et al. 1996). The variable spectrum of clinical severity has been directly linked to cell surface expression of PLP and DM20 in heterologous cells (Gow and Lazzarini 1996, Thomson et al. 1997), as illustrated also in Figure 10.2. Mutations within the *PLP1*-specific region of the gene (resulting in aberrant PLP but normal DM20) are associated with a milder clinical phenotype and no oligo-dendrocyte death, whereas most other mutations affect trafficking of both PLP and DM20 and are associated with more severe PMD and increased oligodendrocyte death (Schneider

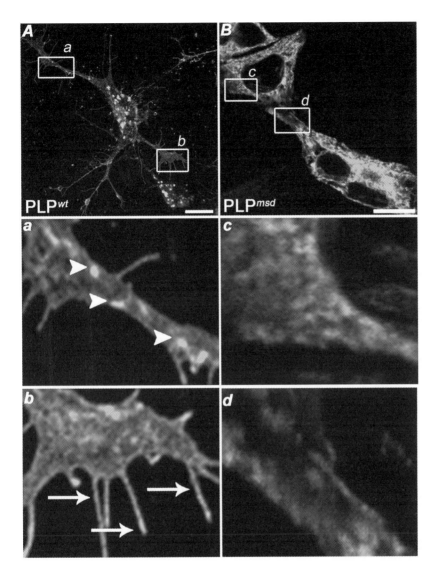

Fig. 10.2. PMD-causing mutations of PLP are retained in the endoplasmic reticulum of transfected cells. *A*: Wild-type proteolipids (PLP*wt*) readily traffic to the cell surface of transfected oligodendroglial cells as demonstrated by green fluorescent microspikes at the tips of processes. Glial cells protrude numerous filopodial processes and PLP*wt* accumulates in the endosomal/lysosomal compartment. Magnified insets (*a, b*) of boxed area in *A* show glial processes with endosomal/lysosomal accumulation of PLP (arrowheads) and filopodial protrusions (arrows). Scale bar: 10 μm (left). *B*: Mutant proteins, such as PLP*msd* (A242V substitution) derived from the PMD model *jimpy-msd*, fail to reach the glial cell surface. Glial cells lack any labeled microspikes (magnified insets in *c, d*). Note also the paucity of cellular processes. There is a reticular distribution of EGFP fluorescence, with no accumulation in the endosomal/ lysosomal compartment. Magnifications (*c, d*) of the boxed areas in *B* are located in a close proximity to the cell surface. Note that there is complete absence of fine microspikes. Scale bar: 10 μm (right). (A color version of this figure is available in the Plate section.)

179

et al. 1992, Gow and Lazzarini 1996, Gow et al. 1998). Swanton and colleagues compared a spectrum of clinically distinct *PLP1* mis-sense mutations and revealed a tendency of premature PLP oligomerization in the ER of heterologous cells that again was associated with increasing severity of disease (Swanton et al. 2005). The authors suggested that wild-type PLP forms stable oligomers only after reaching the cell surface, reflected in a long "maturation time" of the protein. In contrast, mutant PLP appears to assemble prematurely into oligomers (already in the ER), which could mask essential signals for the transport to the cell surface (Swanton et al., 2005). The analysis of subcellular trafficking of PLP/DM20 mis-sense mutants in oligodendroglial cells demonstrated distinct defects of mutations that caused mild and severe disease, all of which being associated with impaired cholesterol binding and lipid raft association (Kramer-Albers et al. 2006). PLP associated with severe disease was retained in the ER, whereas PLP associated with milder disease (i.e., rump-shaker) accumulated in the lamp1-positive endosomal/lysosomal compartment. Moreover, mutant PLP associated with severe disease was rapidly degraded and exhibited a high turnover rate compared with wild-type and rumpshaker PLP (Krämer-Albers et al. 2006). Another study with *rumpshaker* mice (kept on different genetic backgrounds) suggested that disease severity is not only caused by differential PLP processing, but possibly different gain-of-function effects involving other proteins of myelin (McLaughlin et al. 2007).

Although mis-sense mutations affect all regions of PLP and DM20, there is an over-representation within the second extracellular loop, suggesting that this region is critical for normal protein conformation and myelin stability. We have recently shown that a subset of disease-associated point mutations in *PLP1* converge mechanistically by perturbing the formation of an intra-molecular disulfide-bridge in PLP/DM20 in the lumen of the ER (Dhaunchak and Nave 2007). Importantly, this disulfide bridge is dispensable for normal PLP/DM20 folding and trafficking, and it is not the substituted amino acid itself that causes retention in the ER. But when the unpaired cysteine becomes sterically exposed (as a result of a substitution in the protein's loop region) it engages in intermolecular crosslinks with PLP itself or other proteins. Abnormal PLP adducts fail to oligomerize and become the primary cause of ER retention, and thus oligodendrocyte dysfunction and death in vivo. ER retention of PLP may cause further abnormal protein crosslinks (Swanton et al. 2003). Indeed, normal trafficking of mutant PLP/DM20 is restored by removal of the critical cysteine residues. While this model is likely to explain PMD when caused by single substitutions in EC2 (presently 30 documented natural mutations), it is unlikely to explain many other mutants, many of which map into transmembrane domains and may act by premature oligomerization, as discussed before (Swanton et al. 2005).

The role of a heptapeptide sequence of PLP as a novel retention signal (within the PLP-specific region) was proposed by Southwood et al. (2007). The analysis of transfected fibroblasts led the authors to conclude that mild PMD mutations cause protein retention in the ER, which is (partially) dependent on the presence of the cytoplasmically exposed heptapeptide K-G-R-G-S-R-G. In contrast, the retention of proteins associated with severe PMD mutations occurs independently of this peptide.

Taken together, abnormal retention of misfolded protein in the ER of oligodendrocytes underlies the cause of premature cell death in PMD, and this toxic effect of PLP is modulated

180

by the activation of *chop* and other unidentified modifier genes (Gow et al. 1994, Gow and Lazzarini 1996, Gow et al. 1997, Thomson et al. 1997, Cerghet et al. 2001, Southwood et al. 2002, McLaughlin et al. 2007;). A better understanding of these disease-modulating pathways may hopefully lead to therapeutic strategies.

PLP1 M**UTATION AND** A**XONAL** D**EGENERATION**

Although myelin is assembled in the absence of PLP/DM20, the *Plp1*-null mutant mice develop normally and synthesize compact myelin sheaths with only minor ultrastructural abnormalities. A key observation in these mice was the finding of widespread axonal swellings that cause neurodegeration, predominantly of small-caliber axons (Griffiths et al. 1998). Such fiber degeneration is probably secondary to impaired axonal transport (Edgar et al. 2004), and is direct proof that myelinated axons require local oligodendroglial support. Length-dependent axonal degeneration of the CNS, as observed in *Plp1*-null animals, has also been documented in human patients with PMD (Garbern et al. 2002). In a recent study Werner and co-workers, using gel-based proteome analysis, identified three proteins of the septin family that were reduced in abundance, and a virtual absence of nicotinamide adenine dinucleotide (NAD^+)-dependent deacetylase sirtuin 2 (SIRT2) from myelin, when purified from *Plp1*-null mice (Werner et al. 2007). SIRT2 loss in *Plp1*-null mice was post-transcriptional, suggesting that PLP/DM20 is required for its transport into the myelin compartment. Since SIRT2 enzymatic activity is controlled by the NAD^+/NADH ratio, its function might couple axoglial metabolism and the long-term support of axons by oligodendrocytes.

Similar degeneration of axons has also being noted in the CNS of mice lacking the oligodendrocyte-specific *Cnp1* (CNPase) gene (Lappe-Siefke et al. 2003). Thus, several genes may be required by oligodendrocytes to provide axonal support, independent of myelin assembly. The underlying molecular mechanism of axoglial interactions is presently unknown.

Pelizaeus–Merzbacher-like disease

Pelizaeus–Merzbacher-like disease (PMDL) is an autosomal-recessive leukodystrophy that is clinically similar to PMD and can be caused by mutations in the *GJA12* gene (Uhlenberg et al. 2004). However, a genetic screen of a clinically well-characterized cohort of 193 patients with PMLD (from 182 families), identified *GJA12* mutations in only 16 patients (from 14 families), revealing PMLD to be genetically heterogenous (Henneke et al., 2008). Interestingly, in five families only one mutated *GJA12* allele was found. Clinically, PMLD patients are comparable to milder isoforms of PMD (SPG-2) but with better cognition and earlier signs of axonal degeneration. Highly expressed in oligodendrocytes, the *GJA12* gene encodes a 439-amino-acid gap-junction protein (connexin 47; CX47). Although genetic ablation of *Gja12* in mice causes no obvious dysfunction, loss of the human gene has been confirmed as one cause of PMLD (Odermatt et al. 2003, Bugiani et al. 2006, Orthmann-Murphy et al. 2007, Salviati et al. 2007, Wolf et al. 2007). Double-mutant mice lacking both *Gja12* and *Gjp1* (*connexin 32; cx32*) have severe CNS myelin abnormalities causing premature death (Menichella et al. 2003).

Conclusion

A wide range of naturally occurring and genetically engineered animal models of PMD have contributed to our current understanding of the molecular basis of this human myelin disorder and its wide clinical spectrum. Animal models have helped us dissect the cause of disease, including oligodendrocyte death, the toxic effect of misfolded protein, and the loss of axonal support by oligodendrocytes. Since it has been difficult to assign a particular function to PLP/DM20 in CNS myelin, the exact mechanism is still unknown. Currently, there is no cure or treatment for patients with PMD/SPG2 or PMLD. Myelin function might be improved by gene therapy, stem cell transplantation, or novel drugs, all of which can be tested in the wide range of available animal models.

REFERENCES

Al-Saktawi KM, McLaughlin M, Klugmann M, et al. (2003) Genetic background determines phenotypic severity of the Plp rumpshaker mutation. J Neurosci Res 72: 12–24.

Anderson TJ, Schneider A, Barrie JA, et al. (1998) Late-onset neurodegeneration in mice with increased dosage of the proteolipid protein gene. J Comp Neurol 394: 506–519.

Bauer J, Bradl M, Klein M, et al. (2002) Endoplasmic reticulum stress in PLP-overexpressing transgenic rats: gray matter oligodendrocytes are more vulnerable than white matter oligodendrocytes. J Neuropathol Exp Neurol 61: 12–22.

Beesley JS, Lavy L, Eraydin NB, Siman R, Grinspan JB. (2001) Caspase-3 activation in oligodendrocytes from the myelin-deficient rat. J Neurosci Res 64: 371–379.

Billings-Gagliardi S, Adcock LH, Wolf MK. (1980) Hypomyelinated mutant mice: description of jpmsd and comparison with jp and qk on their present genetic backgrounds. Brain Res 194: 325–338.

Billings-Gagliardi S, Kirschner DA, Nadon NL, et al. (1995) Jimpy 4J: a new X-linked mouse mutation producing severe CNS hypomyelination. Dev Neurosci 17: 300–310.

Boison D, Bussow H, D'Urso D, Muller HW, Stoffel W. (1995) Adhesive properties of proteolipid protein are responsible for the compaction of CNS myelin sheaths. J Neurosci 15: 5502–5513.

Boison D, Stoffel W. (1994) Disruption of the compacted myelin sheath of axons of the central nervous system in proteolipid protein-deficient mice. Proc Natl Acad Sci USA 91: 11 709–11 713.

Bongarzone ER, Campagnoni CW, Kampf K, et al. (1999) Identification of a new exon in the myelin proteolipid protein gene encoding novel protein isoforms that are restricted to the somata of oligodendrocytes and neurons. J Neurosci 19: 8349–8357.

Bongarzone ER, Jacobs E, Schonmann V, Campagnoni AT. (2001) Classic and soma-restricted proteolipids are targeted to different subcellular compartments in oligodendrocytes. J Neurosci Res 65: 477–484.

Bugian M, Al Shahwan S, Lamanteam E, et al. (2006) GJA12 mutations in children with recessive hypomyelinating leukoencephalopathy. Neurology 67: 273–279.

Campagnoni AT, Skoff RP. (2001) The pathobiology of myelin mutants reveal novel biological functions of the MBP and PLP genes. Brain Pathol 11: 74–91.

Campagnoni CW, Garbay B, Micevych P, et al. (1992) DM20 mRNA splice product of the myelin proteolipid protein gene is expressed in the murine heart. J Neurosci Res 33: 148–155.

Cerghet M, Bessert DA, Nave KA, Skoff RP. (2001) Differential expression of apoptotic markers in jimpy and in Plp overexpressors: evidence for different apoptotic pathways. J Neurocytol 30: 841–855.

Csiza CK, de Lahunta A. (1979) Myelin deficiency (md): a neurologic mutant in the Wistar rat. Am J Pathol 95: 215–223.

Dautigny A, Mattei MG, Morello D, et al. (1986) The structural gene coding for myelin-associated proteolipid protein is mutated in jimpy mice. Nature 321: 867–869.

Dentinger MP, Barron KD, Csiza CK. (1982) Ultrastructure of the central nervous system in a myelin deficient rat. J Neurocytol 11: 671–691.

Dhaunchak AS, Nave K-A. (2007) A common mechanism of PLP/DM20 misfolding causes cysteine-mediated endoplasmic reticulum retention in oligodendrocytes and Pelizaeus–Merzbacher disease. Proc Natl Acad Sci USA 104: 17 813–17 818.

Diehl HJ, Schaich M, Budzinski RM, Stoffel W. (1986) Individual exons encode the integral membrane domains of human myelin proteolipid protein. Proc Natl Acad Sci USA 83: 9807–9811.

Duncan ID, Hammang JP, Trapp BD. (1987) Abnormal compact myelin in the myelin-deficient rat: absence of proteolipid protein correlates with a defect in the intraperiod line. Proc Natl Acad Sci USA 84: 6287–6291.

Edgar JM, McCulloch MC, Montague P, et al. (2010) Demyelination and axonal preservation in a transgenic mouse model of Pelizaeus–Merzbacher disease. EMBO Mol Med 2(2): 42–50.

Edgar JM, McLaughlin M, Yool D, et al. (2004) Oligodendroglial modulation of fast axonal transport in a mouse model of hereditary spastic paraplegia. J Cell Biol 166: 121–131.

Eicher EM, Hoppe PC. (1973) Use of chimeras to transmit lethal genes in the mouse and to demonstrate allelism of the two X-linked male lethal genes jp and msd. J Exp Zool 183: 181–184.

Ellgaard L, Helenius A. (2003) Quality control in the endoplasmic reticulum. Nat Rev Mol Cell Biol 4: 181–191.

Ellgaard L, Molinari M, Helenius A. (1999) Setting the standards: quality control in the secretory pathway. Science 286: 1882–1888.

Fanarraga ML, Griffiths IR, McCulloch MC, Barrie JA, Kennedy PG, Brophy PJ. (1992) Rumpshaker: an X-linked mutation causing hypomyelination: developmental differences in myelination and glial cells between the optic nerve and spinal cord. Glia 5: 161–170.

Federovitch CM, Ron D, Hampton RY. (2005) The dynamic ER: experimental approaches and current questions. Curr Opin Cell Biol 17: 409–414.

Fuss B, Mallon B, Phan T, et al. (2000) Purification and analysis of in vivo-differentiated oligodendrocytes expressing the green fluorescent protein. Dev Biol 218: 259–274.

Garbern JY. (2007) Pelizaeus–Merzbacher disease: genetic and cellular pathogenesis. Cell Mol Life Sci 64: 50–65.

Garbern JY, Cambi F, Tang XM, et al. (1997) Proteolipid protein is necessary in peripheral as well as central myelin. Neuron 19: 205–218.

Garbern JY, Yool DA, Moore GJ, et al. (2002) Patients lacking the major CNS myelin protein, proteolipid protein 1, develop length-dependent axonal degeneration in the absence of demyelination and inflammation. Brain 125: 551–561.

Gencic S, Hudson LD. (1990) Conservative amino acid substitution in the myelin proteolipid protein of jimpymsd mice. J Neurosci 10: 117–124.

Gow A, Friedrich VL, Jr, Lazzarini RA. (1994) Intracellular transport and sorting of the oligodendrocyte transmembrane proteolipid protein. J Neurosci Res 37:563–573.

Gow A, Gragerov A, Gard A, Colman DR, Lazzarini RA. (1997) Conservation of topology, but not conformation, of the proteolipid proteins of the myelin sheath. J Neurosci 17:181–189.

Gow A, Lazzarini RA. (1996) A cellular mechanism governing the severity of Pelizaeus–Merzbacher disease. Nat Genet 13: 422–428.

Gow A, Southwood CM, Lazzarini RA. (1998) Disrupted proteolipid protein trafficking results in oligodendrocyte apoptosis in an animal model of Pelizaeus–Merzbacher disease. J Cell Biol 140: 925–934.

Greene CE, Vandevelde M, Hoff EJ. (1977) Congenital cerebrospinal hypomyelinogenesis in a pup. J Am Vet Med Assoc 171: 534–536.

Griffiths I, Klugmann M, Anderson T, et al. (1998) Axonal swellings and degeneration in mice lacking the major proteolipid of myelin. Science 280: 1610–1613.

Gutierrez R, Boison D, Heinemann U, Stoffel W. (1995) Decompaction of CNS myelin leads to a reduction of the conduction velocity of action potentials in optic nerve. Neurosci Lett 195: 93–96.

Harding HP, Calfon M, Urano F, Novoa I, Ron D. (2002) Transcriptional and translational control in the Mammalian unfolded protein response. Annu Rev Cell Dev Biol 18: 575–599.

Henneke M, Combes P, Diekmann S, et al. (2008) GJA12 mutations are a rare cause of Pelizaeus–Merzbacher-like disease. Neurology 70: 748–754.

Hirano A, Sax DS, Zimmerman HM. (1969) The fine structure of the cerebella of jimpy mice and their "normal" litter mates. J Neuropathol Exp Neurol 28: 388–400.

Hodes ME, Pratt VM, Dlouhy SR. (1993) Genetics of Pelizaeus–Merzbacher disease. Dev Neurosci 15: 383–394.

Hodes ME, Woodward K, Spinner NB, et al. (2000) Additional copies of the proteolipid protein gene causing Pelizaeus–Merzbacher disease arise by separate integration into the X chromosome. Am J Hum Genet 67: 14–22.

Hurtley SM, Helenius A. (1989) Protein oligomerization in the endoplasmic reticulum. Annu Rev Cell Biol 5: 277–307.

Ikenaka K, Furuichi T, Iwasaki Y, Moriguchi A, Okano H, Mikoshiba K. (1988) Myelin proteolipid protein gene structure and its regulation of expression in normal and jimpy mutant mice. J Mol Biol 199: 587–596.

Inoue K, Lupski JR. (2002) Molecular mechanisms for genomic disorders. Annu Rev Genomics Hum Genet 3: 199–242.

Inoue K, Osaka H, Imaizumi K, et al. (1999a). Proteolipid protein gene duplications causing Pelizaeus–Merzbacher disease: molecular mechanism and phenotypic manifestations. Ann Neurol 45: 624–632.

Inoue K, Osaka H, Sugiyama N, et al. (1996a) A duplicated PLP gene causing Pelizaeus–Merzbacher disease detected by comparative multiplex PCR. Am J Hum Genet 59: 32–39.

Inoue K, Shilo K, Boerkoel CF, et al. (2002) Congenital hypomyelinating neuropathy, central dysmyelination, and Waardenburg–Hirschsprung disease: phenotypes linked by SOX10 mutation. Ann Neurol 52: 836–842.

Inoue K, Tanabe Y, Lupski JR. (1999b). Myelin deficiencies in both the central and the peripheral nervous systems associated with a SOX10 mutation. Ann Neurol 46: 313–318.

Inoue Y, Kagawa T, Matsumura Y, Ikenaka K, Mikoshiba K. (1996b) Cell death of oligodendrocytes or demyelination induced by overexpression of proteolipid protein depending on expressed gene dosage. Neurosci Res 25: 161–172.

Ip CW, Kroner A, Bendszus M, et al. (2006) Immune cells contribute to myelin degeneration and axonopathic changes in mice overexpressing proteolipid protein in oligodendrocytes. J Neurosci 26: 8206–8216.

Johnston AW, Mc KV. (1962) A sex-linked recessive form of spastic paraplegia. Am J Hum Genet 14: 83–94.

Jung M, Sommer I, Schachner M, Nave K-A. (1996) Monoclonal antibody O10 defines a conformationally sensitive cell-surface epitope of proteolipid protein (PLP): evidence that PLP misfolding underlies dysmyelination in mutant mice. J Neurosci 24: 7920–7929.

Kagawa T, Ikenaka K, Inoue Y, et al. (1994) Glial cell degeneration and hypomyelination caused by over-expression of myelin proteolipid protein gene. Neuron 13: 427–442.

Karim SA, Barrie JA, McCulloch MC, et al. (2007) PLP overexpression perturbs myelin protein composition and myelination in a mouse model of Pelizaeus–Merzbacher disease. Glia 55: 341–351.

Karthigasan J, Evans EL, Vouyiouklis DA, et al. (1996) Effects of rumpshaker mutation on CNS myelin composition and structure. J Neurochem 66:338–345.

Kassmann CM, Lappe-Siefke C, Baes M, et al. (2007) Axonal loss and neuroinflammation caused by peroxisome-deficient oligodendrocytes. Nat Genet 39: 969–976.

Kassmann CM, Nave KA. (2008) Oligodendroglial impact on axonal function and survival – a hypothesis. Curr Opin Neurol 21: 235–241.

Kawanishi C, Sugiyama N, Osaka H, et al. (1996) Pelizaeus–Merzbacher disease: a novel mutation in the 5-untranslated region of the proteolipid protein gene. Hum Mutat 7:355–357.

Kleizen, B, Braakman I. (2004) Protein folding and quality control in the endoplasmic reticulum. Curr Opin Cell Biol 16: 343–349.

Klugmann M, Schwab MH, Puhlhofer A, et al. (1997) Assembly of CNS myelin in the absence of proteolipid protein. Neuron 18: 59–70.

Knapp PE, Bartlett WP, Williams LA, Yamada M, Ikenaka K, Skoff RP. (1999) Programmed cell death without DNA fragmentation in the jimpy mouse: secreted factors can enhance survival. Cell Death Differ 6: 136–145.

Knapp PE, Skoff RP, Redstone DW. (1986) Oligodendroglial cell death in jimpy mice: an explanation for the myelin deficit. J Neurosci 6: 2813–2822.

Kobayashi H, Hoffman EP, Marks HG. (1994) The rumpshaker mutation in spastic paraplegia. Nat Genet 7: 351–352.

Koeppen AH, Ronca NA, Greenfield EA, Hans MB. (1987) Defective biosynthesis of proteolipid protein in Pelizaeus–Merzbacher disease. Ann Neurol 21: 159–170.

Komaki H, Sasaki M, Yamamoto T, Iai M, Takashima S. (1999) Connatal Pelizaeus–Merzbacher disease associated with the jimpy(msd) mice mutation. Pediatr Neurol 20: 309–311.

Kramer-Albers EM, Gehrig-Burger K, Thiele C, Trotter J, Nave KA. (2006) Perturbed interactions of mutant proteolipid protein/DM20 with cholesterol and lipid rafts in oligodendroglia: implications for dysmyelination in spastic paraplegia. J Neurosci 26: 11 743–11 752.

Kraus-Ruppert R, Herschkowitz N, Furst S. (1973) Morphological studies on neuroglial cells in the corpus callosum of the Jimpy mutant mouse. J Neuropathol Exp Neurol 32: 197–202.

Lachapelle F, Gumpel M, Baumann N. (1994) Contribution of transplantations to the understanding of the role of the PLP gene. Neurochem Res 19: 1083–1090.

Lappe-Siefke C, Goebbels S, Gravel M, et al. (2003) Disruption of Cnp1 uncouples oligodendroglial functions in axonal support and myelination. Nat Genet 33: 366–374.

Leder C, Schwab N, Ip CW, et al. (2007) Clonal expansions of pathogenic CD8+ effector cells in the CNS of myelin mutant mice. Mol Cell Neurosci 36: 416–424.

Lees M, Brostoff S. (1984) Proteins of myelin. In: Morell P, Ed. Myelin. New York: Plenum, pp. 489–534.

Lees MB, Chao BH, Lin LF, Samiullah M, Laursen RA. (1983) Amino acid sequence of bovine white matter proteolipid. Arch Biochem Biophys 226: 643–656.

Macklin WB, Campagnoni CW, Deininger PL, Gardinier MV. (1987a) Structure and expression of the mouse myelin proteolipid protein gene. J Neurosci Res 18: 383–394.

Macklin WB, Gardinier MV, King KD, Kampf K. (1987b) An AG–GG transition at a splice site in the myelin proteolipid protein gene in jimpy mice results in the removal of an exon. FEBS Lett. 223: 417–421.

Mastronardi FG, Ackerley CA, Arsenault L, Roots BI, Moscarello MA. (1993) Demyelination in a transgenic mouse: a model for multiple sclerosis. J Neurosci Res 36: 315–324.

McLaughlin M, J.A. Barrie JA, S. Karim S, et al. (2006) Processing of PLP in a model of Pelizaeus–Merzbacher disease/SPG2 due to the rumpshaker mutation. Glia 53: 715–722.

McLaughlin M, Karim SA, Montague P, et al. (2007) Genetic background influences UPR but not PLP processing in the rumpshaker model of PMD/SPG2. Neurochem Res 32: 167–176.

Meier C, Bischoff A. (1974) Dysmyelination in "jimpy" mouse. Electron microscopic study. J Neuropathol Exp Neurol 33: 343–353.

Meier C, Bischoff A. (1975) Oligodendroglial cell development in jimpy mice and controls. An electron-microscopic study in the optic nerve. J Neurol Sci 26: 517–528.

Menichella DM, Goodenough DA, Sirkowski E, Scherer SS, Paul DL. (2003) Connexins are critical for normal myelination in the CNS. J Neurosci 23: 5963–5973.

Merzbacher L. (1910) Eine eigenarige familiär-hereditare Erkrankungsform (Aplasia axialis extra-corticalis congenita). Z Neurol Psychiatr 3: 1–138.

Morello D, Dautigny A, Pham-Dinh D, Jolles P. 1986. Myelin proteolipid protein (PLP and DM-20) transcripts are deleted in jimpy mutant mice. EMBO J 5: 3489–3493.

Mothes W, Heinrich SU, Graf R, et al. (1997) Molecular mechanism of membrane protein integration into the endoplasmic reticulum. Cell 89: 523–533.

Nadon NL, Duncan ID. (1995) Gene expression and oligodendrocyte development in the myelin deficient rat. J Neurosci Res 41: 96–104.

Nadon NL, Duncan ID, Hudson LD. (1990) A point mutation in the proteolipid protein gene of the 'shaking pup' interrupts oligodendrocyte development. Development 110: 529–537.

Naidu S, Dlouhy SR, Geraghty MT, Hodes ME. (1997) A male child with the rumpshaker mutation, X-linked spastic paraplegia/Pelizaeus–Merzbacher disease and lysinuria. J Inherit Metab Dis 20: 811–816.

Nave K, Boespflug-Tanguy O. (1996) X-linked developmental defects of myelination: From mouse mutants to human genetic diseases. Neuroscientist 2: 33–43.

Nave KA, Lai C, Bloom FE, Milner RJ. (1986) Jimpy mutant mouse: a 74-base deletion in the mRNA for myelin proteolipid protein and evidence for a primary defect in RNA splicing. Proc Natl Acad Sci USA 83: 9264–9268.

Nave KA, Lai C, Bloom FE, Milner RJ. (1987) Splice site selection in the proteolipid protein (PLP) gene transcript and primary structure of the DM-20 protein of central nervous system myelin. Proc Natl Acad Sci USA 84: 5665–5669.

Odermatt B, Wellershaus K, Wallraff A, et al. (2003) Connexin 47 (Cx47)-deficient mice with enhanced green fluorescent protein reporter gene reveal predominant oligodendrocytic expression of Cx47 and display vacuolized myelin in the CNS. J Neurosci 23: 4549–4559.

Orthmann-Murphy JL, Enriquez AD, Abrams CK, Scherer SS. (2007) Loss-of-function GJA12/Connexin 47 mutations cause Pelizaeus–Merzbacher-like disease. Mol Cell Neurosci 34: 629–641.

Patil C, Walter P. (2001) Intracellular signaling from the endoplasmic reticulum to the nucleus: the unfolded protein response in yeast and mammals. Curr Opin Cell Biol 13: 349–355.

Pearsall GB, Nadon NL, Wolf MK, Billings-Gagliardi S. (1997) Jimpy-4J mouse has a missense mutation in exon 2 of the Plp gene. Dev Neurosci 19: 337–341.

Pelizaeus F. (1885) Uber eine eigenthüümliche Form Spastischer Lähmung mit Cerebralerschinerungen auf hereditärer Grundlage (Multiple Sklerose)..Arch Psychiatr Nervenkr 16: 698–710.

Pfeiffer SE, Warrington AE, Bansal R. (1993) The oligodendrocyte and its many cellular processes. Trends Cell Biol 3: 191–197.

Phillips RJ. (1954) Jimpy, a new totally sexlinked gene in the house mouse. Z Indukt Abstamm Vererbungsl 86: 322–326.

Popot JL, Pham Dinh D, Dautigny A. (1991) Major myelin proteolipid: the 4-alpha-helix topology. J Membr Biol 120: 233–246.

Pribyl TM, Campagnoni C, Kampf K, Handley VW, Campagnoni AT. (1996a). The major myelin protein genes are expressed in the human thymus. J Neurosci Res 45: 812–819.

Pribyl TM, Campagnoni CW, Kampf K, et al. (1996b). Expression of the myelin proteolipid protein gene in the human fetal thymus. J Neuroimmunol 67: 125–130.

Raskind WH., Williams CA, Hudson LD, Bird TD. (1991) Complete deletion of the proteolipid protein gene (PLP) in a family with X-linked Pelizaeus–Merzbacher disease. Am J Hum Genet 49:1355–1360.

Readhead C, Schneider A, Griffiths I, Nave KA. (1994) Premature arrest of myelin formation in transgenic mice with increased proteolipid protein gene dosage. Neuron 12: 583–595.

Rosenbluth J, Nave KA, Mierzwa A, Schiff R. (2006) Subtle myelin defects in PLP-null mice. Glia 54: 172–182.

Rutkowski DT, Kaufman RJ. (2004) A trip to the ER: coping with stress. Trends Cell Biol 14: 20–28.

Saher G, Brugger B, Lappe-Siefke C, et al. (2005) High cholesterol level is essential for myelin membrane growth. Nat Neurosci 8: 468–475.

Salviati L, Trevisson E, Baldoin MC, et al. (2007) A novel deletion in the GJA12 gene causes Pelizaeus–Merzbacher-like disease. Neurogenetics 8: 57–60.

Saugier-Veber P, Munnich A, Bonneau D, et al. (1994) X-linked spastic paraplegia and Pelizaeus–Merzbacher disease are allelic disorders at the proteolipid protein locus. Nat Genet 6:257–262.

Schneider A, Lander H, Schulz G, et al. (2005) Palmitoylation is a sorting determinant for transport to the myelin membrane. J Cell Sci 118: 2415–2423.

Schneider A, Montague P, Griffiths I, et al. (1992) Uncoupling of hypomyelination and glial cell death by a mutation in the proteolipid protein gene. Nature 358: 758–761.

Seeman P, Paderova K, Benes V, Jr, Sistermans EA. (2002) A severe connatal form of Pelizaeus Merzbacher disease in a Czech boy caused by a novel mutation (725C>A, Ala242Glu) at the 'jimpy(msd) codon' in the PLP gene. Int J Mol Med 9: 125–129.

Sidman RL, Dickie MM, Appel SH. (1964) Mutant mice (Quaking and Jimpy) with deficient myelination in the central nervous system. Science 144: 309–311.

Simons M, Kramer EM, Macchi P, et al. (2002) Overexpression of the myelin proteolipid protein leads to accumulation of cholesterol and proteolipid protein in endosomes/lysosomes: implications for Pelizaeus–Merzbacher disease. J Cell Biol 157: 327–336.

Simons M, Kramer EM, Thiele C, Stoffel W, Trotter J. (2000) Assembly of myelin by association of proteolipid protein with cholesterol- and galactosylceramide-rich membrane domains. J Cell Biol 151: 143–154.

Sistermans EA, de Coo RF, De Wijs IJ, van Oost BA. (1998) Duplication of the proteolipid protein gene is the major cause of Pelizaeus–Merzbacher disease. Neurology 50: 1749–1754.

Sistermans EA, de Wijs IJ, de Coo RF, Smit LM, Menko FH, and van Oost BA. (1996) A (G-to-A) mutation in the initiation codon of the proteolipid protein gene causing a relatively mild form of Pelizaeus–Merzbacher disease in a Dutch family. Hum Genet 97: 337–339.

Skoff RP. (1982) Increased proliferation of oligodendrocytes in the hypomyelinated mouse mutant-jimpy. Brain Res 248: 19–31.

Skoff RP, Ghandour MS. (1995) Oligodendrocytes in female carriers of the jimpy gene make more myelin than normal oligodendrocytes. J Comp Neurol 355: 124–133.

Southwood C, Olson K, Wu CY, Gow A. (2007) Novel alternatively spliced endoplasmic reticulum retention signal in the cytoplasmic loop of Proteolipid Protein-1. J Neurosci Res 85: 471–478.

Southwood CM, Garbern J, Jiang W, Gow A. (2002) The unfolded protein response modulates disease severity in Pelizaeus–Merzbacher disease. Neuron 36: 585–596.

Spassky N, Goujet-Zalc C, Parmantier E, et al. (1998) Multiple restricted origin of oligodendrocytes. J Neurosci 18: 8331–8343.

Sporkel O, Uschkureit T, Bussow H, Stoffel W. (2002) Oligodendrocytes expressing exclusively the DM20 isoform of the proteolipid protein gene: myelination and development. Glia 37: 19–30.

Stecca B, Southwood CM, Gragerov A, Kelley KA, Friedrich, VL, Jr, Gow A. (2000) The evolution of lipophilin genes from invertebrates to tetrapods: DM-20 cannot replace proteolipid protein in CNS myelin. J Neurosci 20: 4002–4010.

Stoffel W, Hillen H, Giersiefen H. (1984) Structure and molecular arrangement of proteolipid protein of central nervous system myelin. Proc Natl Acad Sci USA 81: 5012–5016.

Stoffel W, Subkowski T, Jander S. (1989) Topology of proteolipid protein in the myelin membrane of central nervous system. A study using antipeptide antibodies. Biol Chem Hoppe Seyler 370: 165–176.

Swanton E, High S, Woodman P. (2003) Role of calnexin in the glycan-independent quality control of proteolipid protein. EMBO J 22: 2948–2958.

Swanton E, Holland A, High S, Woodman P. (2005) Disease-associated mutations cause premature oligomerization of myelin proteolipid protein in the endoplasmic reticulum. Proc Natl Acad Sci USA 102: 4342–4347.

Thomson CE, Montague P, Jung M, Nave KA, Griffiths IR. (1997) Phenotypic severity of murine Plp mutants reflects in-vivo and in-vitro variations in transport of PLP isoproteins. Glia 20: 322–332.

Tosic M, Dolivo M, Amiguet P, Domanska-Janik K, Matthieu JM. (1993) Paralytic tremor (pt) rabbit: a sex-linked mutation affecting proteolipid protein-gene expression. Brain Res.625: 307–312.

Uhlenberg B, Schuelke M, Ruschendorf F, et al. (2004) Mutations in the gene encoding gap junction protein alpha 12 (connexin 46.6) cause Pelizaeus–Merzbacher-like disease. Am J Hum Genet 75: 251–260.

Vermeesch MK, Knapp PE, Skoff RP, Studzinski DM, Benjamins JA. (1990) Death of individual oligo-dendrocytes in jimpy brain precedes expression of proteolipid protein. Dev Neurosci 12: 303–315.

Wahle S, Stoffel W. (1998) Cotranslational integration of myelin proteolipid protein (PLP) into the membrane of endoplasmic reticulum: analysis of topology by glycosylation scanning and protease domain protection assay. Glia 24: 226–235.

Weimbs T, Stoffel W. (1992) Proteolipid protein (PLP) of CNS myelin: positions of free, disulfide-bonded, and fatty acid thioester-linked cysteine residues and implications for the membrane topology of PLP. Biochemistry 31: 12 289–12 296.

Weimbs T, Stoffel W. (1994) Topology of CNS myelin proteolipid protein: evidence for the nonenzymatic glycosylation of extracytoplasmic domains in normal and diabetic animals. Biochemistry 33: 10 408–10 415.

Werner HB, Kuhlmann K, Shen K, et al. (2007) Proteolipid protein is required for transport of sirtuin 2 into CNS myelin. J Neurosci 27: 7717–7730.

Wight PA, Duchala CS, Readhead C, Macklin WB. (1993) A myelin proteolipid protein-LacZ fusion protein is developmentally regulated and targeted to the myelin membrane in transgenic mice. J Cell Biol 123: 443–454.

Wolf NI, Cundall M, Rutland P, et al. (2007) Frameshift mutation in GJA12 leading to nystagmus, spastic ataxia and CNS dys-/demyelination. Neurogenetics 8: 39–44.

Woodward K, Kendall E, Vetrie D, Malcolm S. (1998) Pelizaeus–Merzbacher disease: identification of Xq22 proteolipid-protein duplications and characterization of breakpoints by interphase FISH. Am J Hum Genet 63: 207–217.

Woodward K, Palmer R, Rao K, Malcolm S. (1999) Prenatal diagnosis by FISH in a family with Pelizaeus–Merzbacher disease caused by duplication of PLP gene. Prenat Diagn 19: 266–268.

Yool D, Klugmann M, Barrie JA, McCulloch MC, Nave KA, Griffiths IR. (2002) Observations on the structure of myelin lacking the major proteolipid protein. Neuropathol Appl Neurobiol 28: 75–78.

11
THERAPEUTIC APPROACHES IN LEUKODYSTROPHIES

Ali Fatemi and Charles Peters

Introduction
The severity of the manifestations of genetic disorders of myelin continues to be a significant challenge, but while curative therapy does not exist for many of these disorders, inroads are now being made using newer technologies. In this chapter, we will discuss the accomplishments and unresolved issues.

CHALLENGES TO TRIAL DESIGN IN LEUKODYSTROPHIES
The evaluation of therapeutic interventions in leukodystrophies has been hampered by multiple factors. Due to the rarity of these diseases, investigators often face the challenge of insufficient sample sizes and power for a controlled trial. The natural course is often incompletely understood and there is a persistent danger that sweeping generalizations overtake actual knowledge. There is often considerable phenotypic variability in disease severity, with genotypic analysis that may not correlate with disease progression, making stratification of patients difficult. The therapeutic windows may be very brief due to the devastating and rapid course of these disorders, giving urgency to undertake therapies. The pathophysiology of most leukodystrophies is still poorly understood, further hampering the optimization of therapy.

While clinical severity scales based on qualitative assessment of symptoms/signs have been used for decades as markers for disease progression and outcome, they are often insensitive to small changes, and are dependent on the skills and experience of the examiner.

In contrast, with the wide use of magnetic resonance imaging (MRI) and other advanced neuroimaging methods, visualization of disease manifestations has become readily available at a macroscopic level for all leukodystrophies. Modern MRI modalities such as diffusion tensor imaging, magnetic resonance spectroscopic imaging, magnetization transfer imaging, and perfusion MRI are being employed as measures of disease in therapeutic trials for leukodystrophies.

Despite these challenges, several therapeutic approaches are available for selected leukodystrophies, and clinical trials are ongoing.

Cell-based therapies
Advances in immunomodulation and stem cell technology have opened the door to a wide range of cell-based interventions over the last 30 years. In fact, bone marrow and cord blood hematopoietic cell transplantations have been conducted for many neurometabolic diseases

(Peters and Steward 2003). From the favorable results in Hurler syndrome (Krivit et al. 1995), it was expected that most storage disorders could be effectively treated by hematopoietic cell transplantation (HCT). However, with time and experience, benefit from HCT appeared to be limited to selected subsets of patients with neurometabolic diseases including early stages of X-linked adrenoleukodystrophy (X-ALD), and probably some cases of metachromatic leukodystrophy (MLD) and globoid cell leukodystrophy (GLD). While beneficial effects have been shown with these interventions, the mechanisms of action are still poorly understood.

Numerous factors play a role in cell-based therapy, including the type of cells used, the route of transplantation, the age of the patient, the pathophysiology of the underlying condition, and the status of the immune system. Principally, the earlier in disease course that treatment is initiated, the more likely it is that it will be beneficial (Weinberg 2005). Furthermore, an additional challenge in the field of HCT remains the occurrence of primary and secondary graft failures and mixed donor chimerism, and sometimes-lethal complications of this procedure (Uckan et al. 2005).

Currently, a number of different stem cell sources exist (Fig. 11.1). Embryonic stem cells, neural stem cells, as well as glial-restricted precursor cells have been transplanted directly into the central nervous system (CNS) in a number of rodent white matter disease models such as experimental allergic encephalitis (EAE) and transverse myelitis in rats, and the myelin-deficient *shiverer* mouse (van Bekkum 2004, Goldman et al. 2008). These studies have shown that such stem cells can differentiate into more mature cells, specifically into astrocytes and oligodendrocytes, and improve the clinical picture to varying degrees. However, their engraftment seems to be highly dependent on the pathophysiology of the underlying condition; the microenvironment of the injured tissue may release factors that determine the fate of exogenous cells (Taylor et al. 2006, Givogri et al. 2008). Another observation regarding embryonic and neural stem cells has been the relatively high incidence of tumor formation after their direct CNS transplantation (Correia et al. 2005, Blum and Benvenisty 2008). Finally, since direct transplantation of cells into the CNS is invasive in a clinical setting, researchers are investigating systemic routes of introducing genetically modified stem cells and bypassing the blood–brain barrier (Young et al. 2004).

Cells derived from human CD34+ cells, which were isolated from either cord blood or peripheral blood, migrated into the brain after infusion into non-obese diabetic immune-deficient mice (Asheuer et al. 2004). Both cord blood- and peripheral blood-derived CD34+ cells differentiated into perivascular and ramified microglia (Fig. 11.2). Furthermore, there are controversial reports suggesting that a small percentage of the peripherally transplanted cells migrate into the CNS and become neurons (Garbuzova-Davis et al. 2003, Walczak et al. 2004). While remarkable effects have been reported after bone marrow transplantation (BMT) or umbilical cord blood transplantation (UCBT), the number of exogenous cells detected in the CNS is minuscule and therefore transdifferentiation into neurons or oligodendrocytes or cell–cell fusion is unlikely to play a major role in the overall beneficial effect of BMT or UCBT (Zigova et al. 2002, Nikolic et al. 2008). Another plausible hypothesis is that bone marrow or cord blood hematopoietic cells ameliorate the disease by correcting the biochemical abnormality through expression of the deficient gene (Matzner

189

Potential Stem Cells with Neural Capability

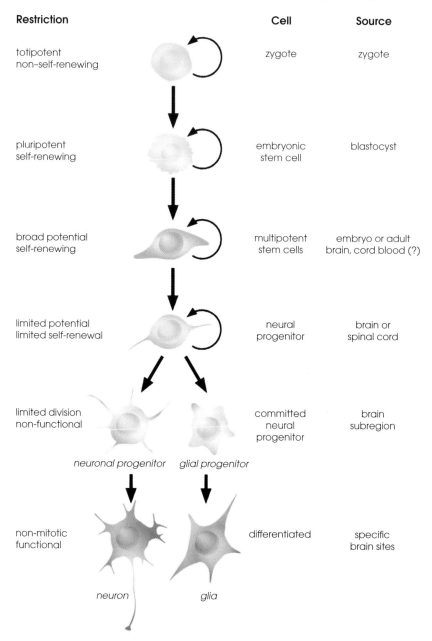

Restriction		Cell	Source
totipotent non–self-renewing		zygote	zygote
pluripotent self-renewing		embryonic stem cell	blastocyst
broad potential self-renewing		multipotent stem cells	embryo or adult brain, cord blood (?)
limited potential limited self-renewal		neural progenitor	brain or spinal cord
limited division non-functional		committed neural progenitor	brain subregion
	neuronal progenitor *glial progenitor*		
non-mitotic functional		differentiated	specific brain sites
	neuron *glia*		

Fig. 11.1. List of stem cells that can give rise to neurons and macroglial cells, presented as a hierarchy beginning with the most primitive multipotent stem cell and concluding with the most restricted. (Adapted with permission from Gage FH. Mammalian neural stem cells. Science 2000; 287: 1433–1438.)

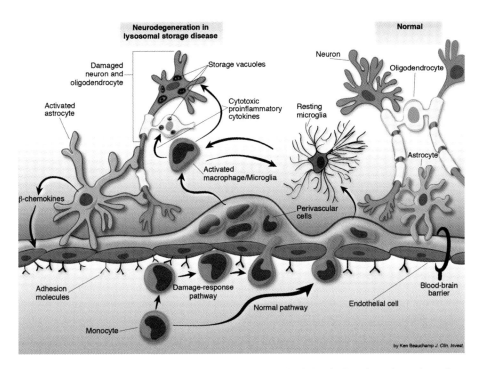

Fig. 11.2. Microglia and macrophages pass through the blood–brain barrier into the perivascular regions and can take up residence in the parenchyma as resting ramified cells. When nervous system damage occurs such as in a lysosomal storage disorder to the left, cytokines and chemokines are released by activated macrophages/microglia leading to upregulation of adhesion molecules on endothelial cells, resulting in migration of more systemic monocytes from the blood into perivascular regions. After hematopoietic stem cell transplantation, donor macrophages and microglia which migrate to the CNS have the opportunity to transfer the needed lysosomal enzyme to deficient cells at sites of damage. (Reprinted with permission from Prioa RL and Wu Y, Blood to brain to the rescue, J Clin Invest 2004; 113: 1108–1110.)

et al. 2000). A study by Schoenberger et al. (2007) demonstrated positive adrenoleukody-strophy protein (ALDP) staining in different CNS cells types of a deceased X-ALD patient after receiving HCT. The authors postulated that this phenomenon was due to transcytosis of the ALDP between the transplanted and host cells.

Several strategies have been proposed to potentiate and accelerate endogenous repair. One approach increases the number of cycling cells through the use of growth factors, for example, platelet-derived growth factor (Siebzehnrubl et al. 2009), glial growth factor-2 (Kingham et al. 2007), neurotrophin-3, and epidermal growth factor (Dasari et al. 2007). Another approach enhances oligodendrocyte differentiation and myelin production by oligotrophic growth factors, such as insulin growth factor-1, lymphocyte inhibitory factor, or ciliary neurotrophic factor, thereby stimulating the stem cell niche in the adult subventricular zone in order to increase the production of oligoneogenic progenitor cells (Broughton et al. 2007).

It is possible that stem cells may have a beneficial effect without directly migrating to the CNS. First, a number of studies have shown that stem cells, such as cord blood hematopoietic cells, can release growth factors including glial cell line-derived neurotrophic factor, and brain-derived neurotrophic factor, which may help with endogenous repair mechanisms such as stimulation of the endogenous stem cell niche (McGuckin et al. 2004). Stem cells may also play a role in immunomodulation (Vendrame et al. 2005, Pluchino and Martino 2008, Bai et al. 2009, Pluchino et al. 2009).

The first indication of an anti-inflammatory effect of neural progenitor cells (NPCs) was noted when these cells were transplanted intraventricularly in rats with acute EAE (Pluchino et al. 2003): In Lewis rats with EAE induced by injections of spinal cord homogenates, there was an acute, reversible paralytic disease that was the result of disseminated CNS inflammation, which occurred without demyelination or axonal injury. Cell transplantation attenuated the inflammatory brain process and clinical severity of disease. Follow-up studies examined the effect of NPC transplantation in the MOG35-55 peptide–induced EAE in C57BL/6 mice, a model with an acute paralytic disease due to a T cell-mediated autoimmune process that causes severe axonal injury and demyelination (Pluchino et al. 2005): neurosphere-derived pluripotent precursor transplants attenuated the inflammatory process, reduced acute axonal injury, reduced chronic axonal loss and demyelination, and improved the clinical performance of the animal.

Cell culture experiments showed a striking inhibition of EAE-derived T-cell activation. The suppressive effect of neural precursors on T cells was accompanied by significant suppression of pro-inflammatory cytokines. The relevance of this neural precursor–T-cell interaction was demonstrated, as intravenously administered NPCs were transiently found in peripheral lymphoid organs, where they interacted with T cells to reduce their disease-causing potential. In this setting, intravenously injected neural precursors did not cross the blood–brain barrier and their effect was mediated by peripheral immunosuppression, resulting in reduced immune cell infiltration into the CNS and consequently less CNS damage (Fig. 11.3). These findings suggest that the beneficial clinical and pathological effects of NPC transplantation are related, in part, to immunomodulatory and anti-inflammatory properties.

Current animal studies aim to understand mechanisms of action of cell transplantation and develop genetically modified cells that would be able to overcome the hurdles of systemic transplantation and engraftment. Others have focused on transplantation of autologous hematopoietic stem cells genetically modified to express the missing protein to circumvent immune related problems associated with allogeneic HCT (Cartier and Aubourg 2008). Promising in concept, these strategies are now ready to be tested in phase I/II clinical trials. Finally, one should mention the very recent description of induced pluripotent stem cells, which are derived from somatic cells (such as skin or blood cells) and transformed into stem cells by transfection of certain stem cell-associated genes via viral vectors (Yamanaka 2008). These cells have in many ways characteristics of embryonic stem cells and could potentially serve as an autologous source of stem cells for each individual.

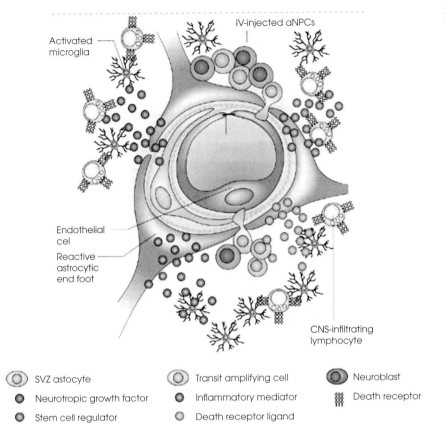

Activated microglia

IV-injected aNPCs

Endothelial cel

Reactive astrocytic end foot

CNS-infiltrating lymphocyte

⊚ SVZ astocyte	⊚ Transit amplifying cell	⊚ Neuroblast
● Neurotropic growth factor	◐ Inflammatory mediator	▓ Death receptor
◑ Stem cell regulator	○ Death receptor ligand	

Fig. 11.3. Peripherally injected neural progenitor cells or neuroblasts alter the CNS immune response by crosstalk. After intravenous injection in rats, these cells selectively migrate to and accumulate in the inflammatory perivascular areas in the CNS, which contain blood-borne inflammatory lymphocytes, activated microglia, reactive astrocytes and inflamed endothelial cells. Depending on the environmental cues, a neuroblast may either remain in the niche in an undifferentiated state promoting apoptosis of neighboring inflammatory cells, or move out of the niche and differentiate. The microenvironment of the injured area is the main determinant in this process. (Modified with permission from Martino et al. Nature Reviews Neuroscience 2006; 7: 395–406.)

GLOBOID CELL LEUKODYSTROPHY

Krabbe disease, also known as globoid cell leukodystrophy (GLD), is caused by mutations in the gene encoding galactosylceramidase and leads to accumulation of psychosine (Wenger et al. 1974). The first definitive report on HCT for GLD described 5 cases (4 late-onset and 1 infantile patients with Krabbe disease) (Krivit et al. 1998). The outcomes may be summarized:

(1) Galactosylceramidase activity levels normalized in lymphoblasts;
(2) normal, stable neuropsychological function maintained in 3 late-onset disease patients;

(3) "improvement in demyelination" shown on MRI of the brain;

(4) Cerebrospinal fluid protein (CSF) levels normalized in all cases, except for an infant who still had a CSF protein level over 150 mg/dl at follow-up, although this was decreased from greater than 550 mg/dl at baseline.

The effect of UCBT in patients with symptomatic infantile GLD and in minimally asymptomatic or presymptomatic infants with GLD has been evaluated (Escolar et al. 2005). While symptomatic infants with infantile GLD did not improve or stabilize, there were suggestions of a beneficial effect in 11 minimally or presymptomatic newborns who received UCBT between 12 and 44 days of age, when compared with their untreated siblings. Upon follow-up at a median age of 3.0 years, the infants that were presymptomatic at the time of transplantation, had age-appropriate cognitive function and receptive language skills. Serial MRI studies demonstrated progressive central myelination. Although the children from this cohort were better neurologically than they would have been had they followed the typical fulminant course of early infantile Krabbe disease, reports suggest that the majority of presymptomatic children receiving transplantation for Krabbe disease have developed motor and language deterioration (Duffner et al. 2009). Additional follow-up is needed to assess long-term outcomes in these patients with unprecedented survival.

METACHROMATIC LEUKODYSTROPHY

Metachromatic leukodystrophy (MLD) is a neurodegenerative lysosomal disease caused by a defect of the enzyme arylsulfatase A, which disrupts the degradation of sulfatides in neurons and glial cells (Gieselmann 2008; see also Chapter 8). The experience with HCT for MLD extends over two decades. Published and unpublished data have shown that it has not been effective in symptomatic patients with the late-infantile form of the disease and may even accelerate its progression (Malm et al. 1996, Bredius et al. 2007). Several reports suggest that bone marrow and cord blood transplantation arrest the progression in patients with the juvenile or adult MLD phenotype (Gorg et al. 2007, Pierson et al. 2008). Evaluation of these results is problematic due to the relatively short follow-up and the variability of progression in untreated patients. While it appears that stabilization of neuropsychological function eventually occurs, deterioration in peripheral nervous system function continues in long-term survivors. Several presymptomatic patients have received transplants (Martin et al. 2006). Longer follow-up is required to assess effectiveness.

X-LINKED ADRENOLEUKODYSTROPHY

X-linked adrenoleukodsytrophy (X-ALD) is the most common leukodystrophy and is caused by mutations in the *ABCD1* gene encoding a peroxisomal ATP-Binding Cassette Transporter, leading to accumulation of very long chain fatty acids (VLCFAs) in the brain, adrenal glands, testis, and plasma (Moser et al. 2004; see also Chapter 5). Hematopoietic stem cell transplantation (HSCT) provides an important therapeutic modality for the cerebral inflammatory forms of X-ALD (Mahmood et al. 2007). Either bone marrow cells (for BMT) or umbilical cord cells (for UCBT) are utilized. Aubourg et al. (1990) were the first to report stabilization and reversal of neurological manifestation in an 8-year-old boy who had early evidence of cerebral involvement. This patient was reported as still well, nearly 20 years later (P. Aubourg, personal communication). Shapiro et al. (2000) reported long-term stabilization of MRI demyelination and neuropsychological function in boys who had received BMT. There was a tendency for deterioration prior to ultimate stabilization in visual processing as seen in the performance IQ scores of boys with a posterior pattern of demyelination. Interestingly, VLCFA concentrations significantly decreased but remained elevated long term, suggesting that VLCFA levels are not an optimal surrogate marker for this treatment. A report of the international HSCT experience provides follow-up on 126 X-ALD patients who were treated between 1982 and 1999 (Peters et al. 2004). This study provides important guidelines for the selection of patients for HSCT. The overall 5-year survival was 56% compared with estimated 45% survival in untreated patients. Transplant-related mortality was 14%. Outcome with respect to mortality, morbidity, and quality of life was unsatisfactory for patients who were already severely involved at the time of HCT; therefore, the procedure is not recommended for them. In contrast, 5-year survival was 92% in a group of patients with early-stage cerebral disease defined as having minimal neuro-logical deficits (i.e., 0–1) and neuroradiological involvement (MRI severity score <9) (Fig. 11.4). Consequently, HSCT can be strongly recommended for them. The article by C. Peters and colleagues (Peters et al. 2004) provides a detailed discussion of the outcomes and indications for HSCT (Table 11.1).

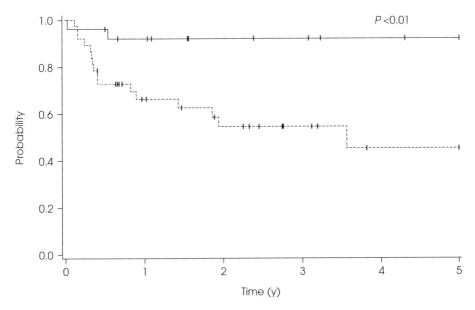

Fig. 11.4. Kaplan–Meier estimate of survival for cerebral X-linked adrenoleukodystrophy following hematopoietic cell transplantation by number of neurological deficits and MRI severity score before transplantation. Solid line indicates patients with 0 to 1 neurological deficits and MRI severity score of less than 9 ($n = 25$). Dashed line indicates patients with two or more neurological deficits or MRI severity score of 9 or greater ($n = 37$). Ticks on probability lines indicate dates of censoring at last follow-up. (Reprinted with permission from Peters C. et al. Blood 2004; 104: 881–888.)

TABLE 11.1
Characteristics of 94 patients with cerebral X-adrenoleukodystrophy (X-ALD) who underwent hematopoietic cell transplantation (HCT)

	Related donor (n = 42)	Unrelated donor (n = 52)	Total (n = 94)
Year of HCT, no. (%)			
Before 1990	5 (12)	0 (0)	5 (5)
1991 to 1995	24 (56)	20 (38)	44 (46)
1996 to 1999	13 (31)	32 (62)	45 (48)
Median age at HCT, y (range)	9.1 (5.2–15.6)	8.9 (4.9–18.6)	9.0 (4.9–18.6)
Reason for diagnosis, no. (%)*			
Family history	11 (29)	17 (35)	28 (33)
X-ALD signs and symptoms	27 (71)	31 (65)	58 (67)
Unknown	4	4	8
Stem cell source and HLA matching			
Marrow/UCB	42/0	40/12	82/12
Matched	33/0	27/4	60/4
Mismatched	9/0	13/8	22/8
Preparative regimen, no. (%)			
Chemotherapy only	31 (74)	17 (33)	48 (51)
Bu/Cy	30 (97)	17 (100)	47 (98)
Bu only	1 (3)	0	1 (2)
Chemotherapy and radiation	11 (26)	35 (67)	46 (49)
Cy/TBI, brain-sparing at 1400 cGy	5 (45)	13 (37)	18 (39)
Bu/Cy/TBI at 300–1200 cGy	1 (9)	9 (26)	10 (22)
Cy/TBI at 1200–1400 cGy	1 (9)	8 (23)	9 (20)
Bu/Cy/TLI at 150–750 cGy	2 (18)	1 (3)	3 (7)
Cy/TAI at 600 cGy	1 (9)	1 (3)	2 (4)
VP-16/Ara-C/Cy/TBI at 1200 cGy	1 (9)	1 (3)	2 (4)
Other	0	2 (6)	2 (4)
GVHD prophylaxis			
CSA/MP, no. (%)	24 (57)	29 (56)	53 (56)
No. with/no. without ATG	3/21	12/17	15/38
CSA/MTX, no. (%)	9 (21)	8 (15)	17 (18)
No. with/no. without ATG	2/7	6/2	8/9
Other, no. (%)	9 (21)	15 (29)	24 (26)
Graft manipulation by elutriation, no. *yes* / no. *no*	3/39	15/37	18/76

UCB indicates umbilical cord blood; Bu, busulfan; Cy, cyclophosphamide; GVHD, graft-versus-host disease; HLA, human leukocyte antigen; TBI, total body irradiation; TLI, total lymphoid irradiation; TAI, total abdominal irradiation; VP-16, etoposide; Ara-C, cytosine arabinoside; CSA, cyclosporin; MP, methylprednisolone; and ATG, antithymocyle globulin.

* Percentages were calculated only for patients with a known reason.

Source: Reprinted with permission from Peters C. et al. Blood 2004; 104: 881–888.

The neuropsychological functional outcomes of boys after HSCT was assessed and reported based upon their MRI demyelination pattern (Table 11.2). Baseline performance IQ scores after HCT and mean changes in them were significantly lower and greater, respectively, in boys with a posterior pattern of demyelination.

At this time, HSCT is not recommended for asymptomatic patients with normal MRI

TABLE 11.2
Comparison of neuropsychological functional outcomes according to MRI pattern of demyelination following hematopoietic cell transplantation (HCT) for cerebral X-linked adrenoleukodystrophy

	Parietal-occipital lobes, *n* = 25	Frontal lobes or pyramidal tracts, *n* = 7	Total, *n* = 32	No neuropsychological function assessment after HCT because of death, *n* = 29	*P*
VIQ*					
Baseline (range)	99 (59–127)	89 (70–107)	**98 (59–127)**	**92 (74–124)**	NS
After HCT (range)	82 (46–123)	79 (57–113)	80.5 (46–123)	–	–
Mean change (CI)	**–13.7** (–20.5 to –6.8)	**–6.4** (–17.8 to 4.9)	**–12.1** (–17.1 to –7.1)	–	**0.25**
PIQ*					
Baseline (range)	96 (45–122.5)	92 (61–100)	**94.5 (45–122.5)**	**77.5 (45–138)**	**<0.01**
After HCT (range)	64 (45–122.5)	93 (54–108)	73 (45–122.5)	–	–
Mean change (CI)	**–21.6** (–30.6 to –12.6)	**0.4** (–6.8 to 7.7)	**–16.8** (–24.6 to –8.9)	–	**0.03**

* VIQ and PIQ baseline evaluations and those after HCT: median (range). Bold denotes statistical comparisons and corresponding *P* values. VIQ indicates verbal intelligence quotient; PIQ, performance intelligent quotient; CI, 95% confidence interval; NS, not significant.

Source: Reprinted with permission from Peters C. et al. Blood 2004; 104: 881–888.

or for those with pure adrenomyeloneuropathy. The mechanism of the beneficial effect of HSCT remains incompletely understood.

PELIZAEUS–MERZBACHER DISEASE

Pelizaeus–Merzbacher disease is an X-linked hypomyelinating disorder of the CNS, most frequently caused by duplication of chromosome Xq22 including the region encoding the dosage-sensitive proteolipid protein 1 (PLP1) gene. *Shiverer*, *jimpy*, *Trembler*, and protein zero (P0) deficient mice have served as animal models for this disorder. Congenitally hypomyelinated *shiverer* mice fail to generate compact myelin and die by 18 to 21 weeks of age. Using multifocal anterior and posterior fossa delivery of sorted fetal human glial progenitor cells into the immune deficient, myelin deficient neonatal *shiverer rag*2 (/) mice, Goldman and colleagues achieved whole neuraxis myelination of the engrafted hosts, which in a significant fraction of cases rescued this otherwise lethal phenotype (Windrem et al. 2008). Interestingly, the transplanted mice exhibited greatly prolonged survival with progressive resolution of their neurological deficits, and substantial myelination in multiple regions was accompanied by the acquisition of normal nodes of Ranvier and transcallosal conduction velocities, ultrastructurally normal and complete myelination of most axons, and a restoration of a substantially normal neurological phenotype. In this study the resultant mice were cerebral chimeras, with murine gray matter but a predominantly human white matter glial composition (Fig. 11.5). Very recently a phase I clinical trial has been initiated to determine the safety of human-cadaver-derived neural stem cell transplantation in patients with Pelizaeus–Merzbacher disease.

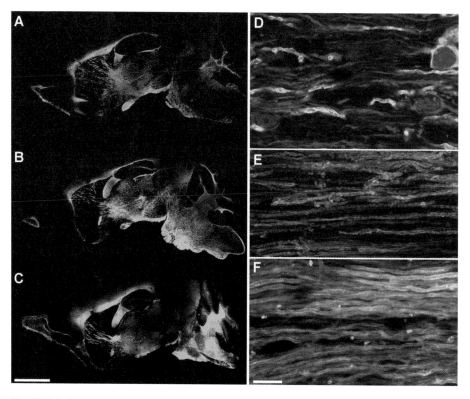

Fig. 11.5. A–C: Myelin Basic Protein (MBP) staining of *shiverer* mice that were transplanted with human glial precursor cell on the first day of life. Images are shown at 20 weeks (**A**); 35 weeks (**B**); and 52 weeks (**C**). While the untreated *shiverer* mouse has no MBP staining, the transplanted animals already demonstrate myelination in major white-matter regions of the brain at 20 weeks. **B:** At 35 weeks, the area of dense myelination has expanded into the mid-brain and hindbrain. **C:** By 1 year, myelin was well distributed, and myelination appeared complete, throughout the forebrain and hindbrain. **D–F:** Corresponding confocal optical sections of transplanted *shiverer* mouse corpus callosum taken at 20 weeks (**D**), 35 weeks (**E**), and 52 weeks (**F**), immunolabeled for neurofilament (red) and myelin basic protein (green), which reveal the progressive increase in axonal ensheathment with time. Scale bars: 2.5 mm (**A–C**), 10 μm (**D–F**). (Modified with permission from Windrem MS et al. Neonatal chimerization with human glial progenitor cells can both remyelinate and rescue the otherwise lethally hypomyelinated shiverer mouse. Cell Stem Cell. 2008; 2: 553–565.) A color version of this figure is available in the Plate section.

Enzyme replacement therapy

Roscoe O. Brady speculated in 1966 that if an enzyme were insufficiently active, one might attempt to purify it and inject it into patients to see if it would provide therapeutic benefit (Brady, 1966, 1967). The first investigation along this line was the intravenous injection of hexosaminidase A, which had been isolated from human urine, into an infant with Sandhoff disease (Johnson et al. 1973). (Such patients accumulate the ganglioside, GM2, in the brain and globoside in peripheral tissues and the blood.) A significant reduction of globoside occurred in the circulation shortly after infusing the enzyme (Johnson et al. 1973). None of the injected enzyme reached the brain. The patient experienced pyrexia following infusion. There was no change in the patient's clinical condition. To date, enzyme replacement therapy (ERT) has provided no reported clear benefits in patients who have a leukodystrophy. However, given its promise, ERT is under investigation in metachromatic and globoid cell leukodystrophies.

Recent therapeutic studies in the mouse model of MLD are highly encouraging. Transplantation of hematopoietic stem cells over-expressing arylsulfatase A led to a remarkable correction of neuropathological changes (Matzner et al. 2002). Matzner et al. (2005) reported the unexpected and surprising findings that IV administration of purified arylsulfatase A improved nervous system pathology and function in the MLD. However, mice can develop anti-arylsulfatase A antibodies, which impede sulfatide clearance without inhibiting enzyme activity (Matzner et al. 2008). The neutralizing effect of antibodies was reproduced in cell culture models of MLD by demonstrating that mouse immune serum reduces the ability of arylsulfatase A to clear sulfatide from cultured enzyme-deficient Schwann and kidney cells (Matzner et al. 2008). A single center, open-label phase I/II ERT trial in patients with late-infantile MLD was recently completed in Denmark and the results have not yet been published, the sponsor of the study released a statement in Summer 2010 that the production of the intravenous drug has been suspended.

Enzyme replacement has been discussed as a potential therapeutic for Krabbe disease. Lee et al. observed an increase in lifespan, an attenuation of the early failure to thrive, and an improvement in the gait of animals treated with recurrent intraperitoneal administration of galactocerebrosidase, but failed to prevent the later precipitous decline occurring just before death (Lee et al. 2009). While it is likely that much of the clinical benefit observed in the treated animals was due to peripheral improvements, the investigators were able to detect a small amount of enzyme in the brain and a resultant reduction in psychosine levels. No clinical trials have been published on the use of ERT in patients with Krabbe disease. However, there is precedent for combining ERT with hematopoietic stem cell transplantation, which is presently done for patients with Hurler syndrome (Boelens 2006). Whether a combined strategy will result in improved outcomes in MLD and GLD awaits further studies.

Gene therapy

Since leukodsytrophies are, by definition, genetic diseases, the ultimate treatment goal would be to correct the genetic defect. Gene transfer technology relies on the delivery of DNA to target cells and expression of the protein it encodes for therapeutic or protective purposes. Transfer of the correct gene could provide direct metabolic correction of specific cells. Multiple vehicles have been proposed for the transfer of genes into the CNS including viral vectors and in-vitro transduced stem cells (Fig. 11.6).

The most important element for successful gene delivery is the selection of an efficient and safe vector system. Viral vectors have the ability to introduce their genetic material into recipient cells, and have been widely used as gene delivery systems (Sands and Haskins 2008). The desired properties of a viral vector include replication deficiency, non-immunogenicity, non-toxicity and the ability to deliver its genetic material to the nucleus

A Correction by in-vivo gene therapy

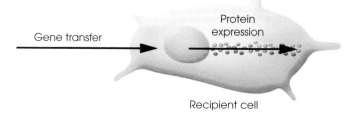

Gene transfer

Protein expression

Recipient cell

B Cross-correction by ex-vivo gene therapy

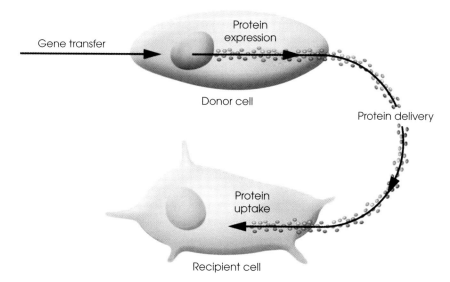

Gene transfer

Protein expression

Donor cell

Protein delivery

Protein uptake

Recipient cell

Fig. 11.6. A: In-vivo gene therapy is based on direct gene transfer into the cells requiring the replacement therapy. **B**: For ex-vivo gene therapy, the gene transfer is performed in a cell type outside the body, and the genetically modified cells are injected into the deficient recipient. The genetically modified cells can then circulate within the bloodstream, migrate into the CNS and cross-correct the genetic defect by protein transfer. (Reprinted from Neumann H, Microglia: a cellular vehicle for CNS gene therapy. J Clin Invest 2006; 116: 2857–2860.)

of a target cell. The recombinant adeno-associated virus (AAV) is a helper-dependent single-stranded DNA parvovirus, whose genome contains only the sequences necessary and sufficient for packaging and integration (Mandel and Burger 2004). All viral genes encoding other wild-type viral proteins are removed to avoid toxicity and immunogenicity. AAV vectors are very promising viral systems for gene delivery in the CNS because they can transduce post-mitotic cells (Mandel and Burger 2004).

There are several serotypes of AAV that can be used for gene transfer in the CNS, with each of them possessing distinct properties regarding their regional pattern of transduction and their cellular tropism. The most widely used is the AAV-2 serotype, which shows specific expression to neurons. Apart from AAV-2, serotypes 1, 4 and 5 have also been tested. More specifically, AAV-5-mediated transfer in the striatum transduces both neurons and astrocytes at the site of infection, but also at more distant sites, such as the septal region and the neocortex (Taymans et al. 2007). Therefore, AAV-5-type vectors may be used in cases in which broader expression of the gene product is desired. AAV-4-mediated gene transfer in the striatum exhibits selectivity to ependymal cells, whereas AAV-1 transduction efficiency is higher with wider distribution in striatal neurons, although AAV-1 may also transduce glial and ependymal cells (Liu et al. 2005).

AAV-mediated gene transfer approaches have been designed for the treatment of many neurological disorders. To date, AAV-mediated gene transfer has several applications that include increased expression of a missing or dysfunctional protein: aspartoacylase (McPhee et al. 2006) for Canavan disease; delivery of neuroprotective or trophic agents (Mandel and Burger 2004); inactivation of a gene (delivery of shRNA via AAV for silencing of the huntingtin gene – Franich et al. 2008), control of neuronal firing, and induction of neuronal cell death (in cases of CNS tumors, delivery of anti-oncogenic or anti-angiogenic agents – Gupta 2000).

Haug and Braun-Falco (2005) have reported that AAV-based vectors restored fatty aldehyde dehydrogenase activity in fibroblast cell lines from patients with Sjögren–Larsson syndrome, a leukodystrophy in which the dehydrogenase is deficient.

AAV-based vectors have been successfully used leading to long-lasting expression of human arylsulfatase A in the brain of the MLD mouse model (Iwamoto et al. 2009). Arylsulfatase A delivery rapidly reversed sulfatide storage and prevented neuropathological abnormalities and neuromotor impairment in this animal model.

Canavan disease was the first neurodegenerative disorder to be treated by gene therapy (McPhee et al. 2006). Patients received intracranial infusions via six cranial burr holes. AAV-2-mediated intraparenchymal delivery of the human aspartoacylase cDNA was achieved. The immune response and safety profiles were monitored in the follow-up of ten patients. Following recombinant AAV-2 administration, there was no evidence of AAV-2-neutralizing antibody titers in serum for the majority of patients tested (7/10). In a subset (3/10) of the patients, low to moderately high levels of AAV-2-neutralizing antibody with respect to baseline were detected. In all patients, there were minimal systemic signs of inflammation or immune stimulation. In those with catheter access to the lateral ventricle of the brain, CSF was examined and there was a complete absence of neutralizing antibody titers, with no overt signs of brain inflammation. So far, no definitive changes in clinical course have been reported.

Another group of viruses that can achieve high transduction efficiency for non-dividing cells are recombinant lentiviral vectors. The most commonly used lentiviral vector is derived from the human immunodeficiency virus 1 (HIV-1) (Lai and Brady 2002), but recombinant vectors based on feline, equine, or simian lentiviruses have been developed as well (Valori et al. 2008). These vectors are well-tolerated after injection in rodent brains (Valori et al. 2008). They provide sustained transgene expression for extended periods and have a large cloning capacity (Lundberg et al. 2008). These features make lentiviral vectors suitable for use in the CNS. These vectors were shown to express the transgene mainly in neurons and to a lesser extent also in glial cells when injected into the adult rat brain using viral promoters such as the human cytomegalovirus (Lundberg et al. 2008).

Ex-vivo gene therapy of hematopoietic stem cells has been discussed as potential therapy for the treatment of diseases that globally affect the CNS. In 1994, transplantation of murine bone marrow cells, which had been transduced with a murine retroviral vector that expressed the glucocerebrosidase gene (which is deficient in Gaucher disease), resulted in the replacement of 20% of microglia with donor-derived microglia that expressed the glucocerebrosidase gene for 3 to 4 months after transplantation(Krall et al. 1994). In 2001, an HIV-1-derived lentivirus vector was used to transduce ex-vivo murine bone marrow cells, which were re-injected into irradiated mice (Priller et al. 2001); this study demonstrated that recruitment of bone marrow-derived microglia that expressed the green fluorescent protein (GFP) reporter gene was specifically attracted to sites of neuronal damage. The lentiviral transfer of genes into CD34+ cells before infusion did not modify the differentiation of human CD34+ cells into microglia and allowed new transgenic proteins to be expressed in these cells (Asheuer et al. 2004). Aubourg and co-workers used a modified HIV-based vector that included the human *ALD* cDNA under the elongation factor 1 alpha promoter control. Transplantation of immune-deficient (non-obese diabetic severe combined immune deficiency, NOD/SCID) mice with these transfected cells led to successful engraftment of these cells, and recombinant ALD protein was expressed in 30 to 85% of bone marrow cells from recipient mice (Benhamida et al. 2003).

Recently, Cartier and Aubourg (2008) have reported on a pilot clinical study employing ex-vivo gene transfer of hematopoietic stem cells in two patients with X-ALD. Mobilized peripheral blood CD34+ cells were collected from two boys with X-ALD and transduced ex vivo with a lentiviral vector expressing the recombinant *ABCD1* gene. It was found that 50% and 30%, respectively, of the transduced CD34+ cells expressed the ALD protein. These transduced cells were then re-infused into the affected boys after full myeloablation. Hematopoietic recovery occurred at day 15 post-transplantation, and the procedure was uneventful. The percentage of corrected lymphocytes and monocytes in the peripheral blood of treated patients remained stable.

While these studies are encouraging, there are still many hurdles to overcome with gene therapy. The main difficulty is the route and timing of delivery. Given the fact that most leukodystrophies involve either the entire white matter or large areas of the brain, it will be difficult to achieve successful gene transfer without invasive surgery, which may cause additional injury to the CNS. Also, it is unlikely that gene therapy will be effective if the disease is at an advanced stage, but little research has been pursued to answer this question. Finally, there is also significant concern about the safety of viral gene transfer. It is possible that the insertion of viral genes into host cells may lead to undesired modulation of the genome, leading to abnormal cell function and further injury.

Other therapeutic approaches

Lorenzo Oil

"Lorenzo Oil" is a 4 : 1 mixture of glyceryl trioleate and glycerylerucate (Moser et al. 2007). It has the biochemical effect of normalizing the plasma levels of VLCFAs in patients with X-ALD within 4 weeks, probably by inhibiting endogenous VLCFA synthesis (Moser et al. 2007). A recent study by Moser and colleagues reported that administration of Lorenzo Oil to asymptomatic boys who had a normal brain MRI significantly reduced their risk of developing childhood cerebral X-ALD (Moser et al. 2005). It is recommended that asymptomatic patients with normal brain MRI who are less than 8 years of age be placed on a carefully supervised program of Lorenzo Oil and dietary therapy. Adrenal function and brain MRI must be monitored at 6-month intervals. Lorenzo Oil does not alter significantly the neurological progression in X-ALD patients who already have evidence of inflammatory cerebral involvement (Moser 1999). A double-blinded placebo-controlled study of Lorenzo Oil therapy in men and women with pure adrenomyeloneuropathy is in progress. Other pharmacological therapeutic approaches have shown therapeutic potential in preclinical studies and preliminary clinical trials. These include 4-phenylbutyrate (Gondcaille et al. 2005), lovastatin (Pai et al. 2000, Weinhofer et al. 2003, Engelen et al. 2008), arginine butyrate (McGovern et al. 2003), and N-acetylcysteine (Tolar et al. 2007).

Vitamin K for Metachromatic Leukodystrophy

Vitamin K has an essential role in biosynthesis of sulfatides and other sphingolipids in the brain (Sundaram et al. 1996). Since sphingolipid accumulates in MLD, administering warfarin, a vitamin K antagonist, may ameliorate the phenotype in this leukodystrophy by decreasing the amount of sphingolipid storage in neuronal cells (Sundaram and Lev 1988). This is being evaluated in a therapeutic trial.

Cerebrotendinous Xanthomatosis

There is compelling evidence that oral administration of chenodeoxycholic acid (CDCA) at a dosage of 750 mg/day benefits patients with cerebrotendinous xanthomatosis (Dotti et al. 2004). CDCA is one of the normal bile acids that is not produced in patients with this disease, because of the enzymatic defect. CDCA administration reduces the levels of cholestanol in plasma and CSF, the excretion of urinary bile alcohols, and bile alcohol glucuronides (Keren and Falik-Zaccai 2009). CDCA is reported to improve somatosensory evoked and motor evoked potentials, visual and brainstem auditory evoked responses, brain MRI abnormalities, and osteoporosis. There are several reports that it halted or slowed neurological progression. Beneficial effects are most evident when therapy is started when deficits are minimal (van Heijst et al. 1998). Biochemical and DNA screening of at-risk relatives now permits identification of asymptomatic persons with cerebrotendinous xanthomatosis. It is possible that CDCA therapy will reduce or prevent later disability.

Addition of statins to the regimen may further decrease cholestanol levels (Dotti et al. 2004), though additional clinical benefits have not been demonstrated. Reduction of cholestanol levels can also be achieved with low-density lipoprotein-apheresis (Mimura et al. 1993), but this relatively invasive therapy would require repeated administration and therefore should be considered only in patients who have not responded to pharmacological therapy.

LITHIUM AND ACETATE FOR CANAVAN DISEASE

Canavan disease is an autosomal recessive disorder involving the gene encoding aspartoacylase leading to accumulation of *N*-acetylaspartate (Surendran et al. 2003; see also Chapter 9). The underlying pathological mechanisms have been unclear. Aspartoacylase converts *N*-acetylaspartate to L-aspartate and acetate in brain oligodendrocytes, and *N*-acetylaspartate has been proposed to participate in lipid synthesis via the aspartate pathway (Baslow and Guilfoyle 2009). Based upon the hypothesis that acetate deficiency limits synthesis of myelin lipids, Namboodiri and colleagues suggested dietary supplementation with oral glyceryltriacetate as a potential treatment (Moffett et al. 2007). However, the success of oral supplementation will depend on the ability of acetate to be absorbed in the intestine, transported across the blood–brain barrier, and taken up by oligodendrocytes. Lithium administration induces a decrease in *N*-acetylaspartate in the brain of the tremor rats, the animal model for Canavan disease (Baslow et al. 2002) and in one patient (Janson et al. 2005). There is an ongoing clinical trial combining lithium and acetate to determine whether this combination therapy will improve outcomes.

Future development

It is crucial to mention that advancement in therapeutics will depend upon international multicenter collaborations, an idea that was strongly promulgated by Hugo Moser. This requires the establishment of a complex infrastructure, which includes electronic databases for clinical, genetic, laboratory, and neuroimaging data. Moser and collaborators showed that such structures could be established with modern, next-generation internet technology and enhance information sharing between institutions. It is expected that with the advancement of computer technology these types of multicenter databases will become feasible and allow the conduct of multiple therapeutic trials.

REFERENCES

Asheuer M, Pflumio F, Benhamida S, et al. (2004) Human CD34+ cells differentiate into microglia and express recombinant therapeutic protein. Proc Natl Acad Sci USA 101: 3557–3562.

Aubourg P, Blanche S, Jambaque I, et al. (1990) Reversal of early neurologic and neuroradiologic manifestations of X-linked adrenoleukodystrophy by bone marrow transplantation. N Engl J Med 322: 1860–1866.

Bai L, Lennon DP, Eaton V, et al. (2009) Human bone marrow-derived mesenchymal stem cells induce Th2-polarized immune response and promote endogenous repair in animal models of multiple sclerosis. Glia 57: 1192–1203.

Baslow MH, Guilfoyle DN. (2009) Are astrocytes the missing link between lack of brain aspartoacylase activity and the spongiform leukodystrophy in canavan disease? Neurochem Res 34: 1523–1534.

Baslow MH, Kitada K, Suckow RF, Hungund BL, Serikawa T. (2002) The effects of lithium chloride and other substances on levels of brain N-acetyl-L-aspartic acid in Canavan disease-like rats. Neurochem Res 27: 403–406.

Benhamida S, Pflumio F, Dubart-Kupperschmitt, A, et al. (2003) Transduced CD34+ cells from adrenoleukodystrophy patients with HIV-derived vector mediate long-term engraftment of NOD/SCID mice. Mol Ther 7: 317–324.

Blum B, Benvenisty N. (2008) The tumorigenicity of human embryonic stem cells. Adv Cancer Res 100: 133–158.

Boelens JJ. (2006) Trends in haematopoietic cell transplantation for inborn errors of metabolism. J Inherit Metab Dis 29, 413–420.

Brady RO. (1966) The sphingolipidoses. N Engl J Med 275: 312–318.

Brady RO. (1967) Enzymatic abnormalities in diseases of sphingolipid metabolism. Clin Chem 13: 565–577.

Bredius RG, Laan LA, Lankester, et al. (2007) Early marrow transplantation in a pre-symptomatic neonate with late infantile metachromatic leukodystrophy does not halt disease progression. Bone Marrow Transplant 39: 309–310.

Broughton SK, Chen H, Riddle A, et al. (2007) Large-scale generation of highly enriched neural stem-cell-derived oligodendroglial cultures: maturation-dependent differences in insulin-like growth factor-mediated signal transduction. J Neurochem 100: 628–638.

Cartier N, Aubourg P. (2008) Hematopoietic stem cell gene therapy in Hurler syndrome, globoid cell leukodystrophy, metachromatic leukodystrophy and X-adrenoleukodystrophy. Curr Opin Mol Ther 10: 471–478.

Correia AS, Anisimov SV, Li JY, Brundin P. (2005) Stem cell-based therapy for Parkinson's disease. Ann Med 37: 487–498.

Dasari VR, Spomar DG, Gondi CS, et al. (2007) Axonal remyelination by cord blood stem cells after spinal cord injury. J Neurotrauma 24: 391–410.

Dotti MT, Lutjohann D, von Bergmann K, Federico A. (2004) Normalisation of serum cholestanol concentration in a patient with cerebrotendinous xanthomatosis by combined treatment with chenodeoxycholic acid, simvastatin and LDL apheresis. Neurol Sci 25: 185–191.

Duffner PK, Caviness VS, Jr, Erbe RW, et al. (2009) The long-term outcomes of presymptomatic infants transplanted for Krabbe disease: report of the workshop held on July 11 and 12, 2008, Holiday Valley, New York. Genet Med 11: 450–454.

Engelen M, Ofman R, Mooijer PA, Poll-The BT, Wanders RJ, Kemp S. (2008) Cholesterol-deprivation increases mono-unsaturated very long-chain fatty acids in skin fibroblasts from patients with X-linked adrenoleukodystrophy. Biochim Biophys Acta 1781: 105–111.

Escolar ML, Poe MD, Provenzale JM, et al. (2005) Transplantation of umbilical-cord blood in babies with infantile Krabbe's disease. N Engl J Med 352: 2069–2081.

Franich NR, Fitzsimons HL, Fong DM, Klugmann M, During MJ, Young D. (2008) AAV vector-mediated RNAi of mutant huntingtin expression is neuroprotective in a novel genetic rat model of Huntington's disease. Mol Ther 16: 947–956.

Garbuzova-Davis S, Willing AE, Zigova T, et al. (2003). Intravenous administration of human umbilical cord blood cells in a mouse model of amyotrophic lateral sclerosis: distribution, migration, and differentiation. J Hematother Stem Cell Res, 12: 255–270.

Gieselmann V. (2008) Metachromatic leukodystrophy: genetics, pathogenesis and therapeutic options. Acta Paediatr Suppl 97: 15–21.

Givogri MI, Bottai D, Zhu HL, et al. (2008) Multipotential neural precursors transplanted into the metachromatic leukodystrophy brain fail to generate oligodendrocytes but contribute to limit brain dysfunction. Dev Neurosci 30: 340–357.

Goldman SA, Schanz S, Windrem MS. (2008) Stem cell-based strategies for treating pediatric disorders of myelin. Hum Mol Genet 17: R76–R83.

Gondcaille C, Depreter M, Fourcade S, et al. (2005) Phenylbutyrate up-regulates the adrenoleukodystrophy-related gene as a nonclassical peroxisome proliferator. J Cell Biol 169: 93–104.

Gorg M, Wilck W, Granitzny B, et al. (2007) Stabilization of juvenile metachromatic leukodystrophy after bone marrow transplantation: a 13-year follow-up. J Child Neurol 22: 1139–1142.

Gupta N. (2000) Current status of viral gene therapy for brain tumours. Expert Opin Investig Drugs 9: 713–726.

Haug S, Braun-Falco M. (2005) Adeno-associated virus vectors are able to restore fatty aldehyde dehydrogenase-deficiency. Implications for gene therapy in Sjogren–Larsson syndrome. Arch Dermatol Res 296: 568–572.

Iwamoto N, Watanabe A, Yamamoto M, et al. (2009) Global diffuse distribution in the brain and efficient gene delivery to the dorsal root ganglia by intrathecal injection of adeno-associated viral vector serotype 1. J Gene Med 11: 498–505.

Janson CG, Assadi M, Francis J, Bilaniuk L, Shera D, Leone P. (2005) Lithium citrate for Canavan disease. Pediatr Neurol 33: 235–243.

205

Johnson WG, Desnick RJ, Long DM, et al. (1973) Intravenous injection of purified hexosaminidase A into a patient with Tay–Sachs disease. Birth Defects Orig Artic Ser 9: 120–124.

Keren Z, Falik-Zaccai TC. (2009) Cerebrotendinous xanthomatosis (CTX): a treatable lipid storage disease. Pediatr Endocrinol Rev 7: 6–11.

Kingham PJ, Kalbermatten DF, Mahay D, Armstrong SJ, Wiberg M, Terenghi G. (2007) Adipose-derived stem cells differentiate into a Schwann cell phenotype and promote neurite outgrowth in vitro. Exp Neurol 207: 267–274.

Krall WJ, Challita PM, Perlmutter LS, Skelton DC, Kohn DB. (1994) Cells expressing human glucocerebrosidase from a retroviral vector repopulate macrophages and central nervous system microglia after murine bone marrow transplantation. Blood 83: 2737–2748.

Krivit W, Lockman LA, Watkins PA, Hirsch J, Shapiro EG. (1995) The future for treatment by bone marrow transplantation for adrenoleukodystrophy, metachromatic leukodystrophy, globoid cell leukodystrophy and Hurler syndrome. J Inherit Metab Dis 18: 398–412.

Krivit W, Shapiro EG, Peters C, et al. (1998) Hematopoietic stem-cell transplantation in globoid-cell leukodystrophy. N Engl J Med 338: 1119–1126.

Lai Z, Brady RO. (2002) Gene transfer into the central nervous system in vivo using a recombinanat lentivirus vector. J Neurosci Res 67: 363–371.

Lee WC, Courtenay A, Troendle FJ, et al. (2005) Enzyme replacement therapy results in substantial improvements in early clinical phenotype in a mouse model of globoid cell leukodystrophy. FASEB J 19: 1549–1551

Liu G, Martins I.H, Chiorini JA, Davidson BL. (2005) Adeno-associated virus type 4 (AAV4) targets ependyma and astrocytes in the subventricular zone and RMS. Gene Ther 12: 1503–1508.

Lundberg C, Bjorklund T, Carlsson T, et al. (2008) Applications of lentiviral vectors for biology and gene therapy of neurological disorders. Curr Gene Ther 8: 461–473.

Mahmood A, Raymond GV, Dubey P, Peters C, Moser HW. (2007) Survival analysis of haematopoietic cell transplantation for childhood cerebral X-linked adrenoleukodystrophy: a comparison study. Lancet Neurol 6: 687–692.

Malm G, Ringden O, Winiarski J, et al. (1996) Clinical outcome in four children with metachromatic leukodystrophy treated by bone marrow transplantation. Bone Marrow Transplant 17: 1003–1008.

Mandel RJ, Burger C. (2004) Clinical trials in neurological disorders using AAV vectors: promises and challenges. Curr Opin Mol Ther 6: 482–490.

Martin PL, Carter SL, Kernan NA, et al. (2006) Results of the cord blood transplantation study (COBLT): outcomes of unrelated donor umbilical cord blood transplantation in pediatric patients with lysosomal and peroxisomal storage diseases. Biol Blood Marrow Transplant 12: 184–194.

Matzner U, Hartmann D, Lullmann-Rauch R, et al. (2002) Bone marrow stem cell-based gene transfer in a mouse model for metachromatic leukodystrophy: effects on visceral and nervous system disease manifestations. Gene Ther 9: 53–63.

Matzner U, Harzer K, Learish RD, Barranger JA, Gieselmann V. (2000) Long-term expression and transfer of arylsulfatase A into brain of arylsulfatase A-deficient mice transplanted with bone marrow expressing the arylsulfatase A cDNA from a retroviral vector. Gene Ther 7: 1250–1257.

Matzner U, Herbst E, Hedayati, et al. (2005) Enzyme replacement improves nervous system pathology and function in a mouse model for metachromatic leukodystrophy. Hum Mol Genet 14: 1139–1152.

Matzner U, Matthes F, Weigelt C, et al. (2008) Non-inhibitory antibodies impede lysosomal storage reduction during enzyme replacement therapy of a lysosomal storage disease. J Mol Med 86: 433–442.

McGovern MM, Wasserstein MP, Aron A, Perrine SP. (2003) Biochemical effect of intravenous arginine butyrate in X-linked adrenoleukodystrophy. J Pediatr 142: 709–713.

McGuckin CP, Forraz N, Allouard Q, Pettengell R. (2004) Umbilical cord blood stem cells can expand hematopoietic and neuroglial progenitors in vitro. Exp Cell Res 295: 350–359.

McPhee SW, Janson CG, Li C, et al. (2006) Immune responses to AAV in a phase I study for Canavan disease. J Gene Med 8: 577–588.

Mimura Y, Kuriyama M, Tokimura Y, et al. (1993) Treatment of cerebrotendinous xanthomatosis with low-density lipoprotein (LDL)-apheresis. J Neurol Sci 114: 227–230.

Moffett JR, Ross B, Arun P, Madhavarao CN, Namboodiri AM. (2007) N-Acetylaspartate in the CNS: from neurodiagnostics to neurobiology. Prog Neurobiol 81: 89–131.

Moser H, Dubey P, Fatemi A. (2004) Progress in X-linked adrenoleukodystrophy. Curr Opin Neurol 17: 263–269.

Moser HW. (1999) Treatment of X-linked adrenoleukodystrophy with Lorenzo's oil. J Neurol Neurosurg Psychiatry 67: 279–280.

Moser HW, Moser AB, Hollandsworth K, Brereton NH, Raymond GV. (2007) "Lorenzo's oil" therapy for X-linked adrenoleukodystrophy: rationale and current assessment of efficacy. J Mol Neurosci 33: 105–113.

Moser HW, Raymond GV, Lu SE, et al. (2005) Follow-up of 89 asymptomatic patients with adrenoleukodystrophy treated with Lorenzo's oil. Arch Neurol 62: 1073–1080.

Nikolic WV, Hou H, Town T, et al. (2008) Peripherally administered human umbilical cord blood cells reduce parenchymal and vascular beta-amyloid deposits in Alzheimer mice. Stem Cells Dev 17: 423–439.

Pai GS, Khan M, Barbosa E, et al. (2000) Lovastatin therapy for X-linked adrenoleukodystrophy: clinical and biochemical observations on 12 patients. Mol Genet Metab 69: 312–322.

Peters C, Charnas LR, Tan Y, et al. (2004) Cerebral X-linked adrenoleukodystrophy: the international hematopoietic cell transplantation experience from 1982 to 1999. Blood 104: 881–888.

Peters C, Steward CG. (2003) Hematopoietic cell transplantation for inherited metabolic diseases: an overview of outcomes and practice guidelines. Bone Marrow Transplant 31: 229–239.

Pierson TM, Bonnemann CG, Finkel RS, Bunin N, Tennekoon GI. (2008) Umbilical cord blood transplantation for juvenile metachromatic leukodystrophy. Ann Neurol 64: 583–587.

Pluchino S, Martino G. (2008) Neural stem cell-mediated immunomodulation: repairing the haemorrhagic brain. Brain 131: 604–605.

Pluchino S, Quattrini A, Brambilla E, et al. (2003) Injection of adult neurospheres induces recovery in a chronic model of multiple sclerosis. Nature 422: 688–694.

Pluchino S, Zanotti L, Brambilla E, et al. (2009) Immune regulatory neural stem/precursor cells protect from central nervous system autoimmunity by restraining dendritic cell function. PLoS One 4: e5959.

Pluchino S, Zanotti L, Rossi B, et al. (2005) Neurosphere-derived multipotent precursors promote neuroprotection by an immunomodulatory mechanism. Nature 436: 266–271.

Priller J, Flugel A, Wehner T, et al. (2001) Targeting gene-modified hematopoietic cells to the central nervous system: use of green fluorescent protein uncovers microglial engraftment. Nat Med 7: 1356–1361.

Sands MS, Haskins ME. (2008) CNS-directed gene therapy for lysosomal storage diseases. Acta Paediatr Suppl 97: 22–27.

Schonberger S, Roerig P, Schneider DT, Reifenberger G, Gobel U, Gartner J. (2007) Genotype and protein expression after bone marrow transplantation for adrenoleukodystrophy. Arch Neurol 64: 651–657.

Shapiro E, Krivit W, Lockman L, et al. (2000) Long-term effect of bone-marrow transplantation for childhood-onset cerebral X-linked adrenoleukodystrophy. Lancet 356: 713–718.

Siebzehnrubl FA, Jeske I, Muller D, et al. (2009). Spontaneous in vitro transformation of adult neural precursors into stem-like cancer cells. Brain Pathol 19: 399–408.

Sundaram KS, Fan JH, Engelke JA, Foley AL, Suttie JW, Lev M. (1996) Vitamin K status influences brain sulfatide metabolism in young mice and rats. J Nutr 126: 2746–2751.

Sundaram KS, Lev M. (1988) Warfarin administration reduces synthesis of sulfatides and other sphingolipids in mouse brain. J Lipid Res 29: 1475–1479.

Surendran S, Michals-Matalon K, Quast MJ, et al. (2003) Canavan disease: a monogenic trait with complex genomic interaction. Mol Genet Metab 80: 74–80.

Taylor RM, Lee JP, Palacino JJ, et al. (2006) Intrinsic resistance of neural stem cells to toxic metabolites may make them well suited for cell non-autonomous disorders: evidence from a mouse model of Krabbe leukodystrophy. J Neurochem 97: 1585–1599.

Taymans JM, Vandenberghe LH, Haute CV, et al. (2007) Comparative analysis of adeno-associated viral vector serotypes 1, 2, 5, 7, and 8 in mouse brain. Hum Gene Ther 18: 195–206.

Tolar J, Orchard PJ, Bjoraker KJ, Ziegler RS, Shapiro EG, Charnas L. (2007) N-acetyl-L-cysteine improves outcome of advanced cerebral adrenoleukodystrophy. Bone Marrow Transplant 39: 211–215.

Uckan D, Cetin M, Yigitkanli I, et al. (2005) Life-threatening neurological complications after bone marrow transplantation in children. Bone Marrow Transplant 35: 71–76.

Valori CF, Ning K, Wyles M, Azzouz M. (2008) Development and applications of non-HIV-based lentiviral vectors in neurological disorders. Curr Gene Ther 8: 406–418.

Van Bekkum DW. (2004) Stem cell transplantation for autoimmune disorders. Preclinical experiments. Best Pract Res Clin Haematol 17: 201–222.

Van Heijst AF, Verrips A, Wevers RA, Cruysberg JR, Renier WO, Tolboom JJ. (1998) Treatment and follow-up of children with cerebrotendinous xanthomatosis. Eur J Pediatr 157: 313–316.

Vendrame, M., Gemma, C., De Mesquita, D., et al. (2005) Anti-inflammatory effects of human cord blood cells in a rat model of stroke. Stem Cells Dev 14: 595–604.

Walczak P, Chen N, Hudson JE, et al. (2004) Do hematopoietic cells exposed to a neurogenic environment mimic properties of endogenous neural precursors? J Neurosci Res 76: 244-254.

Weinberg KI. (2005) Early use of drastic therapy. N Engl J Med 352: 2124-2126.

Weinhofer I, Forss-petter S, Zigman M, Berger J. (2003) Cholesterol regulates ABCD2 gene expression: implications for X-linked adrenoleukodstrophy. Adv Exp Med Biol 544: 331–332.

Wenger DA, Sattler M, Hiatt W. (1974) Globoid cell leukodystrophy: deficiency of lactosyl ceramide beta-galactosidase. Proc Natl Acad Sci USA, 71: 854–857.

Windrem MS, Schanz, SJ, Guo, M, et al. (2008) Neonatal chimerization with human glial progenitor cells can both remyelinate and rescue the otherwise lethally hypomyelinated shiverer mouse. Cell Stem Cell 2: 553-565.

Yamanaka S. (2008) Induction of pluripotent stem cells from mouse fibroblasts by four transcription factors. Cell Prolif 41(Suppl 1): 51–56.

Young PP, Fantz CR, Sands MS. (2004) VEGF disrupts the neonatal blood–brain barrier and increases life span after non-ablative BMT in a murine model of congenital neurodegeneration caused by a lysosomal enzyme deficiency. Exp Neurol 188: 104–114.

Zigova T, Song S, Willing AE, et al. (2002) Human umbilical cord blood cells express neural antigens after transplantation into the developing rat brain. Cell Transplant 11: 265–274.

12
CLINICAL APPROACH TO IDENTIFICATION OF LEUKOENCEPHALOPATHIES

Sakkubai Naidu, Genila Bibat and Doris Lin

Introduction

Abnormalities of brain white matter are among the most prevalent neurological disorders of the brain in childhood, with many still remaining as unclassified leukoencephalopathies. Clinical judgment has been revolutionized by magnetic resonance imaging (MRI), which allows early detection of disorders associated with white matter abnormalities. Combined clinical, neuroimaging, biochemical, and neuropathological evaluations have led to the discovery of novel infantile, childhood, and adult-onset forms of leukoencephalopathy with specific genetic and biochemical defects. Precise phenotypic and molecular definition should permit understanding of biological mechanisms, aid development of therapies, and provide diagnostic and prenatal testing. However, one cannot always note classic features of a known disease as there may be inconsistencies in the disease progression even within the same family, leading to phenotype–genotype variations. The importance of recognizing these disorders cannot be overemphasized as some familial conditions, although not treatable at present, may have or soon include gene defects with which to provide prenatal testing. The prevalence of leukoencephalopathies in pediatric neurology is unknown, but they most commonly present in the first few years of life as shown in our series of patients (Fig. 12.1). This chapter proposes to present general guidelines, without being exhaustive, for approaching childhood onset leukoencephalopathies and to provide an algorithm for diagnostic work-up. Recent lists of leukoencephalopathies (Costello et al. 2009, Kohlschutter et al. 2010) would help to expand the inventory of disorders.

In considering MRI changes in the white matter, one should first be cognizant of age-associated alterations in normal myelination, especially in those under 5 years of age (van der Knaap and Valk 2005). MRI abnormalities in white matter can manifest not only in disorders of myelin affected by diseased oligodendroglia, such as Krabbe disease, but also by astrocytes as in Alexander disease and axons as in Canavan disease. Therefore, MRI changes may reflect involvement of any of these glial or neuronal cells. MRI changes in white matter may be minimal or static (arrested myelination, gliosis), may show progressive improvement (delayed myelination), worsening (degeneration), or may have specific anatomical localization in certain disease entities (e.g., mitochondrial disorders). The abnormalities on MRI are generally diffuse and symmetric in metabolic/genetic conditions, or asymmetric as observed more often in acquired diseases. Such anatomic localizations

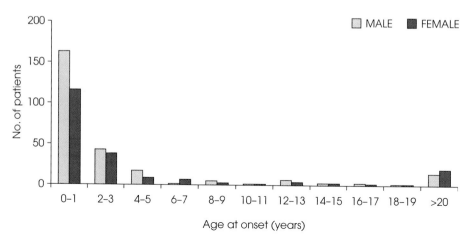

Fig. 12.1. Age at onset and sex differences for leukoencephalopathies.

despite their frequency, however, are not specific to a disease since many conditions may have overlapping MRI features as shown in Figure 12.2A–C. The clinical signs and symptoms are crucial in differentiating the disorders and will guide appropriate diagnostic investigations.

A systematic approach is essential to eliminate known causes of white matter abnormalities. The examination should include both clinical and biochemical assessments which, when combined with MRI evaluations, provide valuable diagnostic clues.

1. Detailed developmental history should be obtained to define acquisition or loss of skills, age and pattern of onset; namely, acute, insidious, or episodic progression of symptoms, which identifies similarities to known disorders, and determines whether the condition is static or progressive.
2. Dysmorphic features of the face, fingers, toes, extremities, spine, or internal organs are a useful guide to prenatal onset, which may be seen in metabolic disorders such as peroxisome biogenesis defects and possible association with known gene defects or cytogenetic abnormalities as in occulo-dento-digital dysplasia due to *GJA1* defect (Paznekas et al. 2003) or 18q- defects, respectively (Angelicheva et al. 1999).
3. Measurement of head circumference and velocity of head growth, especially in the first 2 years of life when there is a rapid increase in head circumference, to identify megalencephaly or microcephaly, is an essential part of the neurological examination, and a vital diagnostic clue to contributing factors.
4. Neurological examination for focal deficits, hypotonia or increased tone, long tract signs, or cerebellar involvement helps identify anatomical regions that are maximally affected.
5. Fundoscopy for retinal changes recognizes causes such as intrauterine infections, or conditions associated with retinitis (e.g., mitochondrial dysfunction, peroxisomal disorders, neuronal ceroid lipofuscinosis), cherry red spots (ganglioside storage), or

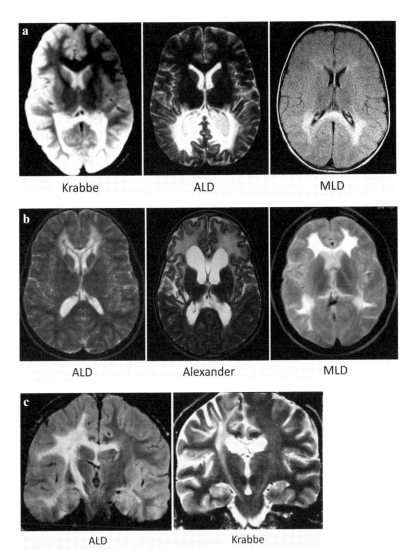

Krabbe   ALD   MLD

ALD   Alexander   MLD

ALD   Krabbe

Fig. 12.2. A: Similar pattern of white matter signal abnormality predominantly involving the parietal–occipital regions and splenium of corpus callosum in three different leukodystrophies: Krabbe disease (axial T2WI), cerebral adrenoleukodystrophy (ALD) (axial T2WI), and late-infantile metachromatic leukodystrophy (MLD) (axial FLAIR). All three conditions have normocephaly and show posterior preponderance, but ALD also has contrast enhancement at the edge of the lesion and skin hyperpigmentation from adrenal insufficiency. **B:** Similar pattern of white matter signal abnormality predominantly involving the frontal regions and sometimes genu of corpus callosum in three different leukodystrophies: ALD (axial T2WI), Alexander disease (axial T2WI), and MLD (axial PD). The anterior preponderance seen in approximately 17% of ALD patients is indistinguishable by MRI from a patient with juvenile MLD. The juvenile MLD patient, however, does not demonstrate signs of adrenal insufficiency. Alexander disease is usually marked by macrocephaly. **C:** Similar pattern of hyperintense signal abnormality involving the right corticospinal tract and parietal white matter in two different leukodystrophies: ALD (coronal PD) and Krabbe disease (axial T2WI).

211

optic pallor (metachromatic leukodystrophy – MLD). Electroretinogram helps to identify retinal degeneration (NCL, mitochondrial disorders).

6. Cutaneous pigmentary or vascular nevi are important in identifying congenital developmental anomalies such as neurofibromatosis or hypomelanosis of Ito.

7. Organomegaly warrants consideration of storage disorders in the absence of infections or hematological conditions.

8. Many white matter abnormalities are associated with peripheral nerve involvement, for which neurophysiological examinations or nerve biopsies provide valuable leads.

9. Biochemical assessments often cover a broad exploration of thyroid function, plasma amino acids, urine organic acids, and lactate to identify mitochondrial dysfunction. Further investigations are guided by the clinical picture and MRI lesions.

10. The endemic nature of certain disorders should be taken into consideration, for example: Salla disease due to increased free N-acetyl neuraminic acid, commonly seen in patients of Scandinavian descent (Erikson et al. 2002); Nasu Hakola disease (polycystic lipomembranous osteodysplasia with sclerosing leukoencephalopathies – PLOSL), which presents with loss of myelin, basal ganglia calcification, and bone cysts, resulting from mutations in two genes *TREM2* and *DAP12* (Klunemann et al. 2005) and is seen in those from Japan and Scandinavian countries; Tay–Sachs disease even in the non-Jewish populations (Park et al. 2010); and megalencephalic leukoencephalopathy with cysts (MLC1) in the Agarwal community from India (Gorospe et al. 2004).

In our review of 460 patients with leukoencephalopathies we noted a striking relationship of leukoencephalopathies to age at onset and sex (see Fig. 12.1). Interestingly, in the majority of children symptoms arise before 5 years of age, when myelination is active, and males were more commonly affected.

Clinical features
Compared with neuronal diseases, cognitive decline or seizures as initial symptoms are less prominent in leukoencephalopathies, although they may certainly follow. Acute onset of disease is often due to infectious causes as with viral infections caused by human T-cell leukemia virus infection (Pandit 2009) or cytomegalovirus (CMV), post-infectious as in acute disseminated encephalomyelitis (ADEM, Fig. 12.3A) (Menge et al. 2005), or immune-mediated etiology as in multiple sclerosis (Banwell et al. 2007). On the other hand, some inherited disorders could be precipitated by infection or other illness, for example, vanishing white matter (VWM) disease, an autosomal recessive disorder (Labauge et al. 2007), matrilineally inherited mitochondrial disorders (Leverve 2007), or hemophagocytic lympho-histiocytosis, which may be inherited or triggered by infections (Janka 2007, Ohno et al. 2009). A more recently recognized autosomal dominant condition called acute necrotizing encephalomyelitis is precipitated by infections, resembles encephalitis except for being recurrent, and is associated with a defect in the Ran-binding protein gene, *RANBP2* (Fig. 12.3B) (Neilson et al. 2009). Progression of the illness causing white matter changes may be slow, as in Krabbe disease or MLD (see Chapters 6 and 8), or intermittent, as in progres-

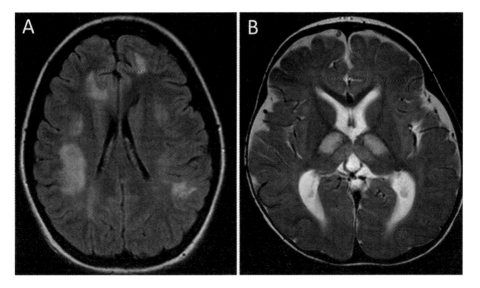

Fig. 12.3. A: Acute disseminated encephalomyelitis (ADEM) in a previously healthy 16-year-old woman who presented acutely with fever, hypotension, and disorientation. Axial FLAIR image shows multifocal hyperintensity in the cerebral white matter bilaterally. She had complete recovery from the acute illness after 8 weeks without any neurological sequelae. **B:** Autosomal dominant acute necrotizing encephalomyelitis in a 2-year-old boy who presented with encephalopathy. His brother had a similar clinical history. Axial T2WI shows bilateral symmetric hyperintense signal abnormality in the thalami. The changes are typically localized to the thalamus and brainstem, but are also common in external capsule, claustrum, temporal lobes, and limbic structures. The child's clinical and MRI presentation, in addition to the family history, resembles those with a defect in the RANBP2 gene. (Image courtesy of Dr Maya Thomas, Vellore, India.)

sive cavitating leukoencephalopathy (Naidu et al. 2005), VWM disease (Pronk et al. 2006), and mitochondrial disorders (Haas et al. 2007).

DYSMORPHIC CONDITIONS

Clinicians become aware upon entering the examination room if there is overt dysmorphism in the patient. Recognition of metabolic disorders with dysmorphism is important as therapeutic approaches are becoming available in some, such as enzyme replacement therapy in mucopolysaccharidosis II (Martin et al. 2008). Other conditions associated with noticeable dysmorphic features include congenital defects of glycosylation, or peroxisome biogenesis defects, but the degree of dysmorphism may vary. Dysmorphism and white matter abnormalities are also seen in chromosomal abnormalities as in 18q- defects (Angelicheva et al.1999). Molecular defects have been detected in leukoencephalopathies with dysmorphism, such as oculodentodigital dysplasia due to mutations in the connexin 43 (*GJA1*) gene (Paznekas et al. 2003) and Sotos disease with *NSD1* gene defects (Kurotaki et al. 2002). Dysmorphism with early onset seizures and cystic changes on MRI are seen in molybdenum cofactor deficiency. Macrocrania with leukoencephalopathies is common in Canavan disease, MLC1, Alexander disease, and Soto disease.

213

SPASTICITY

Spasticity in the lower extremities more than in the upper extremities is a common feature in most white matter diseases. Many present with associated dystonic posturing and rigidity, as seen in Krabbe disease or MLD. Of the disorders presenting with leukoencephalopathy and spastic paraparesis, adrenolekodystrophy, spastic paraplegia 11 (Stevanin et al. 2007) and adult-onset autosomal-dominant leukodystrophy linked to 5q23.2-q23.3 are prominent (Meijer et al. 2008).

EYE ABNORMALITIES

The eye is considered to be a window to the brain (Poll-The et al. 2003) making fundoscopic examination an integral part of the neurological evaluation. White matter abnormalities with retinal pigmentary defects are seen in peroxisome biogenesis disorders (Folz and Trobe 1991), mitochondrial disorders (Crimi et al. 2003), and neuronal ceroid lipofuscinosis (NCL) (Weleber et al. 2004). Retinal degenerative changes are also seen in conditions associated with intrauterine infections such as toxoplasmosis, rubella, and CMV. Cherry-red spots noted in lysosomal disorders (Biswas et al. 2008) may or not be associated with leukoencephalopathy as in Tay–Sachs disease, but is reported as an unusual finding in a patient with Krabbe disease (Naidu et al. 1988). Cherry-red spots and leukoencephalopathy occur with corneal clouding in GMI gangliosidosis, and Niemann–Pick type 1 disease (Di et al. 2005). Hypomyelination with cataracts is associated with hyccin gene defect (gene is also referred to as FAM126A) (Zara et al. 2006), mucolipidosis IV (Smith et al. 2002), and Wilson disease in which Kaiser–Fleisher rings are present (Taly et al. 2009).

CUTANEOUS NEVI

Pallister Killian, caused by mosaic tetrasomy of chromosome 12p with intellectual disabilities, dysmorphism, epilepsy, and cutaneous stripes from the mosaicism, has periventricular white matter abnormalities (Saito et al. 2006). Neurofibromatosis type 1 is known to have patchy white matter changes that improve over time (Lopes Ferraz Filho et al. 2008).

ORGANOMEGALY

Hepatosplenomegaly is common in storage disorders that are associated with white matter abnormalities. Common lysosomal storage diseases, or peroxisome biogenesis disorders, which tend to manifest organomegaly are described below under metabolic conditions. These conditions are distinguished from infectious processes by the acute onset of illness and the hematological responses to infection.

PERIPHERAL NERVE INVOLVEMENT

Neuropathy may be obvious in the form of pes cavus, or may be more subtle and recognizable only by electrophysiological studies or nerve biopsy. Common conditions associated with leukoencephalopathy and neuropathy include Krabbe disease (Siddiqi et al. 2006), MLD (Ramakrishnan et al. 2007), neuroaxonal dystrophy (Goebel 1999), and hyccin deficiency (Zara et al. 2006). Pelizaeus–Merzbacher disease (PMD) (Shy et al. 2003) and PMD-like disease caused by mutations in gap junction protein alpha-12 gene or connexin

46.6 (*GJC2* gene) are seen with prominent hypomyelination and neuropathy (Uhlenberg et al. 2004). The mitochondrial disorders, in particular the neurogastrointestinal encephalomy-opathy, present with leukoencephalopathy and neuropathy (Marti et al. 2002).

CEREBROSPINAL FLUID ANALYSIS

Specific CSF biomarkers can identify degenerative processes, mitochondrial dysfunction, infectious etiologies, or altered immune response. Elevated levels of protein and patho-logically abnormal protein are features in lysosomal storage disorders such as MLD and Krabbe disease, and GM1 gangliosidosis (Satoh et al. 2007, Broekman et al. 2009). Despite the progressive nature of the white matter lesions in adrenoleukodystrophy (ALD), it is uncommon to find elevated CSF protein. Increased lactate may be seen in mitochondrial defects, although not essential for the diagnosis of mitochondrial dysfunction. Lactate has also been found to be more elevated in bacterial than in viral infections and test results should be interpreted cautiously when associated with acute onset of illness that may have associated white matter changes (de Almeida et al. 2009). Increased levels of CSF α-interferon or pterin levels were used to confirm the diagnosis of Aicardi–Goutieres syndrome (AGS) until the recent discovery of multiple gene defects causing the disease (Crow et al. 2006a, b). Immunological changes in CSF are useful in differentiating multiple sclerosis or subacute sclerosing panencephalitis from inherited forms of leukoencephalopathy. Recently, Mochel et al. (2009a) reported patients with ataxia and hypomyelination with elevated CSF sialic acid, shown by high-resolution proton nuclear magnetic resonance spectroscopy (MRS), in the absence of elevations in urine and cultured skin fibroblasts. In a separate study, Mochel and colleagues showed two siblings with mild hypomyelination and mental retardation in whom free sialic acid in the CSF was increased without increased urinary excretion. They had a mutation in *SLC17A5*, a gene that encodes sialin, a lysosomal membrane protein that transports sialic acid out of lysosomes. Mutations in *SLC17A5* are responsible for free sialic acid storage disease (Salla disease) (Mochel et al. 2009b). Such observations demonstrate marked clinical variability within known diseases.

SEIZURES

Although leukoencephalopathies are not expected to cause seizures they may be a con-comitant in conditions such as MLD, Krabbe disease, Alexander disease, X-linked ALD, peroxisomal disorders, and MLC1.

Metabolic changes

LYSOSOMAL DISORDERS

Many lysosomal disorders present with abnormal white matter, some of which are demyelinating while others are secondary to hypomyelination. The most common of the demyelinating conditions are MLD, Krabbe disease, and GM1 gangliodidosis. On the other hand, hypomyelination occurs in conditions such as fucosidosis and Salla disease, both of which present with slowly progressive dysmorphic changes and dementia. Fucosidosis, a recessive disorder associated with severe-to-patchy hypomyelination (Prietsch et al. 2008),

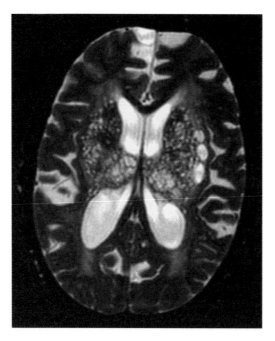

Fig. 12.4. Enlarged perivascular spaces in mucopolysaccharidosis type II (Hunter syndrome). Axial T2WI shows innumerable dilated cystic spaces in the basal ganglia and thalami. There is also diffuse volume loss with enlargement of the ventricular system and cortical sulci. Patchy T2 hyperintense signal abnormality is present in the periventricular white matter.

results from α-L-fucosidase enzyme deficiency causing storage of fucose-containing glycolipids, glycoproteins, and oligosaccharides, and their increased excretion. Fucosidosis is diagnosed by reduced enzyme levels in white cells due to mutations in the *FUCA1* gene (Fukushima et al. 1985). Mucopolysaccharidosis is associated with dysmorphism, dementia, and organomegaly, which result from storage of products that are not subject to cleavage owing to the enzyme defects that cause various types of the disease (Seto et al. 2001, Zafeiriou et al. 2001, Matheus et al. 2004). The MRI shows prolonged T2 relaxation time in white matter and enlarged perivascular (or Virchow–Robin) spaces (Fig. 12.4). The enlarged perivascular spaces results in a peculiar lattice-like or "cribiriform" appearance in the white matter and subcortical regions. These enlarged spaces are presumed to result from an inability to resorb CSF and a form of communicating hydrocephalus rather than storage within the cells (Kara et al. 2008).

PEROXISOMAL DISORDERS

Adrenoleukodystrophy (ALD) is identified by elevations in very long chain fatty acids (VLCFAs) and primary adrenal insufficiency with pigmentation of skin, gums, and nipples, as well as the "bathing-suit" area. In those with cerebral involvement, the MRI can be easily distinguished by the occipital lesions seen in the majority of patients (see Fig. 12.2A), and altered blood–brain barrier noted at the periphery of the white matter lesions in contrast studies. However, in some patients, the lesions may be seen initially in the frontal regions (see Fig. 12.2B), only in the internal capsule, or following tracts as in patients with adult-onset Krabbe disease (see Fig. 12.2C). Younger patients presenting with peroxisome biogenesis defects and MRI changes form a heterogenous group of patients with elevated VLCFAs, varying clinical course, and varying severity (Steinberg et al. 2006).

Mitochondrial diseases are a heterogeneous group of disorders with impaired energy production due to a genetically based abnormality in oxidative phosphorylation. Disorders of mitochondrial metabolism are a common cause of neurological disease with a prevalence of 1 in 5000 (Haas et al. 2007). Depending on the subtype of mitochondrial involvement, the clinical manifestations and regions of white matter involved may vary (Lerman-Sagie et al. 2005). The variable presentation of mitochondrial disorders due to heteroplasmy and nonspecific biomarkers pose diagnostic problems, as noted in leukoencephalopathy with brainstem and spinal cord involvement and lactic acidosis. In this disorder, despite involvement of the nuclear-encoded mitochondrial aspartyl-tRNA synthetase deficiency (Scheper et al. 2007) and MRS evidence for lactic acidosis, there are no changes in blood or fibroblast respiratory enzyme function. This recessive disorder manifests progressive ataxia, spasticity, posterior column dysfunction, milder cognitive deficits, and MRIs showing leukoencephalopathies with involvement of brainstem and spinal tracts. Very often, mitochondrial disorders with childhood onset may present with acute clinical manifestations when associated with infection, which results in increased energy demand.

Magnetic resonance imaging

The presence of increased signal intensity in T2-weighted images and abnormal fluid-attenuated inversion recovery (FLAIR) does not invariably implicate primary myelin-producing oligodendroglial involvement. MRI abnormalities reflect changes in multiple cell types such as myelin in MLD or Krabbe disease, astrocytes in Alexander disease, and neuronal or axonal disease in NCL and Canavan disease, where they cause secondary changes in myelination due to poor neuronal/axonal interaction with myelin (Colello and Pott 1997, Nave 2010)

Demyelination involves destruction or damage of myelin, which can be acquired (e.g., infectious, immune-mediated, toxic) or hereditary (metabolic), while **dysmyelination** is a term used to denote abnormal synthesis or degradation of myelin, most often involving a defect in the myelin biochemical pathway. However, both demyelination and dysmyelination can occur concurrently, and are more clearly defined pathologically, for example, in ALD and Krabbe disease. On MRI, demyelination is identified by increased intensity on FLAIR, sometimes accompanied by contrast enhancement or restricted diffusion.

Hypomyelination may be seen in dysmyelinating conditions and is heterogenous in etiology. Establishment of hypomyelination versus delayed myelination requires serial MRI evaluations, where delayed myelination shows some improvement in myelination, even though it may not reach age-appropriate levels. On MRI, hypomyelination is not conspicuous on FLAIR but demonstrates signal intensity of immature white matter (i.e., T1 isointensity to gray matter and T2 hyperintensity). Hypomyelination encompasses a wide variety of white matter distribution and associated clinical features such as nystagmus in PMD (Fig. 12.5A). In a certain condition termed hypomyelination with atrophy of the basal

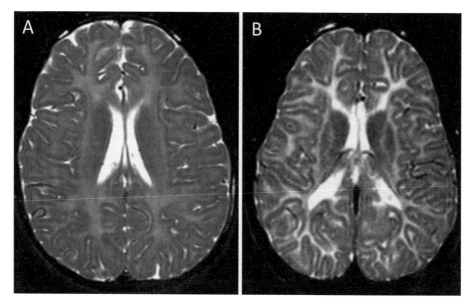

Fig. 12.5. Hypomyelination can be seen in a variety of conditions. **A:** A 6-year-old boy with Pelizaeus–Merzbacher disease, which is caused by a defective gene on the X-chromosome encoding proteolipid protein 1 (PLP1), a constituent of myelin. Axial T2WI shows mild hyperintense signal in the white matter due to diffuse hypomyelination. **B:** A 6-year-old girl with conventional type of Salla disease. Axial T2WI shows homogeneous hyperintensity in the cerebral white matter, including the internal capsules. (Reproduced with permission from AJNR Am J Neuroradiol 1999; 20: 433–443).

ganglia and cerebellum (van der Knaap et al. 2002), there is dementia and progressive rigidity. Reduced cerebral folate levels and 5-methyltetrahydrofolate have been reported in this condition that responded to folinic acid treatment (Mercimek-Mahmutoglu and Stockler-Ipsiroglu 2007). Hypomyelination with cataracts can be seen in hyccin deficiency due to mutations in the FAM126A (DRCTNNB1A) gene (Zara et al. 2006) or mucolipidosis IV identified by gastrin deficiency (Schiffmann et al. 1998). Hypomyelination with abnormal dentition is a well-described condition (Wolf et al. 2005). In Salla disease (Fig. 12.5B), where there is diffuse hypomyelination, the sialuria is due to a transport defect and not secondary to sialidase deficiency. Recently, patients have been described with hypomyelination, cerebellar atrophy, ataxia, peripheral neuropathy, and increased CSF sialic acid, without mutations in the candidate genes in the free sialic acid biosynthesis pathways (Mochel et al. 2009a). Hypomyelination is also seen in association with gene defects such as RRM2B causing a mitochondrial DNA depletion syndrome (Acham-Roschitz et al. 2009) and MCT8, which encodes an integral membrane protein transporter of thyroid hormone (Vaurs-Barriere et al. 2009).

Calcifications
Neovascular responses due to infectious (Fig. 12.6A) or immune disorders result in calcification. Aicardi–Goutieres syndrome (AGS) is a recessive disorder in which multiple gene

defects have been identified to present with similar clinical features of repeated encephalitis-like disease, intracranial calcifications (Fig. 12.6B), and temporal lobe cysts (Fig. 12.7A) (Crow et al. 2006a, b, Rice et al. 2007). AGS and pseudo-TORCH syndrome are the same disorder. Patients may manifest disease early in infancy reminiscent of congenital infection when the defective gene encodes the 3′→5′ exonuclease TREX1. Mutations also occur in three subunits of RNASEH2 including RNASEH2 A, B, and C, where the patients have later onset and occasionally intact neurological function, particularly with RNASEH2B mutations.

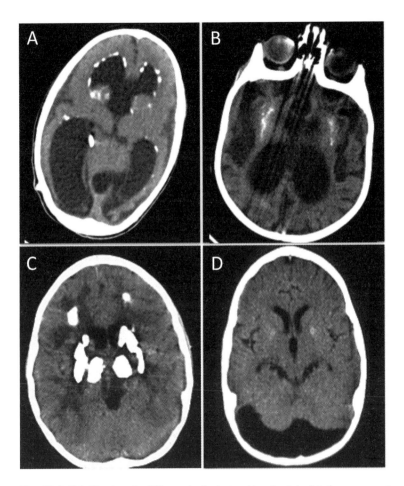

Fig. 12.6. Calcifications in different leukodystrophies, best depicted on non-contrast head CT. **A:** Congenital CMV infection. Multiple calcifications are identified in the periventricular regions and right caudate head. There is also lissencephaly. **B:** Aicardi–Goutieres syndrome in a 1-year-old child. Global volume loss with enlargement of the ventricles and sulci. Dystrophic calcification is identified in the bilateral putamina, which are small. **C:** Labrune disease (LCCC). Coarse calcifications are identified in the bilateral frontal white matter, basal ganglia, and thalami. **D:** Cockayne syndrome. Small areas of calcification are present in the bilateral globus pallidus, and an incidental retrocerebellar arachnoid cyst is seen.

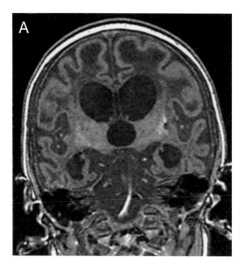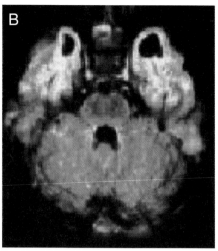

Fig. 12.7. Parenchymal cystic lesions can be seen in Aicardi–Goutieres syndrome (AGS), RNASET2 deficiency, and also in MLC1 (not shown). **A:** Coronal FLAIR shows global atrophy and temporal lobe cysts in a patient with AGS. **B:** Axial T1WI shows cysts in the bilateral temporal tips in another patient with RNASET2 deficiency. Patients with AGS are distinguished by the frequent encephalitic events with calcification in the basal ganglia and cerebellar regions (see Fig. 12.6B, CT of the same patient shown in **A**). Frequent encephalitis is not a feature of RNASET2 deficiency but calcifications may be seen.

Cree encephalitis is allelic with AGS (Crow et al. 2003). AGS was previously identified by the presence of increased α-interferon levels in the CSF (Goutieres et al. 1998). Interestingly, AGS shows overlap with systemic lupus erythematosis at both the clinical and pathological levels and patients with AGS present with features of chillblains (Kolivras et al. 2008). It is hypothesized that in AGS, the defective nucleases fail to remove endogenous nucleic acid species produced during normal cellular processing. This failure results in activation of the immune system with elevation in CSF α-interferon levels, similar to that triggered by viruses to explain the similarities to congenital infections and aspects of lupus erythematosis.

Labrune disease (Fig. 12.6C), also referred to as leukoencephalopathy with cerebral calcifications and cysts (LCCC), is a progressive disorder related to cerebral microangiopathy. Patients develop seizures, increased tone, ataxia, and intellectual deterioration, with age-associated clinical deterioration. MRI shows increasing calcifications and cystic changes in brain parenchyma unlike AGS or congenital infections (Labrune et al. 1996, Nagae-Poetscher et al. 2004).

Patients with Cockayne syndrome (Fig. 12.6D) are divided into two groups, A and B, who present with photosensitivity, deep-set eyes, hearing loss, ataxia, peripheral neuropathy, and intracranial calcifications. Cockayne syndrome occurs secondary to mutations in the excision repair cross-complementing 8 (ERCC8) gene for group A (Henning et al. 1995) and ERCC6 for group B (Mallery et al. 1998), with defects in the repair of transcriptionally active genes. Cockayne syndrome does not present with temporal lobe cysts, and differs from AGS in having neuropathy, hearing loss, and photosensitivity.

A recently described condition with parenchymatous calcifications is due to mutations in the RNASET2 gene, located on chromosome 6. The gene defect results in a condition clinically resembling congenital CMV infection (Fig. 12.6A). Head circumference is normal or microcephalic with significant cognitive delays, behavior problems, and MRI showing temporal lobe cysts. There are no reports of overt infections similar to AGS but comparable mechanisms may be at play (Henneke et al. 2009).

Childhood intrauterine infections such as CMV and toxoplasmosis manifest cerebral calcifications (Hedlund and Boyer 1999). Cysticercosis is caused by infection of the brain by encysted larvae of *Taenia solium*, and is a major cause of seizures in endemic areas (Singhi and Singhi 2009) and the edema surrounding the cysts appears as increased T2 signal intensity on MRI. A condition that overlaps with infectious disease but does not manifest calcifications is the autosomal dominant acute necrotizing encephalopathy (ANE) of infancy, which was originally described in Japan but occurs worldwide (Neilson et al. 2009). It is usually a familial, rapidly progressive, recurrent encephalopathy triggered by common viral infections. While most ANE is sporadic and nonrecurrent, this autosomal-dominant disorder with variable penetrance is identified to be associated with mutations in the Ran-Binding Protein 2 (RANBP2). Some patients with classic disease manifestations did not have mutations in the *RANBP2* and so the disorder with mutations in RANBP2 has been named ANE1. The *RANBP2* encodes a nuclear pore protein located on the cytoplasmic surface of the nuclear pore and plays a complex role throughout the cell cycle. It facilitates protein import and export and, in neurons, is associated with microtubules and mitochondria. Interestingly, the lesions occur in sites similar to that in Wernicke encephalopathy and Leigh encephalopathy. Patients with familial occurrence resembled those with isolated ANE in all respects – namely, seizures, coma, and elevated CSF proteins – however, those with isolated ANE had elevated serum transaminases. Although patients with ANE1 commonly become symptomatic during childhood, some manifested illness during adolescence and adulthood. The incomplete penetrance of the gene is unexplained.

Cystic lesions

Enlarged perivascular spaces (see Fig. 12.4) should be differentiated from parenchymal necrotic or degenerative changes. A well-known condition with megalencephaly, leukoencephalopathy, and cystic changes in the temporal lobes (MLC1), is caused by mutations in the *MLC1* gene (van der Knaap et al. 1995). There are patients with classic clinical and MRI features of MLC in whom the *MLC1* gene mutation is absent, suggesting it is a heterogenous disorder. It is multiethnic in origin but also endemic to the Agarwal community in India (Gorospe et al. 2004). The RNASET2 gene defect (Fig. 12.7B) more recently described by Henneke et al. (2009) also presents with bilateral temporal lobe cystic changes, but without megalencephaly, and bilateral temporal lobe cysts are also seen in AGS (Fig. 12.7). Both these disorders present with intracranial calcifications, unlike MLC1. However, in AGS, repeated episodes of encephalitis and elevated α-interferon levels in the CSF occur that are not reported in those with RNASET2 gene defects. Familial autosomal-dominant disposition to porencephalic cysts and leukoencephalopathy is described with mutations in the collagen 4A1. Because of variable penetrance, non-manifesting carriers may not demonstrate abnormalities (Breedveld et al. 2006), while others may present with recurrent strokes or hemorrhages without porencephaly (Vahedi et al. 2007, Shah et al. 2010)

Progressive cystic lesions may be seen in a recessive disorder of childhood onset termed progressive cavitating leukoencephalopathy (PCL) (Naidu et al. 2005), in which new white matter lesions and cystic degeneration progressively increase over time. In PCL cystic lesions in the corpus callosum are very common. Cystic degenerative changes are also seen in terminal cases of Alexander disease over frontal regions (see Chapter 7). Rarely, cystic lesions are documented in Wilson disease (Sankhyan et al. 2008), although the classic MRI manifestation in that disease involves signal abnormality of the putamen and caudate with hypointensity of the globus pallidus on T2-weighted images, as well as the frequently described "faces of the panda" (Sankhyan et al. 2008). The association of corneal and hepatic involvement with low ceruloplasmin levels differentiates Wilson disease from other cystic degenerative disorders (Taly et al. 2009). A progressive cavitating leukoencephalopathy with variable focal enhancement has been described in mitochondrial complex I deficiency (Schuelke et al. 1999, Wolf et al. 2003, Zafeiriou et al. 2008), complex II deficiency (Brockmann et al. 2002), and complex IV deficiency (Topcu et al. 2000). A severe loss of white matter with cystic degeneration is also part of the recessive disorder VWM disease, which results from mutations in the five subunits of the translation initiation factor eIF2B that is required for translation of RNA to protein, particularly under conditions of stress (Pronk et al. 2006). In VWM disease the MRI shows cerebral white matter loss occupied by CSF, which on MRS shows markedly reduced metabolites with the earliest reduction being in the N-acetyl aspartate peak (Pronk et al. 2006, Dreha-Kulaczewski et al. 2008).

Conclusion

We present an approach to the clinical recognition of leukoencephalopathies and their differentiation from conditions that have a similar clinical course or MRI expression. Although MRI is useful in considering diagnosis it could be limiting, as different genetic disorders may share comparable patterns of cerebral involvement as shown in Figures 12.2, 12.3, 12.5, 12.6, and 12.7. In order to simplify the approach to identifying leukoencephalopathies an algorithm is provided (Appendix 1) that utilizes clinical as well as MRI features. Although the algorithm does not include all disorders with white matter abnormalities, it provides general guidelines, which we hope will direct clinicians to request specific tests in an informed manner.

REFERENCES

Acham-Roschitz, B., Plecko, B., Lindbichler, F., et al. (2009) A novel mutation of the RRM2B gene in an infant with early fatal encephalomyopathy, central hypomyelination, and tubulopathy. Mol Genet Metab 98(3): 300–304 available from: PM:19616983.
Angelicheva D, Turnev I, Dye D, et al. (1999) Congenital cataracts facial dysmorphism neuropathy (CCFDN) syndrome: a novel developmental disorder in Gypsies maps to 18qter. Eur J Hum Genet 7(5): 560–566 available from: PM:10439962.
Banwell B, Ghezzi A, Bar-Or A, Mikaeloff Y, Tardieu M. (2007) Multiple sclerosis in children: clinical diagnosis, therapeutic strategies, and future directions. Lancet Neurol 6(10): 887–902 available from: PM:17884679.

Biswas J. Nandi K, Sridharan S, Ranjan P. (2008) Ocular manifestation of storage diseases. Curr Opin Ophthalmol 19(6): 507–511 available from: PM:18854696.

Breedveld G., de Coo IF, Lequin MH, et al. (2006) Novel mutations in three families confirm a major role of COL4A1 in hereditary porencephaly. J Med Genet 43(6): 490–495 available from: PM:16107487.

Brockmann K, Bjornstad A, Dechent P, et al. (2002) Succinate in dystrophic white matter: a proton magnetic resonance spectroscopy finding characteristic for complex II deficiency. Ann Neurol 52(1): 38–46 available from: PM:12112045.

Broekman ML, Tierney LA, Benn C, Chawla P, Cha JH, Sena-Esteves M. (2009) Mechanisms of distribution of mouse beta-galactosidase in the adult GM1-gangliosidosis brain. Gene Ther 16(2): 303–308 available from: PM:18818671.

Colello RJ, Pott U. (1997) Signals that initiate myelination in the developing mammalian nervous system. Mol Neurobiol 15(1): 83–100 available from: PM:9396006.

CostelloDJ, Eichler AF, Eichler FS. (2009) Leukodystrophies: classification, diagnosis, and treatment. Neurologist 15(6): 319–328. Review PMID: 19901710.

Crimi M, Galbiati S, Perini MP, et al. (2003) A mitochondrial tRNA(His) gene mutation causing pigmentary retinopathy and neurosensorial deafness. Neurology 60(7): 1200–1203 available from: PM:12682337.

Crow YJ, Black DN, Ali M, et al. (2003) Cree encephalitis is allelic with Aicardi–Goutieres syndrome: implications for the pathogenesis of disorders of interferon alpha metabolism. J Med Genet 40(3): 183–187 available from: PM:12624136.

Crow YJ, Hayward BE, Parmar R, et al. (2006a) Mutations in the gene encoding the $3'$–$5'$ DNA exonuclease TREX1 cause Aicardi–Goutieres syndrome at the AGS1 locus. Nat Gene 38(8): 917–920 available from: PM:16845398.

CrowYJ, Leitch A, Hayward BE, et al. (2006b) Mutations in genes encoding ribonuclease H2 subunits cause Aicardi–Goutieres syndrome and mimic congenital viral brain infection. Nat Genet 38(8): 910–916 available from: PM:16845400

de Almeida SM, Faria FL. de Goes FK, et al. (2009) Quantitation of cerebrospinal fluid lactic acid in infectious and non-infectious neurological diseases. Clin Chem Lab Med 47(6): 755–761 available from: PM:19527140

Di RM, Rossi A, Parenti G, et al. (2005). Different molecular mechanisms leading to white matter hypomyelination in infantile onset lysosomal disorders. Neuropediatrics 36(4): 265–269 available from: PM:16138252.

Dreha-Kulaczewski SF, Dechent P, Finsterbusch J, et al. (2008) Early reduction of total N-acetyl-aspartate-compounds in patients with classical vanishing white matter disease. A long-term follow-up MRS study. Pediatr Res 63(4): 444–449 available from: PM:18356755.

Erikson A, Aula N, Aula P, Mansson JE. (2002) Free sialic acid storage (Salla) disease in Sweden. Acta Paediatr 91(12): 1324–1327 available from: PM:12578289.

Folz SJ, Trobe JD. (1991) The peroxisome and the eye. Surv Ophthalmol 35(5): 353–368 available from: PM:1710072.

Fukushima H, de Wet JR, O'Brien JS. (1985) Molecular cloning of a cDNA for human alpha-L-fucosidase. Proc Natl Acad Sci USA 82(4): 1262–1265 available from: PM:2983333.

Goebel HH. (1999) Extracerebral biopsies in neurodegenerative diseases of childhood. Brain Dev 21(7): 435–443 available from: PM:10522518.

Gorospe JR, Singhal BS, Kainu T, et al. (2004) Indian Agarwal megalencephalic leukodystrophy with cysts is caused by a common MLC1 mutation. Neurology 62(6): 878–882 available from: PM:15037685.

Goutieres F, Aicardi J, Barth PG, Lebon P. (1998) Aicardi–Goutieres syndrome: an update and results of interferon-alpha studies. Ann Neurol 44(6): 900–907 available from: PM:9851434.

Haas RH, Parikh S, Falk MJ, et al. (2007) Mitochondrial disease: a practical approach for primary care physicians. Pediatrics 120(6): 1326–1333 available from: PM:18055683.

Hedlund GL, Boyer RS. (1999) Neuroimaging of postnatal pediatric central nervous system infections. Semin Pediatr Neurol 6(4): 299–317 available from: PM:10649838.

Henneke M, Diekmann S, Ohlenbusch A, et al. (2009) RNASET2-deficient cystic leukoencephalopathy resembles congenital cytomegalovirus brain infection. Nat Genet 41(7): 773–775 available from: PM:19525954.

Henning KA, Li L, Iyer N, et al. (1995) The Cockayne syndrome group A gene encodes a WD repeat protein that interacts with CSB protein and a subunit of RNA polymerase II TFIIH. Cell 82(4): 555–564 available from: PM:7664335.

223

Janka GE. (2007) Hemophagocytic syndromes. Blood Rev 21(5): 245–253 available from: PM:17590250.

Kara S, Sherr EH, Barkovich AJ. (2008) Dilated perivascular spaces: an informative radiologic finding in Sanfilippo syndrome type A. Pediatr Neurol 38(5): 363–366 available from: PM:18410855.

Klunemann HH, Ridha BH, Magy L, ET AL. (2005) The genetic causes of basal ganglia calcification, dementia, and bone cysts: DAP12 and TREM2. Neurology 64(9): 1502–1507 available from: PM:15883308.

Kohlschütter A, Bley A, Brockmann K, et al. (2010 Leukodystrophies and other genetic metabolic leukoencephalopathies in children and adults. Brain Dev 32(2): 82–89. Review.PMID: 19427149.

Kolivras A, Aeby A, Crow YJ, Rice GI., Sass U, Andre J. (2008) Cutaneous histopathological findings of Aicardi–Goutieres syndrome, overlap with chilblain lupus. J Cutan Pathol 35(8): 774–778 available from: PM:18422690.

Kurotaki N, Imaizumi K, Harada N, et al. (2002) Haploinsufficiency of NSD1 causes Sotos syndrome. Nat Genet 30(4): 365–366 available from: PM:11896389.

Labauge P, Fogli A, Niel F, Rodriguez D, Boespflug-Tanguy O. (2007) [CACH/VWM syndrome and leucodystrophies related to EIF2B mutations]. Rev Neurol (Paris) 163(8–9): 793–799 available from: PM:17878805.

Labrune P, Lacroix C, Goutieres F, de LJ, et al. (1996) Extensive brain calcifications, leukodystrophy, and formation of parenchymal cysts: a new progressive disorder due to diffuse cerebral microangiopathy. Neurology 46(5): 1297–1301 available from: PM:8628470.

Lerman-Sagie T, Leshinsky-Silver E, Watemberg N, Luckman Y, Lev D. (2005) White matter involvement in mitochondrial diseases. Mol Genet Metab 84(2): 127–136 available from: PM:15670718.

Leverve XM. (2007) Mitochondrial function and substrate availability. Crit Care Med 35(9 Suppl): S454–S460 available from: PM:17713393.

Lopes Ferraz Filho JR, Munis MP, Soares SA, et al. (2008) Unidentified bright objects on brain MRI in children as a diagnostic criterion for neurofibromatosis type 1. Pediat Radiol 38(3): 305–310 available from: PM:18231788.

Mallery DL, Tanganelli B, Colella S, et al. (1998) Molecular analysis of mutations in the CSB (ERCC6) gene in patients with Cockayne syndrome. Am J Hum Genet 62(1): 77–85 available from: PM:9443879.

Marti R, Spinazzola A, Nishino I, et al. (2002) Mitochondrial neurogastrointestinal encephalomyopathy and thymidine metabolism: results and hypotheses. Mitochondrion 2(1–2): 143–147 available from: PM:16120316.

Martin R, Beck M, Eng C, et al. (2008) Recognition and diagnosis of mucopolysaccharidosis II (Hunter syndrome). Pediatrics 121(2): e377–e386 available from: PM:18245410.

Matheus MG, Castillo M, Smith JK, Armao D, Towle D, Muenzer J. (2004) Brain MRI findings in patients with mucopolysaccharidosis types I and II and mild clinical presentation. Neuroradiology 46(8): 666–672 available from: PM:15205860.

Meijer IA, Simoes-Lopes AA, Laurent S, et al. (2008) A novel duplication confirms the involvement of 5q23.2 in autosomal dominant leukodystrophy. Arch Neurol 65(11): 1496–1501 available from: PM:19001169.

Menge T, Hemmer B, Nessler S, et al. (2005) Acute disseminated encephalomyelitis: an update. Arch Neurol 62(11): 1673–1680 available from: PM:16286539.

Mercimek-Mahmutoglu S, Stockler-Ipsiroglu S. (2007) Cerebral folate deficiency and folinic acid treatment in hypomyelination with atrophy of the basal ganglia and cerebellum (H-ABC) syndrome. Tohoku J Exp Med 211(1): 95–96 available from: PM:17202777.

Mochel F, Sedel F, Vanderver A, et al. (2009a) Cerebellar ataxia with elevated cerebrospinal free sialic acid (CAFSA). Brain 132(Pt 3): 801–809 available from: PM:19153153.

Mochel F, Yang B, Barritault J, et al. (2009b) Free sialic acid storage disease without sialuria. Ann Neurol 65(6): 753–757 available from: PM:19557856.

Nagae-Poetscher LM, Bibat G, Philippart M, et al. (2004) Leukoencephalopathy, cerebral calcifications, and cysts: new observations. Neurology 62(7): 1206–1209 available from: PM:15079028.

Naidu S, Bibat G, Lin D, et al. (2005) Progressive cavitating leukoencephalopathy: a novel childhood disease. Ann Neurol 58(6): 929–938 available from: PM:16315274.

Naidu S, Hofmann KJ, Moser HW, Maumenee IH, Wenger DA. (1988) Galactosylceramide-beta-galactosidase deficiency in association with cherry red spot. Neuropediatrics 19(1): 46–48 available from: PM:3362311.

Nave KA. (2010) Myelination and the trophic support of long axons. Nat Rev Neurosci 11(4): 275–283 available from: PM:20216548.

Neilson DE, Adams MD, Orr CM, et al. (2009) Infection-triggered familial or recurrent cases of acute necrotizing encephalopathy caused by mutations in a component of the nuclear pore, RANBP2. Am J Hum Genet 84(1): 44–51 available from: PM:19118815.

Ohno T, Ueda Y, Kishimoto W, Arimoto-Miyamoto K, Takeoka T, Tsuji M. (2009) Epstein–Barr virus-induced infectious mononucleosis after two separate episodes of virus-associated hemophagocytic syndrome. Intern.Med 48(13): 1169–1173 available from: PM:19571453.

Pandit L. (2009) Differential diagnosis of white matter diseases in the tropics: An overview. Ann.Indian Acad.Neurol., 12, (1) 12–21 available from: PM:20151003.

Park NJ, Morgan C, Sharma R, et al. (2010) Improving accuracy of Tay Sachs carrier screening of the non-Jewish population: analysis of 34 carriers and six late-onset patients with HEXA enzyme and DNA sequence analysis. Pediatr Res 67(2): 217–220 available from: PM:19858779.

Paznekas WA, Boyadjiev SA, Shapiro RE, et al. (2003) Connexin 43 (GJA1) mutations cause the pleiotropic phenotype of oculodentodigital dysplasia. Am J Hum Genet 72(2): 408–418 available from: PM:12457340.

Poll-The BT, Maillette de Buy Wenniger-Prick LJ, Barth PG, Duran M. (2003) The eye as a window to inborn errors of metabolism. J Inherit Metab Dis 26(2-3): 229–244 available from: PM:12889663.

Prietsch V, Arnold S, Kraegeloh-Mann I, Kuehr J, Santer R. (2008) Severe hypomyelination as the leading neuroradiological sign in a patient with fucosidosis. Neuropediatrics 39(1): 51–54 available from: PM:18504684.

Pronk JC, van, KB, Scheper GC, van der Knaap MS. (2006) Vanishing white matter disease: a review with focus on its genetics. Ment Retard Dev Disabil Res Rev 12(2): 123–128 available from: PM:16807905.

Ramakrishnan H, Hedayati KK, Lullmann-Rauch R, et al. (2007) Increasing sulfatide synthesis in myelin-forming cells of arylsulfatase A-deficient mice causes demyelination and neurological symptoms reminiscent of human metachromatic leukodystrophy. J Neurosci 27(35): 9482–9490 available from: PM:17728461.

Rice G, Patrick T, Parmar R, et al. (2007) Clinical and molecular phenotype of Aicardi–Goutieres syndrome. Am J Hum Genet 81(4): 713–725 available from: PM:17846997.

Saito Y, Masuko K, Kaneko K, et al. (2006) Brain MRI findings of older patients with Pallister–Killian syndrome. Brain Dev 28(1): 34–38 available from: PM:15967614.

Sankhyan N, Sharma S, Kalra V, Garg A, Balkrishnan P. (2008) Cystic white-matter changes in childhood Wilson's disease. Pediatr Neurol 39(4): 281–282 available from: PM:18805369.

Satoh H, Yamato O, Asano T, et al. (2007) Cerebrospinal fluid biomarkers showing neurodegeneration in dogs with GM1 gangliosidosis: possible use for assessment of a therapeutic regimen. Brain Res 1133(1): 200–208 available from: PM:17196562.

Scheper GC, van der Klok T, van Andel RJ, et al. (2007) Mitochondrial aspartyl-tRNA synthetase deficiency causes leukoencephalopathy with brain stem and spinal cord involvement and lactate elevation. Nat Genet 39(4): 534–539 available from: PM:17384640.

Schiffmann R, Dwyer NK, Lubensky IA, et al. (1998) Constitutive achlorhydria in mucolipidosis type IV. Proc Natl Acad Sci USA 95(3): 1207–1212 available from: PM:9448310.

Schuelke M, Smeitink J, Mariman E, et al. (1999). Mutant NDUFV1 subunit of mitochondrial complex I causes leukodystrophy and myoclonic epilepsy. Nat Genet 21(3): 260–261 available from: PM:10080174.

Seto T, Kono K, Morimoto K, et al. (2001) Brain magnetic resonance imaging in 23 patients with mucopolysaccharidoses and the effect of bone marrow transplantation. Ann Neurol 50(1): 79–92 available from: PM:11456314.

Shah S, Kumar Y, McLean B, et al. (2010) A dominantly inherited mutation in collagen IV A1 (COL4A1) causing childhood onset stroke without porencephaly. Eur J Paediatr Neurol 14(2): 182–187 available from: PM:19477666.

Shy ME, Hobson G, Jain M, et al. (2003) Schwann cell expression of PLP1 but not DM20 is necessary to prevent neuropathy. Ann Neurol 53(3): 354–365 available from: PM:12601703.

Siddiqi ZA, Sanders DB, Massey JM. (2006) Peripheral neuropathy in Krabbe disease: electrodiagnostic findings. Neurology 67(2): 263–267 available from: PM:16864819.

Singhi P, Singhi S. (2009) Neurocysticercosis in children. Indian J Pediatr 76(5): 537–545 available from: PM:19466387..

Smith JA, Chan CC, Goldin E, Schiffmann R. (2002) Noninvasive diagnosis and ophthalmic features of mucolipidosis type IV. Ophthalmology 109(3) 588–594 available from: PM:11874766.

Steinberg SJ, Dodt G, Raymond GV, Braverman NE, Moser AB, Moser HW. (2006) Peroxisome biogenesis disorders. Biochim Biophys Acta 1763(12): 1733–1748 available from: PM:17055079.

Stevanin G, Santorelli FM, Azzedine H, et al. (2007). Mutations in SPG11, encoding spatacsin, are a major cause of spastic paraplegia with thin corpus callosum. Nat Genet 39(3): 366–372 available from: PM:17322883.

225

Taly AB, Prashanth LK, Sinha S. (2009) Wilson's disease: an Indian perspective. Neurol India 57(5): 528–540 available from: PM:19934550.

Topcu M, Saatci I, Apak RA., Soylemezoglu F, Akcoren Z. (2000) Leigh syndrome in a 3-year-old boy with unusual brain MR imaging and pathologic findings. AJNR Am J Neuroradiol 21(1): 224–227 available from: PM:10669255.

Uhlenberg B, Schuelke M, Ruschendorf F, et al. (2004) Mutations in the gene encoding gap junction protein alpha 12 (connexin 46.6) cause Pelizaeus–Merzbacher-like disease. Am J Hum Genet 75(2): 251–260 available from: PM:15192806.

Vahedi K, Kubis N, Boukobza M, et al. (2007) COL4A1 mutation in a patient with sporadic, recurrent intracerebral hemorrhage. Stroke 38(5): 1461–1464 available from: PM:17379824.

van der Knaap MS, Barth PG, Stroink H, van, NO, Arts, W.F., Hoogenraad F,Valk J. (1995) Leukoencephalopathy with swelling and a discrepantly mild clinical course in eight children. Ann Neurol 37(3): 324–334 available from: PM:7695231.

van der Knaap MS, Naidu S, Pouwels PJ, et al. (2002) New syndrome characterized by hypomyelination with atrophy of the basal ganglia and cerebellum. AJNR Am J Neuroradiol 23(9): 1466–1474 available from: PM:12372733.

van der Knaap MS, Valk J. (2005) Magnetic Resonance of Myelination and Myelin Disorders, 3rd edn. Berlin Heidelberg New York: Springer.

Vaurs-Barriere C, Deville M, Sarret C, et al. (2009) Pelizaeus–Merzbacher-like disease presentation of MCT8 mutated male subjects. Ann Neurol 65(1): 114–118 available from: PM:19194886.

Weleber RG, Gupta N, Trzupek KM, Wepner MS, Kurz DE, Milam AH. (2004) Electroretinographic and clinicopathologic correlations of retinal dysfunction in infantile neuronal ceroid lipofuscinosis (infantile Batten disease). Mol Genet Metab 83(1-2): 128–137 available from: PM:15464427.

Wolf NI, Harting I, Boltshauser E, et al. (2005) Leukoencephalopathy with ataxia, hypodontia, and hypomyelination. Neurology 64(8): 1461–1464 available from: PM:15851747.

Wolf NI, Seitz A, Harting I, et al. (2003) New pattern of brain MRI lesions in isolated complex I deficiency. Neuropediatrics 34(3): 156–159 available from: PM:12910441.

Zafeiriou DI, Rodenburg RJ, Scheffer H, et al. (2008) MR spectroscopy and serial magnetic resonance imaging in a patient with mitochondrial cystic leukoencephalopathy due to complex I deficiency and NDUFV1 mutations and mild clinical course. Neuropediatrics 39(3): 172–175 available from: PM:18991197.

Zafeiriou DI, Savvopoulou-Augoustidou PA, Sewell A, et al. (2001) Serial magnetic resonance imaging findings in mucopolysaccharidosis IIIB (Sanfilippo's syndrome B). Brain Dev 23(6): 385–389 available from: PM:11578848.

Zara F, Biancheri R, Bruno C, Bordo L. (2006) Deficiency of hyccin, a newly identified membrane protein, causes hypomyelination and congenital cataract. Nat Genet 38(10): 1111–1113 available from: PM:16951682.

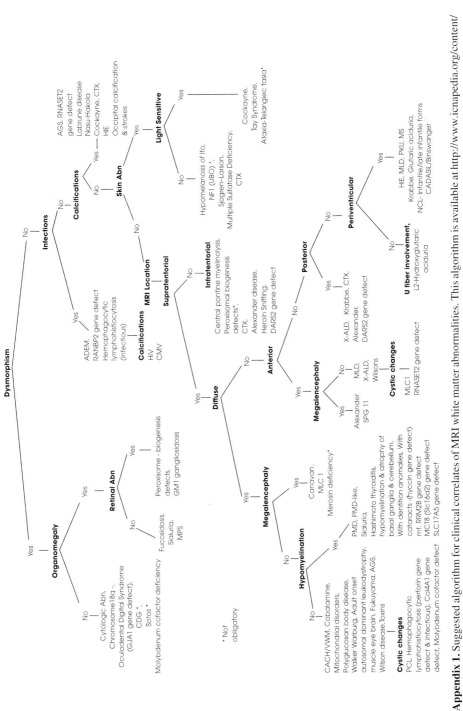

Appendix 1. Suggested algorithm for clinical correlates of MRI white matter abnormalities. This algorithm is available at http://www.ichapedia.org/content/elibrary/978-1-907655-09-8

INDEX

229

230

232

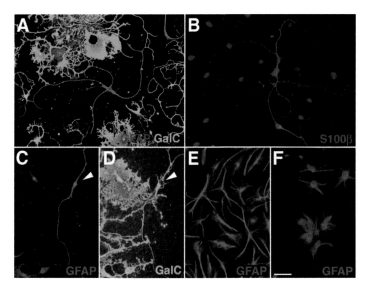

Fig. 3.3. Abnormal astrocytic phenotypes in CACH/VWM disease. Astrocytes derived from a patient with VWM disease show an unusual morphology. Freshly isolated frontal cortex cells have unusually long processes; stained with (**A**) glial fibrillary acidic protein (GFAP) (tetramethylrhodamine isothiocyanate, TRITC), galactosylceramide (GalC) (fluorescein isothiocyanate, FITC), and (**B**) protein S-100b (TRITC). **C**, **D**: Some GFAP+ cells also co-label with GalC, normally a marker for oligodendrocyte lineage cells. **E**: Normal astrocytes derived from BMP-treated human glial precursor cells, GFAP (TRITC). **F**: Primary human post-natal astrocytes derived from temporal lobe of a 17-year-old patient. Scale bars: **A**–**D** 75 μm and **E**, **F** 25 μm. Adopted from Dietrich J. et al. *EIF2B5* mutations compromise GFAP+ astrocyte generation in vanishing white matter leukodystrophy. Nature Medicine 2005; 11(3): 277–283; with permission.

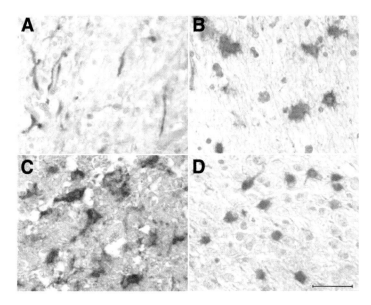

Fig. 3.4. Phenotype of GFAP-positive astrocytes in different neurological conditions. **A**: CACH/VWM disease. **B**: Adrenoleukodystrophy. **C**: Stroke. **D**: Progressive multifocal leukoencephalopathy. Error bar: 50 μm. Adopted from Dietrich J. et al. *EIF2B5* mutations compromise GFAP+ astrocyte generation in vanishing white matter leukodystrophy. Nature Medicine 2005; 11(3): 277–283; with permission.

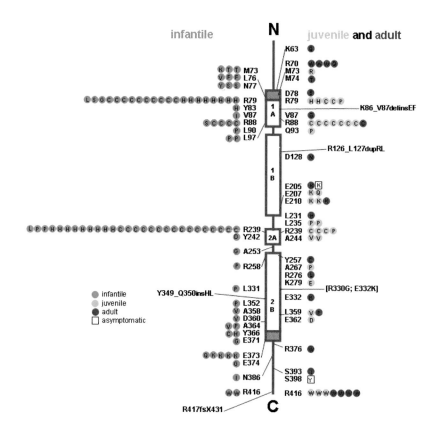

Fig. 7.2. Locations of *GFAP* mutations in Alexander disease in relation to the protein structure. The four open rectangular boxes represent the helical coiled–coil rod domains of GFAP; these structural motifs are highly conserved among most intermediate filament proteins. The solid lines joining these segments are non-helical linker regions, and the solid lines at either end are the non-conserved, random coil, N-terminal and C-terminal regions. The gray box just before segment 1A is a non-conserved prehelical sequence important for initiation of rod formation at the start of 1A; the gray box at the end of 2B represents the highly conserved 365TYRKLLEGEE374 sequence that includes the end of the coiled-coil 2B segment at E371. The wild-type amino acid is indicated next to the structure, and amino acid replacements within symbols on either side. Infantile cases are on the left, shown as blue circles; juvenile and adult cases are on the right, as orange and red circles, respectively, and asymptomatic cases as white squares. Each symbol represents a single patient, except that familial cases, including identical twins, are represented by a single symbol coded for the onset type of the proband. This figure is a modification and update of Figure 24.4 in Brenner et al. (2009).

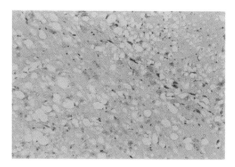

Fig. 9.1 Brain biopsy of a patient with Canavan disease, showing spongy degeneration of the brain. This procedure is no longer necessary, since diagnosis can be made by urine analysis for excessive amount of *N*-acetylaspartic acid.

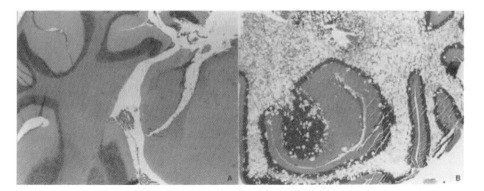

Fig. 9.7. Cerebellum of the knock-out mouse with spongy degeneration of the white matter is seen on the right while on the left is a normal cerebellum.

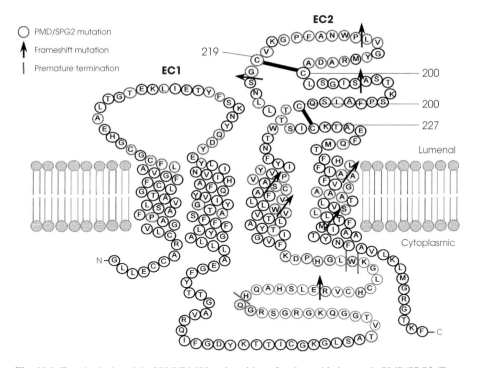

Fig. 10.1. Topological model of PLP/DM20 and position of amino acid changes in PMD/SPG2. Two-dimensional model of proteolipid protein (PLP) (276 residues as black beads) and its splice isoform DM20, lacking 35 residues (marked in gray) from an intracellular loop. The orientation of four trans-membrane domains positions both N- and C-terminus into the glial cytoplasm. Within the second extracellular domain (EC2), the position of two disulfide-bridges is indicated. Positions of amino acids in EC2 which are substituted in patients with Pelizaeus–Merzbacher disease (PMD) are marked in yellow. The single-letter code of the wild-type sequence is shown. Disulfide bonds in extracellular loop 2 (EC2) are critical for PLP folding (Dhaunchak and Nave 2007) and indicated by black lines. Many substitutions within EC2 lead to abnormal PLP crosslinks that result in protein retention in the endoplasmic reticulum and activation of the unfolded-protein response.

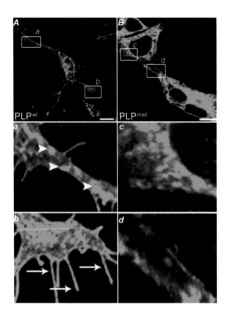

Fig. 10.2. PMD-causing mutations of PLP are retained in the endoplasmic reticulum of transfected cells. *A*: Wild-type proteolipids (PLP^*wt*) readily traffic to the cell surface of transfected oligodendroglial cells as demonstrated by green fluorescent microspikes at the tips of processes. Glial cells protrude numerous filopodial processes and PLP^*wt* accumulates in the endosomal/lysosomal compartment. Magnified insets (*a, b*) of boxed area in *A* show glial processes with endosomal/lysosomal accumulation of PLP (arrowheads) and filopodial protrusions (arrows). Scale bar: 10 μm (left). *B*: Mutant proteins, such as PLP^*msd* (A242V substitution) derived from the PMD model *jimpy-msd*, fail to reach the glial cell surface. Glial cells lack any labeled microspikes (magnified insets in *c, d*). Note also the paucity of cellular processes. There is a reticular distribution of EGFP fluorescence, with no accumulation in the endosomal/ lysosomal compartment. Magnifications (*c, d*) of the boxed areas in *B* are located in a close proximity to the cell surface. Note that there is complete absence of fine microspikes. Scale bar: 10 μm (right).

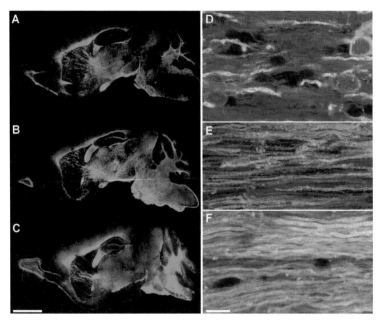

Fig. 11.5. A–C: Myelin Basic Protein (MBP) staining of *shiverer* mice that were transplanted with human glial precursor cell on the first day of life. Images are shown at 20 weeks (**A**); 35 weeks (**B**); and 52 weeks (**C**). While the untreated *shiverer* mouse has no MBP staining, the transplanted animals already demonstrate myelination in major white-matter regions of the brain at 20 weeks. **B:** At 35 weeks, the area of dense myelination has expanded into the mid-brain and hindbrain. **C:** By 1 year, myelin was well distributed, and myelination appeared complete, throughout the forebrain and hindbrain. **D–F:** Corresponding confocal optical sections of transplanted *shiverer* mouse corpus callosum taken at 20 weeks (**D**), 35 weeks (**E**), and 52 weeks (**F**), immunolabeled for neurofilament (red) and myelin basic protein (green), which reveal the progressive increase in axonal ensheathment with time. Scale bars: 2.5 mm (**A–C**), 10 μm (**D–F**). (Modified with permission from Windrem MS et al. Neonatal chimerization with human glial progenitor cells can both remyelinate and rescue the otherwise lethally hypomyelinated shiverer mouse. Cell Stem Cell. 2008; 2: 553–565.)

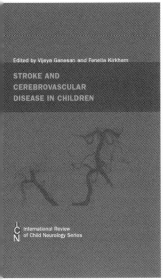

Stroke and Cerebrovascular Disease in Children

VIJEYA GANESAN AND FENELLA KIRKHAM (EDS)
2011 ▪ 368 PAGES ▪ HARDBACK ▪ 280 X 205 MM ▪ 978-1-898683-34-6
£145.00 / €174.00 / US$199.95

This book for the first time summarizes the state of the art in this field. A team of eminent clinicians, neurologists and researchers provide an up-to-the-minute account of all aspects of stroke and cerebrovascular disease in children, ranging from a historical perspective to future directions, through epidemiology, the latest neuroimaging techniques, neurodevelopment, co-morbidities, diagnosis and treatment. The authors' practical approach to the clinical problems makes this essential reading for practising clinicians. It will also be of interest to researchers in the field.

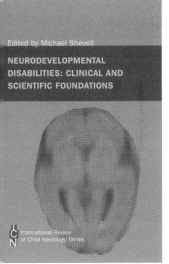

Neurodevelopmental Disabilities: Clinical and Scientific Foundations

MICHAEL SHEVELL (ED)
2009 ▪ 504 PAGES ▪ SOFTBACK ▪ 232 X 152 MM ▪ 978-1-898683-67-4
£75.00 / €90.00 / US$119.95

This book takes a comprehensive approach to addressing the challenges of neurodevelopmental disabilities in child health, with a special focus on global developmental delay and developmental language impairment. It presents the scientific basis of these disorders and their underlying causes. Issues related to medical management, rehabilitation, and eventual outcomes are also addressed in detail. The book has wide appeal to those in paediatrics, developmental paediatrics, child neurology, and paediatric rehabilitation. Some chapters are devoted to the particular issues faced in underdeveloped countries. The book also provides extensive information in a single source relating to often-overlooked areas such as medical management, rehabilitation, public policy, and ethics.

International Reviews of Child Neurology

Published for the International Child Neurology Association by Mac Keith Press www.mackeith.co.uk

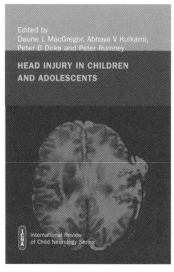

Head Injury in Children and Adolescents

DAUNE L. MACGREGOR, ABHAYA V. KULKARNI, PETER B. DIRKS, & PETER RUMNEY (ED)
2007 ▪ 272 PAGES ▪ HARDBACK ▪ 232 x 152 MM ▪ 978-1-898683-50-6
£60.00 / €72.00 / US$110.00

This is a comprehensive framework for the car needed by children and their families following traumatic brain injury. The contributors review th long-term cognitive and behavioural disabilities both severe, mild traumatic head injurie and provide an overview of new treatments fc children who have had traumatic brain injury, such a neuroprotective strategies, advanced treatment i neurointensive settings and new rehabilitatic techniques. They demonstrate that preventativ measures, with the regulatory and legislative strengt of governments, hold the key to reduction in th incidence of traumatic brain injury.

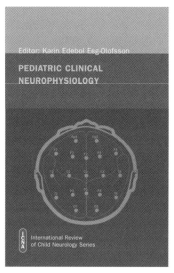

Pediatric Clinical Neurophysiology

KARIN EDEBOL EEG-OLOFSSON (ED)
2007 ▪ 264 PAGES ▪ HARDBACK ▪ 232 x 152 MM ▪ 978-1-898683-48-3
£65.00 / €78.00 / US$119.95

This book introduces clinical neurophysiology and i applications to the paediatric neurologist. It does nc aim at being a textbook of either clinica neurophysiology or paediatric neurology, but bridging these two fields, as a handbook for th clinician. The focus is on the methods applied in th setting of a clinical neurophysiological laboratory Particularly valuable are the examples and referenc values for nerve conduction studies, EMG, evoke potentials, autonomic testing, EEG, and transcrania magnetic stimulation. The book will stimulate readers interest in paediatric clinical neurophysiology in thei daily clinical work.

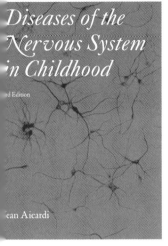

Diseases of the Nervous System in Childhood
THIRD EDITION

JEAN AICARDI WITH MARTIN BAX AND CHRISTOPHER GILLBERG (EDS)
CLINICS IN DEVELOPMENTAL MEDICINE
2009 ▪ 912 PAGES ▪ HARDBACK ▪ 280 X 205 MM ▪ 978-1-898683-59-9
£175.00 / €210.00 / US$335.00

Diseases of the nervous system in infancy and childhood have a profound impact on the lives of patients and their families and are probably the most disruptive of all paediatric ailments. Aicardi's *Diseases of the Nervous System in Childhood* is the essential resource for child neurologists, neurologists, paediatricians, and physicians in developmental medicine. The third edition has been extensively updated to incorporate the tremendous volume of new information since the previous edition, but remains as clinically oriented as its predecessors.

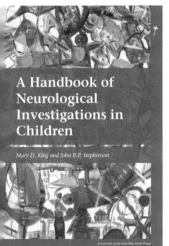

A Handbook of Neurological Investigations in Children

MARY D. KING AND JOHN B.P. STEPHENSON
A PRACTICAL GUIDE FROM MAC KEITH PRESS
2009 ▪ 400 PAEGS ▪ SOFTBACK ▪ 240 X 170 MM ▪ 978-1-898683-69-8
£39.95 / €78.00 / US$48.00

Neurological disorders in children are common: families want to know what is wrong, why it happened, and whether it will happen again. Management and treatment depend on establishing the diagnosis, which usually requires investigations, but the number of possible neurological investigations is now very large indeed, and uncritical investigations may be seriously misleading and often costly. This book, based on the authors' vast combined personal experience, gives practical guidance on how to target any specific condition with the minimum of tests. Throughout, vignettes of real cases help to illustrate the use of the tests in different clinical situations.

Other titles from Mac Keith Press

www.mackeith.co.uk

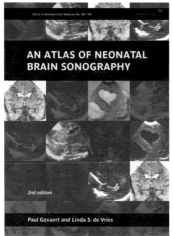

An Atlas of Neonatal Brain Sonography
SECOND EDITION

PAUL GOVAERT AND LINDA S. DE VRIES
CLINICS IN DEVELOPMENTAL MEDICINE No. 182-183
2010 ▪ 420 PAGES ▪ HARDBACK ▪ 280 X 205 MM ▪ 978-1-898683-56-8
£149.50 / €72.00 / US$240.00

This Atlas covers the entire spectrum of brain disea: as studied with ultrasound, illustrated throughout wi superb-quality images. It is aimed at neonatologis and radiologists confronted with everyday clinic questions on the neonatal ward. Most newborn bra disorders can be identified with ultrasound; this boc will therefore be particularly useful in settings wi limited MRI facilities. Prenatal ultrasound specialis will also find it valuable as a postnatal reference their field of interest. Suggestions for differenti diagnosis accompany all the sonographic finding guiding the clinician in proceeding from an abnorm image to a diagnosis.

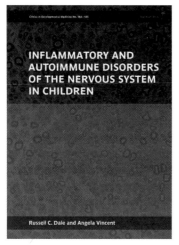

Inflammatory and Autoimmune Disorders of the Nervous System in Children

RUSSELL C. DALE AND ANGELA VINCENT (EDS)
CLINICS IN DEVELOPMENTAL MEDICINE No. 184-185
2010 ▪ 504 PAGES ▪ HARDBACK ▪ 240 X 170 MM ▪ 978-1-898683-66-7
£110.00 / €132.00 / US$199.95

Inflammatory disorders of the nervous syster collectively make up 10-20% of acute paediatr neurology presentations and many are potentiall treatable. Better diagnosis and often simple treatmen could lead to substantial clinical benefit and reductio in long-term disability. This book provides a detaile and comprehensive summary of the childhood disease that are, or are likely to be, caused by the immun system. The authors not only describe these disorder and their treatments comprehensively, helpin paediatricians and paediatric neurologists to improv their understanding and recognition of the condition: but also highlight recent and exciting development that will be of considerable importance in the future.